TIZIANO TESTORI   MASSIMO DEL FABBRO   ROBERTO WEINSTEIN   STEPHEN WALLACE

MAXILLARY SINUS SURGERY

and alternatives in treatment

Quintessence

British Library Cataloguing in Publication Data

Chururgia del seno mascellare e le alternative
terapeutiche. English.
Maxillary sinus surgery and alternatives in treatment.
1. Maxillary sinus--Surgery. 2. Maxillary sinus--Diseases--
Treatment.
I. Title II. Testori, Tiziano.
617.5'2059-dc22

ISBN-13: 9781850971702

Italian edition published by ACME SAS, copyright 2005.

Printing and binding: Bosch-Druck, Landshut/Ergolding
Printed in Germany.

TIZIANO TESTORI   MASSIMO DEL FABBRO   ROBERTO WEINSTEIN   STEPHEN WALLACE

MAXILLARY SINUS SURGERY

and alternatives in treatment

QUINTESSENCE PUBLISHING

London, Berlin, Chicago, Tokyo, Barcelona, Istanbul, Milan, Moscow,
New Delhi, Paris, Beijing, Prague, São Paulo, Seoul and Warsaw

authors

TIZIANO TESTORI

MD, DDS, FICD received his MD degree (1981), DDS degree (1984), and Speciality in Orthodontics (1986) from the University of Milan, Italy. He is Head of the Section of Implant Dentistry and Oral Rehabilitation, Galeazzi Institute (Chairman: Prof. R.L. Weinstein), University of Milan, Italy. He had a Fellowship at the Department of Oral Maxillo-Facial Surgery, School of Dentistry, Loma Linda University, Loma Linda CA (Head: Philip J. Boyne, DMD, MS, DSc) (1991), and a Fellowship at the Division of Oral Maxillo-Facial Surgery, School of Medicine, University of Miami, Miami FL (Head: Robert E. Marx, DDS) (2000). He is a Visiting Professor at New York University, College of Dentistry, USA, and Fellow of the "International College of Dentists" (FICD). He is President of the Italian Society of Oral Surgery and Implantology (SICOI). He is a member of the Periodontology/ Implantology Editorial Board for Practical Procedures & Aesthetic Dentistry (PPAD) (a Montage Media publication), and a member of the Editorial Board of the European Journal of Oral Implantology (Quintessence Publishing Co. Ltd). He acts as referee for Oral Surgery and Implant Dentistry for the National Committee of the Health Ministry for CE programs. He is a reviewer for the Cochrane collaboration, Oral Health Group, and founding member of the Italian Section of the ICOI (International College of Oral Implantologists). He is an active member of the European Board of Oral Surgery (EFOSS), and active member and lecturer for the Academy of Osseointegration (AO), American Academy of Periodontology (AAP) and American Association of Oral and Maxillofacial Surgeons (AAOMFS). He is author of over 200 scientific and clinical papers for professional journals.

MASSIMO DEL FABBRO

Born in Milano, Italy in 1964. Degree in Biology (1989) at the University of Milan. Ph.D. in Human Physiology (1994) at the University of Milan. Post-doctoral fellowship (1995-1997) at the Institute of Physiology, University of Milan. In 1999-2002 he obtained a grant for the project "Physiopathology of Periodontal and Peri-implant soft tissues" at the Department of Medicine, Surgery and Dentistry, University of Milan. Since 2002 he has been a Researcher in Dentistry, Oral Surgery & Medicine at the faculty of Medicine of the University of Milan. His scientific interests are in the fields of physiopathology of periodontal and peri-implant tissues, biology of osseointegration, regenerative techniques, tissue engineering, biomedical statistics, and methodology of research. He is Head of the Section of Oral Physiology at the Department of Health Technologies (Chair: Prof. R. Weinstein), IRCCS Istituto Ortopedico Galeazzi, University of Milan. He is author and co-author of over 80 papers in the fields of periodontology, implant dentistry, endodontics and physiology.

ROBERTO WEINSTEIN

Born in Varese in 1948, graduated in Medicine in 1972 and specialized in Clinical Dentistry in 1974 at the University of Milan, Italy. A student of Giorgio Vogel, in 1981 he became a University Researcher, in 1988 he became an Associate Professor at the University of Modena, and in 1990 he became a Tenured Professor at the University of Milan. He has been Head of the Dental Clinic at the Orthopaedic Institute Galeazzi in Milan since 2002, where he is also the Scientific Director. He has also been the Head of the Odontostomatology School of Specialization and has held the Chair for the Undergraduate course in Dentistry and Dental Prosthesis Work. He is Past President and Founder of the SIOH (Società Italiana di Odontostomatologia per Handicappati) and Past President of the Italian Society of Periodontology.

STEPHEN WALLACE

Graduated in Dental Medicine in 1967 from New York University, College of Dentistry, certificate in Periodontology in 1971 at Boston University. He is an Associate Professor at the Department of Oral Implantology, New York University, Periodontics and Implant Dentistry, and divides his time between teaching and clinical research. He is a fellow of the International Congress of Oral Implantologists (ICOI) and the American Academy of Periodontology (AAP) and the Academy of Osseointegration (AO). He is the author of over 50 scientific papers on grafting biomaterials and on surgical procedures for maxillary sinus lifting. An internationally renowned speaker, he practises in Waterbury, Connecticut, focusing his work in the areas of periodontology and implantology.

the following have contributed to the creation of this book:

ALESSANDRO BAJ
MD, Specialist in Maxillofacial Surgery, Visiting Professor at the Postgraduate Program in Maxillofacial Surgery the University of Parma, Visiting Professor at the Undergraduate Program School of Dentistry at the University of Milan, Department of Clinical Maxillofacial Surgery, Chairman Prof. A.B. Giannì, Istituto Galeazzi, Milan, Italy.

GIANMARCO BELLONI
MD, Specialist in Radiology, First-level Executive at the Diagnostic Radiology Imaging Department, ARS Medical Clinic Group Lugano, Ticino, CH, Italy.

FRANCESCA BIANCHI
Doctor of Dental Surgery (DDS), Tutor at the Implantology and Oral Rehabilitation Department, Head Dr T. Testori. School of Dentistry, Chairman Prof. R.L. Weinstein. Department of Health Technologies Istituto Ortopedico Galeazzi IRCCS, University of Milan, Italy.

MATTEO CAPELLI
Doctor of Dental Surgery (DDS), Tutor at the Implantology and Oral Rehabilitation Department, Head Dr T. Testori. School of Dentistry, Chairman Prof. R.L. Weinstein. Department of Health Technologies Istituto Ortopedico Galeazzi IRCCS, University of Milan, Italy.

FRANCO CARLINO
MD, Specialist in Maxillofacial Surgery, Fellow at the Clinical Maxillofacial Surgery Department, Chair Prof. A.B. Giannì, Istituto Ortopedico Galeazzi IRCCS, Milan, Italy.

GIORGIO CASTELLAZZI
MD, Specialist in Radiology, Department of Diagnostic & Interventional Radiology, Istituto Ortopedico Galeazzi IRCCS, Milan, Italy.

GIAMPIERO CORDIOLI
MD, Specialist in General Surgery, Specialist in Dental Medicine and Dental Prostheses, Director of the Dental Clinic, University of Padua, Italy.

LUCA FRANCETTI
Associate Professor, Head of the Periodontology Department, School of Dentistry, Chairman Prof. R.L. Weinstein. Department of Health Technologies, Istituto Ortopedico Galeazzi IRCCS, University of Milan, Italy.

LUCA FUMAGALLI
Doctor of Dental Surgery (DDS), Tutor at the Implantology and Oral Rehabilitation Department, Head Dr T. Testori. School of Dentistry, Chairman Prof. R.L. Weinstein. Department of Health Technologies, Istituto Ortopedico Galeazzi IRCCS, University of Milan, Italy.

FABIO GALLI
MD, Head of the section of Implant Prosthetic Dentistry. Implantology and Oral Rehabilitation Department, Head Dr T. Testori. School of Dentistry, Chairman Prof. R.L. Weinstein. Department of Health Technologies, Istituto Ortopedico Galeazzi IRCCS, University of Milan, Italy.

ALDO BRUNO GIANNÌ
MD, Specialist in Maxillofacial Surgery, University of Milan, Director of the Postgraduate Program in Maxillofacial Surgery, University of Milan, Italy. Director of Department of Maxillofacial Surgery, Department of Health Technologies Istituto Ortopedico Galeazzi IRCCS, University of Milan, Italy.

ZEINA MAJZOUB
MD, Specialist in Odontostomatology and in Periodontology, Boston University, USA. Director of the Clinical Research Department, Lebanese University, Beirut, Lebanon.

MARIO MANTOVANI   MD, Visiting Professor at University of Milan, Italy, Specialist in Otorhinolaryngology and Cervical-facial Pathologies, Specialist in Plastic Surgery, Specialist in Maxillofacial Surgery. Otorhinolaryngology Clinic at the University of Milan, Ospedale Maggiore Policlinico IRCCS, Milan.

GIANPIERO MASSEI   MD, Specialist in Maxillofacial Surgery, Specialist in Plastic Surgery, Chairman of the Biocra Society, private practice in Turin, Italy.

RICCARDO MONTEVERDI   MD, Specialist in Maxillofacial Surgery. Visiting Professor at the Undergraduate Program School of Dentistry at the University of Milan, Department of Clinical Maxillofacial Surgery, Chairman Prof. A.B. Giannì, Istituto Galeazzi, Milan, Italy.

ANDREA PARENTI   Doctor of Dental Surgery (DDS), Tutor at the Implantology and Oral Rehabilitation Department, Head Dr T. Testori. School of Dentistry, Chairman Prof. R.L. Weinstein. Department of Health Technologies, Istituto Ortopedico Galeazzi IRCCS, University of Milan, Italy.

FRANCO PERONA   Medical Doctor MD, Specialist in Radiology, Director Department of Diagnostic & Interventional Radiology, IRCCS Istituto Ortopedico Galeazzi, Milan, Italy. Professor at the School of Radiology, Faculty of Medicine, University of Milan.

PIETRO SALVATORI   Medical Doctor MD, Specialist in Maxillofacial Surgery, Specialist in Otorhinolaryngology, Head of the Cervical-Maxillofacial Surgery Unit, Istituto Ortopedico Galeazzi, Milan, Italy.

FRANCESCO SANTORO   Medical Doctor MD, Specialist in Otorhinolaryngology, Otorhinolaryngology Department, at S. Anna Hospital, Como, Italy, Director Prof. R. Spinelli.

SILVIO TASCHIERI   Medical Doctor MD, Specialty in Dentistry (DDS), Visiting Professor and Head of the Department of Endodontics and Endodontic Surgery, School of Dentistry, Chairman Prof. R.L. Weinstein. Department of Health Technologies, Istituto Ortopedico Galeazzi IRCCS, University of Milan, Italy.

OLIVEIRA TOMIC   Medical Doctor MD, Specialist in Plastic Surgery, Department of Clinical Maxillofacial Surgery, Chairman Prof. A.B. Giannì, Department of Health Technologies, Istituto Ortopedico Galeazzi IRCCS, University of Milan, Italy.

CONCEZIONE TOMMASINO   Associate Professor of Anesthesia and Intensive Care, University of Milan, Italy. Head of the Anesthesiology Department for Dental Medicine. San Raffaele Hospital, Milano, Italy.

PAOLO TRISI   Doctor of Dental Surgery (DDS), Scientific Director of the BioCra (Biomaterial Clinical Research Association, Pescara). Head of the Biomaterials Department, School of Dentistry, Chairman Prof. R.L. Weinstein. Department of Health Technologies, Istituto Ortopedico Galeazzi IRCCS, University of Milan, Italy.

PASCAL VALENTINI — Doctor of Dental Surgery (DDS). Head of Post-graduate Program in Implantology, Department of Health Science and Human Biology, University of Corsica, Pasquale Paoli Corte, France. Associate Clinical Professor Loma Linda University, Loma Linda, CA, USA.

TOMASO VERCELLOTTI — Medical Doctor MD, Specialty in Dentistry (DDS), Visiting Professor in Maxillofacial Surgery, University of Genoa, Italy, Otorhinolaryngology Clinic, Chair Prof. A. Salami.

FRANCESCO ZUFFETTI — Medical Doctor MD, Specialty in Dentistry (DDS), Tutor at the Implantology and Oral Rehabilitation Department, Head Dr T. Testori. School of Dentistry, Chairman Prof. R.L. Weinstein. Department of Health Technologies Istituto Ortopedico Galeazzi IRCCS, University of Milan, Italy.

contents

foreword

In recent years, the focus has shifted to new aspects of implantology. The 1980s was the decade of osseointegration, the 90s were the years of guided bone regeneration and the current decade is that of esthetic techniques, load-bearing, and the simplification of operational procedures. These various aspects often overlap, and it is usually in the decade that follows that the key problems are finally resolved and new protocols are drawn up.

Maxillary sinus elevation techniques have played an important part in clinical research since the reference publication by Philip Boyne in 1980. Today, after 25 years of studies by doctors and researchers, more than 1000 scientific articles are available that deal exclusively with the subject of maxillary sinus augmentation.

The idea for this book originated at the Consensus Conference on Maxillary Sinus Surgery of the Italian Society of Oral Surgery, which was held in Montecatini in November 2001. Taking their idea from the conference, the authors of this book began to work together closely, creating a new, up-to-date text that brings together the most recent scientific discoveries and the most innovative clinical protocols, together with the possible alternatives to maxillary sinus augmentation techniques. This book seeks to present the various approaches used for maxillary sinus augmentation, as presented at the Consensus Conference in Montecatini, together with a thorough analysis of all the protocols, based on the evidence.

'Maxillary Sinus Surgery and Alternatives in Treatment' reports the clinical experience and the efforts of research carried out by a prestigious group of clinicians and researchers who analyze maxillary sinus elevation from every possible angle. The surgical procedures are presented with the support of basic scientific knowledge and other medical specialities, thanks to the large number of multi-disciplinary research contributions. No aspect related to maxillary sinus surgery has been neglected: endoscopic, radiological, anesthesia and conscious sedation techniques are all presented in the form of operational protocols.

The rational basis and specific clinical indications for each graft material are shown, in addition to relative histologic data.

Both traditional and innovative techniques for maxillary sinus surgery are discussed, together with the clinical criteria that support them. The chapters on alternative therapies, piezoelectric surgery and the application of PRP in maxillary sinus surgery are particularly innovative. The chapters on short-term and long-term complications and the review of literature are also extremely interesting.

The book begins with anatomy, otorhinolaryngological implications and bone healing, and goes on to cover diagnosis, surgery and patient-monitoring. This allows students and experts to enter the world of modern implantology via a consistent training path.

This publication thus manages to combine the goals of a student text book with a valid tool for the development of professional clinical experts.

Finally, my appreciation goes to all the authors who, thanks to their efforts, have created a book that will contribute to improving our patients' health, the ultimate goal for which all doctors must strive.

Dennis Tarnow

CHAIRMAN OF DEPARTMENT OF PERIODONTICS AND
IMPLANT DENTISTRY
NEW YORK UNIVERSITY

preface

Writing a scientific book is always an exciting, unforgettable journey for the authors, for several reasons.

The first is connected to the tool used to divulge their thoughts: printed matter. It may seem obsolete to use this means of communication in the age of the Internet, but using printing, the greatest invention of all time, to communicate scientific knowledge is one of the greatest adventures that Man can face.

The second reason is an inherent part of the profession of lecturer that we authors practice: the possibility of communicating the subject of our research is a decisive moment in our professional life.

Last, but not least, is the possibility of offering the scientific community a further chance for debate and comparison which, we hope, this book may encourage.

We hope that the readers can share our journey and our belief in scientific progress.

Roberto L. Weinstein
Stephen S. Wallace
Massimo Del Fabbro
Tiziano Testori

acknowledgements

My sincere thanks go to Giovanna, my lifelong companion and esteemed colleague, and to Veronica, my beloved daughter who, through their silent strength, have supported me, accepting my lack of attention and company.

My thanks must also go to my teachers, who taught me that one can only truly treat the patients who come to us to cure their health through knowledge, dedication, discipline, professional ethics and the humility to feel like a student for life.

My deepest esteem and gratitude go to the masters who welcomed me to their professional surgeries and their university institutes. Ennio Giannì and Antonino Salvato taught me a multidisciplinary and dental medical approach. Melvyn H. Harris, Philip J. Boyne and Robert E. Marx, from the oral surgery field, have been milestones in my professional life, together with Myron Nevins, Richard J. Lazzara, Dennis P. Tarnow and Arun K. Garg, with their teachings on periodontal and implantology fields.

My gratitude also goes to all the authors who have allowed this book to be published, thanks to their scientific contribution, to Massimo Del Fabbro for his dedication and willingness while the book was being created, in addition to his contribution as the author of important chapters.

Special thanks go to Roberto L. Weinstein, a friend, expert and modern master who, with his volcanic mind, inspired, coordinated and led the writing of this volume.

I would also like to thank Paolo Bellizzomi and his editorial team for their excellent revision work that allowed us to create a modern, easy-to-consult text.

Last, but not least, my thanks to all the colleagues who have believed in us, buying the book in the hope that it will aid the better care of their patients.

Tiziano Testori

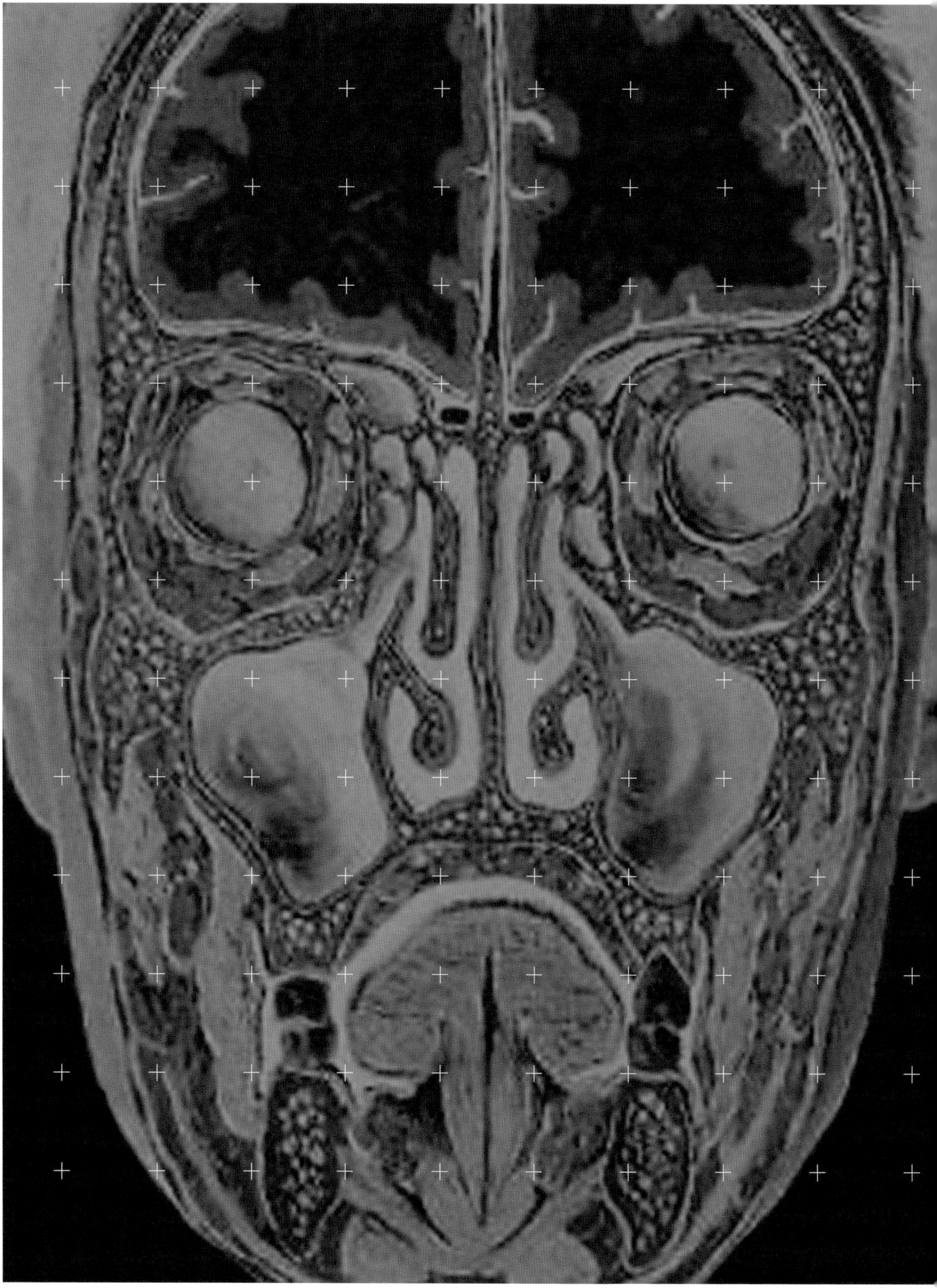

M. DEL FABBRO

Introduction and background

01

01

The use of osseointegrated implants is currently an efficient, reliable method for short- and long-term treatment of patients affected by part or total edentulism. The rate of success and predictability of implant treatment depends on several factors, but is generally rather high.

The goal, however, is to extend this rehabilitative method to a large number of patients, including those with low quality and/or quantity of bone. In the past, an inadequate volume and a low quality of bone tissue were contraindications to implant treatment.

In particular, due to the low bone quality and the tendency for progressive resorption after tooth loss, the posterior maxilla has always been a high-risk area for rehabilitation with implant-supported fixed prostheses, atrophic alveolar ridges and/or a highly pneumatized maxillary sinus, conditions that imply a limited amount of residual bone, the task becomes even more difficult. One solution is resorting to reduced length implants, but in this case particular clinical parameters must exist to avoid biomechanical problems due to the poor implant/crown ratio between the length of the implant and that of the restoration.

In these cases, implants require careful planning and may need pre-prosthetic surgery involving bone grafting of the maxillary sinus (or antrum of Highmore), which is aimed at correcting bone quantity defects and creating optimal conditions for inserting implants in the posterior areas of the jawbone.

From a historical point of view, oral implantology tried initially to overcome the problem of lack of bone support in the posterior areas by using prostheses with distal extensions supported by implants inserted anteriorly, or by combining long implants in the anterior areas with short implants in the posterior areas. This approach can still be considered valid for some clinical cases, after a careful diagnostic evaluation.

For many years, dental and maxillofacial surgeons avoided complex operations requiring access to the maxillary sinus from the oral cavity unless it was absolutely necessary.

In 1984, based on clinical and experimental evidence, Brånemark showed how the the apical end of an osseointegrated implant can be inserted into the maxillary sinus (and in the nasal sinus) without altering the state of health of the sinus region, on the condition that the Schneiderian membrane, the ciliated mucosa lining the walls of the maxillary sinus, remains intact. These experiments were meant to show how a bone graft is not always necessary for implant treatment in the posterior areas of the atrophic jawbone. However, the failure rate for this procedure reported by Brånemark was rather high (up to 70%), in an observation period that ranged from 5 to 10 years of functional loading.

Further experimental evidence on macaques (*Macaca fascicularis*) proved that implants with the apical end protruding up to 5 mm in the maxillary sinus can easily be subjected to occlusal load for over one year, in the same way as implants inserted into bone grafts (Boyne 1993). One of the key factors for success seems to be the correct distribution of occlusal loads among the implants inserted in the posterior areas of the jawbone, and other implants or natural teeth. It is known, however, that long-term success of endosseous implants depends on the degree of osseointegration and this in turn depends on both primary stability, due to the compactness of bone cortex and bone quality, and on secondary stability that is the result of the progressive growth of bone tissue around the entire surface of the implant. Even though an implant inserted into reduced height and width bone, with one end jutting out in to the antrum, may have good primary stability if the cortex is adequately compact, it will have limited anchorage, therefore it will be extremely difficult to obtain osseointegration over the whole surface (essential for the "duration" of the implant). Also, crestal bone loss may occur progressively over the years, further reducing the implant's stability.

Therefore, in case of defective bone quality, it is of utmost importance to increase the quantity of bone that can accommodate an endo-osseous implant of suitable length in the posterior-lateral areas of the maxilla, by means of a maxillary sinus floor elevation. The indication for sinus elevation, together with marked pneumatisation, is therefore the need to incorporate suitably long implants to improve anchorage in an area that is subjected to high functional loads.

There are also some important techniques that can aid the incorporation of the graft and the healing of the site with the formation of new bone tissue. Some of these are: a conservative surgical technique, aimed at maximum preservation of the vascular bed in the muscosa and the periosteum; the prevention of overheating the site (by cauterisation or the use of high-speed burs); aseptic technique; rigid fixation of the graft in the site that will accommodate the implants if block grafts are used.

Maxillary sinus reconstructions using bone grafts to correct traumatic defects such as the surgical reduction of fractures of the maxilla, the orbit, the nasal septum or alveolar processes have been carried out for several years and a large amount of literature is available on this matter. In contrast, operations involving bone grafts in the maxillary sinus in the presence of an atrophic posterior jawbone, aimed at allowing the insertion of dental implants in this region, are relatively infrequent, or were so until about 20 years ago.

In recent years there has been a growing diffusion of maxillary sinus elevation procedures associated with implantology. This is also testified by the growing number of scientific papers published on this matter, making this procedure a necessary technique in the treatment of atrophic jawbones.

The first documented experiences of bone grafts in the maxillary sinus, together with reconstructions using prostheses, date back to the late 1960s, attributed to Philip J. Boyne. He had to carry out "secondary alveolar osteoplasty" operations on the alveolar processes of the maxilla, in order to increase the inter-arch space in patients who needed total prostheses with rather expanded maxillary tuberosities that interfered with the opposing arch. As the patients all had marked pneumatization of the maxillary sinuses, with reduced bone height, it was necessary first to carry out a bone graft on the sinus floor augmentation to increase bone depth. Boyne augmented the maxillary sinus floor with a cortico-cancellous graft harvested from the iliac crest, using the spongiosa cortex with the Caldwell-Luc technique, after separating the mucosa. After about 3 months, Boyne carried out the osteoplasty operation on each patient, without the risk of penetrating the maxillary sinus, owing to the high volume of bone present after the graft. Without this procedure, the patients would not have been able to receive rehabilitation through prostheses.

Later, in the 1970s, the same surgical procedure for lifting the maxillary sinus for pre-prosthetic rehabilitation purposes was carried out, though rarely, on patients with highly pneumatized sinuses, who needed to undergo implantation procedures using blade implants. There are few reports published from this period, however. The first paper concerning the treatment of patients with endosseous implants associated with maxillary sinus elevation operations was published in 1980 by Boyne and James. The maxillary sinus was accessed via antrostomy in order to create a "bone window". The latter was then delicately pushed and turned inside the antrum, a maneuver that necessitated the partial separation of the Schneiderian membrane from the sinus floor. The bone graft was then inserted below the membrane and the opening was closed. The material used for the graft was generally autogenous bone, and the blade implants were inserted in a subsequent operation, some months after the sinus elevation procedure. Prosthetic reconstructions comprised fixed or removable prostheses, placed in the edentulous areas of the posterior regions of the maxilla.

In the same period, Tatum and collaborators worked a lot on this type of operation, trying to develop and improve new surgical procedures that were aimed at obtaining an increase in bone depth in the posterior maxilla. Tatum was one of the main proponents of the maxillary sinus elevation technique for implant purposes using autogenous bone grafts taken from the iliac crest (Tatum 1977, 1986).

Later, with the diffusion of osseointegrated implants that were originally developed by Branemark and his collaborators from the Swedish school, some of the requisites for implant treatment were modified.

Progress in the field of biomaterials and the refinement of techniques and protocols for the rehabilitation of edentulism using osseo-integrated implants contributed to increase the success rate and the predictability of implant treatment. There has therefore been a huge diffusion of the use of osseointegrated implants in clinical practice and an expansion of research on innovative surgical techniques.

Over the years, various techniques have been proposed for maxillary sinus augmentation, which differ in the surgical protocol (the method and anatomic site for carrying out the antrostomy); in the autogenous bone harvesting site (intraoral, extraoral, depending on the amount of bone that is needed for the operation); in the type of graft material used (autogenous, alloplastic bone); in the timing of implant surgery in relation to the maxillary sinus floor elevation (simultaneous, i.e. during the same surgical procedure, or later, during a further surgical session); in the use or non-use of resorbable or non-resorbable membranes; and in the extent of the elevation of the sinus membrane. This heterogeneity, which is often present in the refinement stage of any innovative surgical procedure, shows how the method for sinus augmentation has not yet been optimized. Of course, this does not mean that there can only be one, unchangeable type of perfect technique. Instead, the ideal method is based on solid principles, but at the same time the type of surgical procedure should be chosen and adapted depending on the patient's specific needs and characteristics.

Alongside the bone graft procedures, new regenerative techniques have been developed in recent years, and are currently being investigated. Some examples are the use of growth factors, bone morphogenetic proteins (such as BMP-2 and BMP-7; Boyne et al. 1997; Boyne 2005), osteogenetic distraction, platelet-rich plasma (PRP; Kassolis et al. 2000; Froum et al. 2002); and (the arrangement of) cellular cultures (of osteoblasts and fibroblasts) for the *in vitro* generation of a bone matrix. Progress in tissue engineering has provided a considerable contribution to the development of these methods, but many of them are still at the initial experimental stage and currently there are insufficient case studies to justify their diffusion and wide-scale use, in contrast to bone grafting procedures. Many multi-center studies are currently being performed on BMPs, embedded in collagen-based substrata, concerning their use during maxillary sinus reconstruction for implant purposes. They are powerful osteoinductive materials capable of inducing neo-osteogenesis without the need for bone grafting. It has been proved that BMPs can completely repair large-scale mandibular defects, and the first experiments on the maxillary sinuses have proved to be rather promising (Boyne et al. 1997).

A systematic analysis of the literature over the last 20 years, described in a later chapter, shows how maxillary sinus floor elevation, associated with implants, is an efficient and predictable surgical technique, regardless of the method used. There is, in fact, a 92% average survival rate of implants inserted on bone grafts in the maxillary sinus. This data confirms what emerged from the *Consensus Conference* on sinus grafting in 1996, which collected retrospective data from 3000 implants over an observation period of up to 10 years. The average success rate reported at the Consensus Conference, considering implants with at least 3 years of functional load, was found to be 90%.

There are over 1400 reported studies on maxillary sinus grafting. The majority are studies with a low to medium level of evidence (clinical case series, retrospective analyses), but prospective randomized controlled clinical trials are rare. With so many suitable techniques, there is a need for studies with a higher level of evidence.

REFERENCES

1 **Beirne O.R.**
Material choices for sinus lifts.
Sel. Read. Oral Maxillofac. Surg. 1999; 7: 1-20.

2 **Boyne P.J.**
Lectures to postgraduate Course. US Navy Dental School,
National Naval Medical Center, Bethesda, MD, 1965-1968.

3 **Boyne P.J., James R.A.**
Grafting of the maxillary sinus floor with autogenous marrow and bone.
J. Oral Maxillofac. Surg. 1980; 38: 613-617.

4 **Boync P.J.**
Analysis of performance of root-form endosseous implants placed in the maxillary sinus.
J. Long Term. Eff. Med. Impl. 1993; 3: 143-159.

5 **Boyne P.J., Lily C.J., Marx R.E., et al.**
De novo bone induction by recombinant human bone morphogenetic protein-2 (rhBMP-2) in maxillary sinus floor augmentation.
J. Oral Maxillofac. Surg. 2005; 63: 1693-1707.

6 **Boyne P.J., Marx R.E., Nevins M., Triplett G., Lazaro E., Lilly L.C., Alder M., Nummikoski P.**
A feasibility study evaluating rhBMP-2/absorbable collagen sponge for maxillary sinus floor augmentation.
Int. J. Periodontics Restorative Dent. 1997; 17: 11-25.

7 **Brånemark P.J.**
An experimental and clinical study of osseointegrated implants penetrating the nasal cavity and maxillary sinus.
J. Oral Maxillofac. Surg. 1984; 42: 497-505.

8 **Froum S.J., Wallace S.S., Tarnow D.P., Cho S.C.**
Effect of platelet-rich plasma on bone growth and osseointegration in human maxillary sinus grafts: three bilateral case reports.
Int. J. Periodontics Restorative Dent. 2002; 22: 45-53.

9 **Jensen O.T., Shulman L.B., Block M.S., Iacono V.J.**
Report of the Sinus Consensus Conference of 1996.
Int. J. Oral Maxillofac. Implants 1998; 13: 11-41.

10 **Kassolis J.D., Rosen P.S., Reynolds M.A.**
Alveolar ridge and sinus augmentation utilizing platelet-rich plasma in combination with freeze-dried bone allograft: case series.
J. Periodontol. 2000; 71: 1654-1661.

11 **Misch C.E.**
Maxillary sinus augmentation for endosteal implants: organized alternative treatment plans.
Int. J. Oral Implantol. 1987; 4: 49-58.

12 **Summers R.B.**
The osteotome technique: part 3-Less invasive methods of elevating the sinus floor.
Compendium 1994; 15: 698, 700, 702-704.

13 **Tatum O.H.**
Maxillary sinus grafting for endosseous implants.
Lecture, Alabama Implant Study Group, Annual Meeting.
Birmingham AL, USA, 1977.

14 **Tatum O.H.**
Maxillary and sinus implant reconstruction.
Dent. Clin. North Am. 1986; 30: 207-229.

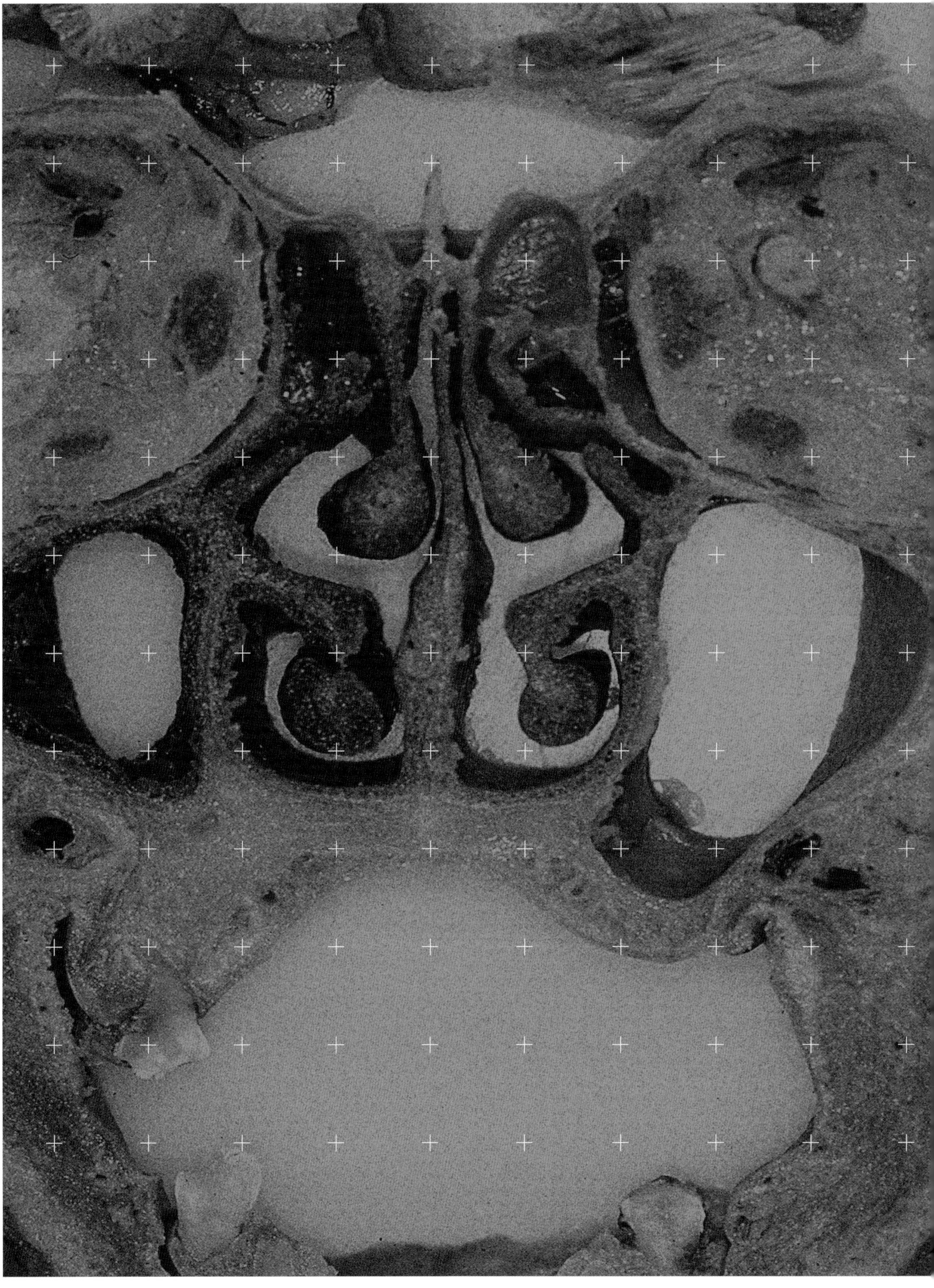

M. DEL FABBRO
T. TESTORI

Anatomy of the maxillary sinus

02

02

BASIC ANATOMY

The maxillary sinus begins to develop between the second and third month of pregnancy, with an evagination of the nasal passage lateral wall mucosa. At birth, it is about 0.1 to 0.2 cm³ in size and remains small until eruption of the permanent teeth (Van den Bergh et al. 2000). Development, in terms of pneumatization (the increase of the volume of air contained in it), is completed by adolescence, although its volume may increase further after tooth loss in the posterior maxilla.

The maxillary sinus is the largest of the paranasal cavities, which include the ethmoidal, frontal and sphenoidal sinuses and which usually occupies a large part of the maxillary bone. It is an air cavity with a quadrangular pyramidal shape with various walls: a medial wall facing the nasal cavity, a posterior wall facing the maxillary tuberosity, a mesio-vestibular wall for the presence of the canine fossae, an upper wall which is the orbit floor, and finally, a lower wall that is next to the alveolar process and which is the bottom of the maxillary sinus itself (McGowan et al. 1993). The maxillary sinus communicates with the homolateral nasal fossa by means of a natural ostium located antero-superiorly on the medial surface, which drains into the middle meatus

(May et al. 1990). All paranasal sinuses communicate with the nasal fossae and therefore also, indirectly, with each other **FIG. 1A-B, 2A-C**. They serve mainly to humidify and heat the air we breathe in. They also contribute to reducing the weight of our facial bones, protect the base of the skull against trauma, thermally insulate the upper nerve centers and influence phonation by acting as an indirect resonance box (Blanton & Biggs 1969; Ritter & Lee 1978).

The two bone walls most often involved in maxillary sinus surgery are the mesio-vestibular wall and the medial wall.

The mesio-vestibular wall is usually made up of a thin cortex (thickened bone walls are occasionally found) containing the neurovascular bundle: the arterial anastomosis between the upper, infra-orbital posterior-alveolar artery and the infra-orbital nerve that permeates and innervates the anterior teeth, if present, and related periodontal tissues **FIG. 3A-C**. In some cases it may be 2 mm thick, especially in brachytype patients with an increased cross-facial diameter. A variation in thickness or an interruption cannot normally be detected in an orthopantograph. Pre-existing thicknesses can be evaluated prior to surgery only by means of a CT scan. Lack of bone cortex areas can be found, with a consequent direct contact between vestibular mucosa and sinus mucosa **FIG. 4A-C**. The posterior teeth are innervated by neurovascular branches coming from the maxillary tuberosity (de Mol Van Otterloo 1994). This anatomic aspect has consequences due to the narrow space available for antrostomy surgery. An apical surgical approach to any viable teeth may cause a high risk of tooth necrosis (Van den Bergh et al. 2000).

The medial wall is rectangular and forms the bone septum that separates the maxillary sinus from the nasal cavity. The lower portion corresponds to the lower meatus of the nasal cavity (Chanavaz 1990).

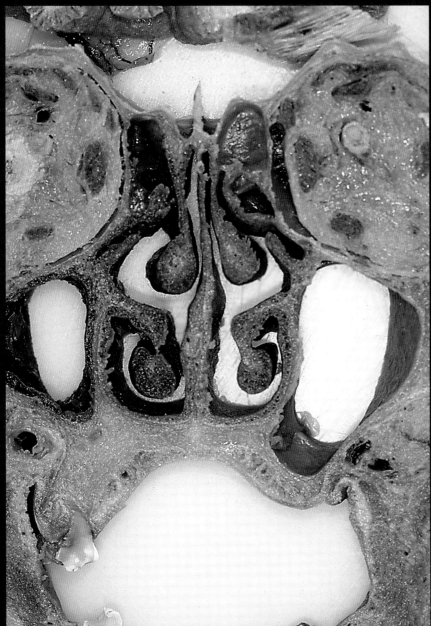

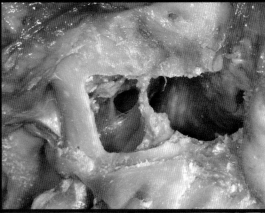

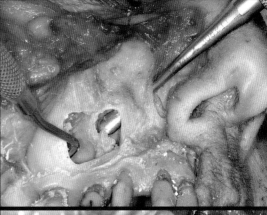

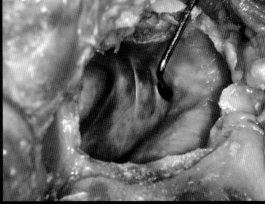

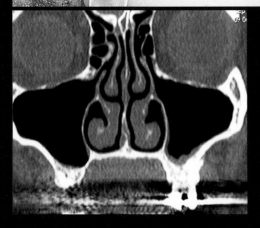

1 A → ANTERIOR SECTION OF THE MAXILLARY SINUSES. HYPERPNEUMATIZATION OF THE LEFT SINUS AND ATROPHY OF THE ALVEOLAR RIDGE FURTHER TO THE LOSS OF TEETH CAN BE NOTED.

1 B → CT ANTERIOR SECTION OF MAXILLARY SINUSES. THE OSTEOMEATAL COMPLEX CAN BE SEEN.

2 A-B → RATIO OF THE MAXILLARY SINUS. THE PROBE ENTERS FROM THE PYRIFORM OPENING AND REACHES THE MEDIAL WALL OF THE SINUS (LATERAL WALL OF THE NASAL CAVITY).

2 C → CLOSE-UP OF OSTIUM. THIS FORAMEN IS NORMALLY A 6 MM BY 3.5 MM OVAL.

An accessory ostium may be found on this wall in the maxillary sinus **FIG. 5A-B**; it is important to know about this occurrence, as during an operation to lift the floor of the maxillary sinus, the mucosa must not be detached up to this point. The sinus floor includes the alveolar process of the jawbone and part of the hard palate. It is normally located about 1 cm below the floor of the nasal fossae (McGowan et al. 1993). In adults with a full set of teeth, the floor of the maxillary sinus is the strongest of the bone walls surrounding the cavity. It has various recesses and depressions near to the first molar and premolar teeth (alveolar recesses).

As a person gets older, the sinus floor is resorbed and tends to form dehiscences around the roots, so that the root ends jut out into the cavity, only covered by the Schneiderian membrane and by a small bone cortex flap, which is sometimes missing. The area surrounding the roots may remain for many months after a tooth has been extracted and it is necessary to be extremely careful during the separation of the membrane from these exposed apices as it may easily tear.

SINUS MEMBRANE

The inner walls of the sinus are covered by a mucous membrane (Schneiderian membrane), which is covered by pseudo-stratified columnar ciliated epithelium formed by basal cells, columnar cells and goblet cells fixed to the basal membrane: there are serum-mucosa glands in the lamina directly underneath, especially next to the ostium opening. This epithelium continues from the nasal respiratory epithelium. Normally the thickness of the Schneiderian membrane varies from 0.13 mm to 0.5 mm. **FIG. 6A-B**.

The membrane can, however, undergo pathologies that cause it to thicken, due to inflammation, which may result in sinusitis. It is advisable to fix an appointment with an ENT specialist when membrane thickening of more than 3 to 4 mm is noted **FIG. 7**. Clinically, a pathologic membrane is thickened and gelatinous, especially in cases of hyperplastic-hypertrophic sinusitis **FIG. 8A-D, 9A-B**.

The termination of a pathologic process may result in adherences on the bone below, which become evident through visible fibrotic processes in the membrane **FIG. 10**. The epithelial layer is thinner and has less vascularization than the nasal epithelium. Under normal conditions, the epithelium is kept humid by the continuous secretion of fluid from the goblet cells and the serum-mucosa glands. This epithelium transports the mucus produced towards the sinus ostium and discharge it into the nasal fossae (Stammberger 1986). This process takes place thanks to the 100 to 150 cilia present on each columnar cell, which vibrate at a frequency of about 1000 beats per minute. As it is in direct contact with the air we breathe in, this membrane also acts as an immunologic barrier, although to a lesser extent than the nasal mucosa.

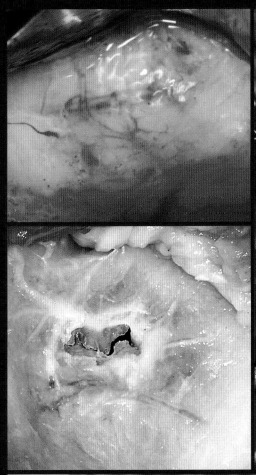

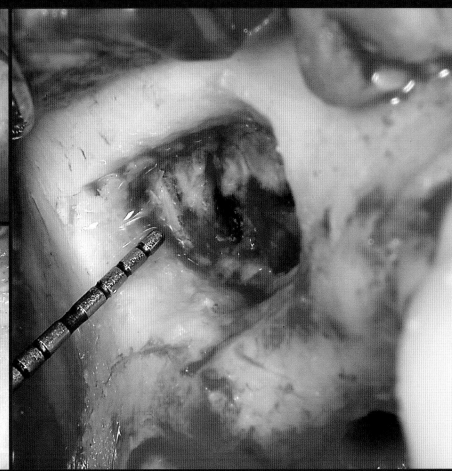

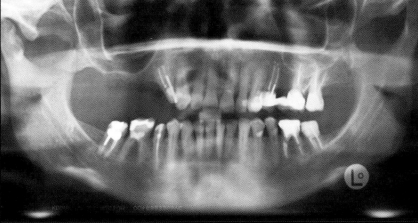

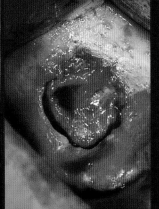

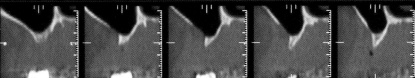

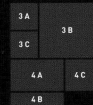

3 A → **LATERAL WALL OF THE MAXILLARY SINUS. THE THINNESS ALLOWS A VIEW OF THE UNDERLYING AERIAL CAVITY AND THE ARTERIAL ANASTOMOSIS.**

3 B → **CLINICAL CASE WITH A THICK LATERAL SINUS WALL.**

3 C → **AUTOPTIC FINDING OF THIN LATERAL WALL, WHICH SHOWS UNDERLYING VASCULARIZATION.**

4 A → **PRESURGICAL ORTHOPANTOGRAPH EXAMINATION. THE MAXILLARY SINUS APPEARS TO BE NORMAL.**

4 B → **CT OF THE MAXILLARY SINUS LATERAL WALL IN THE SAME PATIENT. A TOTAL LACK OF BONE CORTEX CAN BE SEEN DUE TO EARLIER INFLAMMATION PROCESSES.**

4 C → **CLINICAL PHOTO. THE TOTAL LACK OF BONE ON THE MAXILLARY SINUS VESTIBULAR WALL CAN BE NOTED.**

DIMENSIONS

The average size of the maxillary sinus in an adult is: volume about 12 to 15 cm^3 (with large variations, from 3.5 to 35.2 cm^3); height: 36 to 45 mm; length: 38 to 45 mm; width: 25 to 35 mm (Eckert-Mobius 1954; Uchida et al. 1998a and 1998b; Van den Bergh et al. 2000).

The maxillary sinus can therefore vary greatly in size, and it tends to increase in size with age and tooth loss, due to continuous resorption of the walls, both in the antero-posterior, the medio-lateral and the supero-inferior directions. The extent and form of this pneumatization may vary from person to person, and even in the two sinuses of the same person.

In the case of extremely narrow maxillary sinuses, which can only be seen using computed coronal tomography – CCT – it is vital to pay attention during antrostomy as the bone window may not be large enough to allow it to be turned sufficiently inwards, unless it is ground away (Tatum procedure). If this condition is discovered prior to the operation, it may be possible to plan a suitably sized opening, for example wider and lower, to carry out an antrostomy by erosion or to remove the window completely (complete osteotomy).

PROGRESSIVE CHANGE, EDENTULISM AND BONE RESORPTION

In case of maxillary edentulism, the thickness of the bone between the maxillary sinus and the alveolar ridge tends to become visibly thinner, even reaching values of less than 1 mm. This may be due in great part to the absence or reduction of normal masticatory loads (Cawood et al. 1988, 1991). Progressive resorption of the edentulous ridge in the posterior areas of the maxilla follows a well-defined path, which differs from that of the anterior regions and includes repeatable, predictable morphologic changes. There are different stages of resorption, which led Cawood and Howell to set up a classification of the increasing degrees of atrophy, based on the morphologic differences in the residual ridge (Cawood et al. 1988).

This classification is extremely useful for presurgical diagnostic assessment, as the appearance of the ridge morphology is connected to the horizontal and vertical size of bone available for possible implants.

There can be several causes behind resorption of the alveolar ridge. First of all, the intensity, the direction and the regularity of masticatory loads applied to the alveolar process areas play an important role in preserving the bone structures. Teeth are elements that can transfer suitable biomechanical stimuli to the alveolar bone, essential for limiting bone loss, which increases in the period immediately after the avulsion of a tooth, as the result of a bone remodeling process caused by the lack of functional load. Later, vertical bone loss stabilizes on average at about 0.1 mm/year, with large variations depending on the person. This bone resorption may become faster, and bone density will progressively deteriorate due to systemic factors such as hormonal imbalances, metabolic factors, inflammation and certain systemic pathologies. Age and gender may also influence the extent of bone loss.

The sinus floor therefore tends to lower craniocaudally, while the alveolar ridge is resorbed in the opposite direction. The length of time during which teeth are missing is correlated to the extent of alveolar resorption and to the pneumatization of the alveolar process in the maxillary sinus.

Long-term edentulous subjects rarely have a sufficient amount of bone to allow endosseous implants to be inserted, especially in the molar region.

Anatomic studies carried out on cadavers in whom the bone height was equal to the dis-

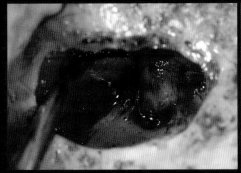
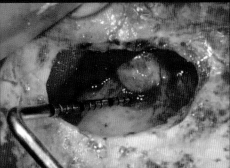
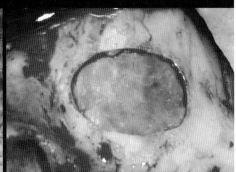

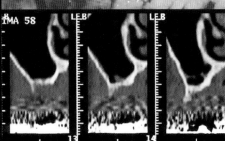

5 A-B → DISCOVERING THE PRESENCE OF AN ADDITIONAL OSTIUM. ALTHOUGH INFREQUENT, THIS POSSIBILITY MUST BE INVESTIGATED AND MANAGED APPROPRIATELY. IT IS THEREFORE NECESSARY TO ISOLATE AND LEAVE THE MUCOSAL TUNNEL WHOLE.

6 A → A THIN SINUS MEMBRANE CAN BE SEEN FURTHER TO ANTROSTOMY.

6 B → PERPENDICULAR CT SECTIONS OF THE MAXILLARY SINUS. THE THICKNESS OF THE MUCOSA IN AN ANTRUM IN A HEALTHY STATE IS ABOUT 0.13 TO 0.5 MM.

7 → PERPENDICULAR CT SECTIONS: SLIGHTLY THICKENED MUCOSA BUT LESS THAN 3 MM, IS NOT A CONTRA-INDICATION FOR SINUS LIFTING IF NO OTHER SYMPTOMS EXIST.

8 A → PERPENDICULAR CT SECTIONS: MEMBRANE WITH THICKENING GREATER THAN 3 TO 4 MM.

8 B-C-D → PATHOLOGICAL MEMBRANE INCREASED IN THICKNESS AND WITH GELATINOUS APPEARANCE.

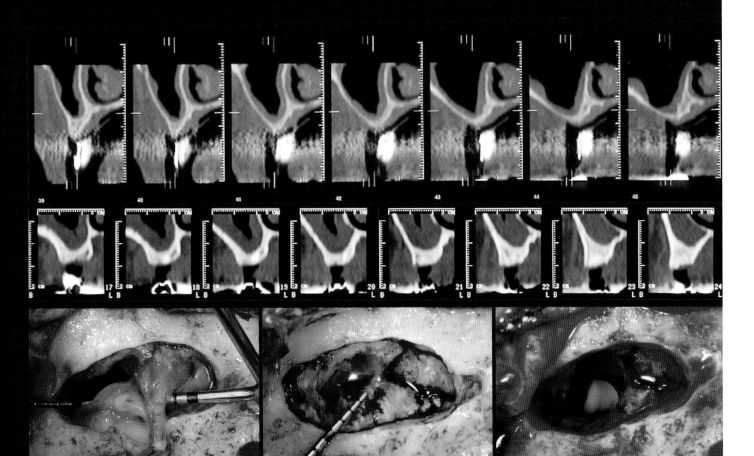

tance between the edge of the alveolar ridge and the maxillary sinus floor, and the width of the residual ridge was 1 mm and 3 mm apically at the ridge edge, found that the limiting factor for a possible insertion of endosseous implants is not so much the width as the height of the residual ridge. Greater bone loss vertically is plausible due to the concurrence of alveolar resorption and sinus pneumatization. The latter, however, seems to have a more important influence on the bone resorption process.

It is this lack of vertical bone in the posterior areas of the maxilla that often makes a preliminary maxillary sinus lifting operation necessary, using bone grafts or other bone regeneration techniques that allow an increase of the vertical height, prior to rehabilitation using implants.

The sinus membrane may undergo thickening after inflammation or allergic phenomena. This increase in thickness may be either generalized or localized to some areas that cause streaks in the membrane. In these cases, an ENT specialist may be required to surgically return the maxillary sinus to a physiologic state before the sinus lift operation can be carried out.

BONY SEPTA

The maxillary sinus normally stretches in an antero-posterior direction from the two regions to the first premolar area. The molar sinuses are often asymmetrical. Inside the cavity, bony septa are often found that originate from the sinus floor and rise for a variable height on the lateral wall. These bone septa, also called Underwood septa **FIG. 11A-B** can be found more often at the first molar or the premolar areas. They are made up of bone cortex in a vestibular-palatal direction that divide the back part of the sinus into multiple compartments known as posterior recesses. Sometimes these reach from the base to the upper sinus wall resulting in two sinuses of a smaller size (Miles 1973).

Incidence of septa varies from 16 to 58% with an average of about 30% (Underwood 1910; Jensen & Greer 1992; Ulm et al. 1995, Kim et al. 2006). The average height of the septa is about 8 mm, with possible values up to 17 mm. They are usually thicker at the base on the sinus floor, and then thin out in the middle. Velasquez-Plata et al (2002) found that septa can be found in all parts of the maxillary sinus, mainly medio-laterally. They are thin and are partly developed vertically. They are generally higher on the medial of the sinus and are rarely found in multiple formation.

It is believed that the formation of septa may be linked to the various phases of sinus pneumatization, and to the fact that maxillary teeth are lost in different periods. On average, molar teeth are lost before premolars and the edentulous area may encounter a resorption process that leads to a difference in level between the two adjacent portions (molar/premolar) on the maxillary sinus floor. The sinus floor is often on two different levels at the front and back of a septum and it is thought that a bony septum may form in the area between the two regressing areas in order to transfer masticatory loads in an optimal manner; the septa would in this way carry out a biomechanical function. After the complete loss of teeth, the septa may gradually disappear (Van den Bergh et al. 2000).

The presence of these septa may cause complications in maxillary sinus elevation surgery. In this case, a tridimensional x-ray diagnosis of septa presence is important for planning the size, shape and position of the antrostomy, and to help later separation of the sinus membrane from the bony septum**FIG. 12, 13A-B, 14A-D, 15A-C, 16A-B**.

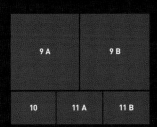

9 A → CT SECTIONS THAT SHOW UP THE RADIOPAQUENESS OF THE LEFT MAXILLARY SINUS AND THE THICKENING OF THE RIGHT MAXILLARY SINUS, PROBABLY DUE TO SINUS INVASION BY ENDOSSEOUS IMPLANTS. IN CASES OF THICKENED MAXILLARY SINUS MEMBRANES, AN EXAMINATION MUST BE CARRIED OUT BY AN ENT SPECIALIST TO CHECK THAT NO COUNTER-INDICATIONS FOR THE OPERATION EXIST.

9 B → PERPENDICULAR CT SECTIONS OF THE SAME PATIENT.

10 → ASPECT OF A MEMBRANE WITH INFLAMMATORY RESULTS. THE STREAKED ASPECT CAN BE SEEN, CAUSED BY FIBROTIC THICKENING.

11 A-B → CLINICAL PHOTOS: PRESENCE OF UNDERWOOD SEPTA INSIDE THE MAXILLARY SINUS.

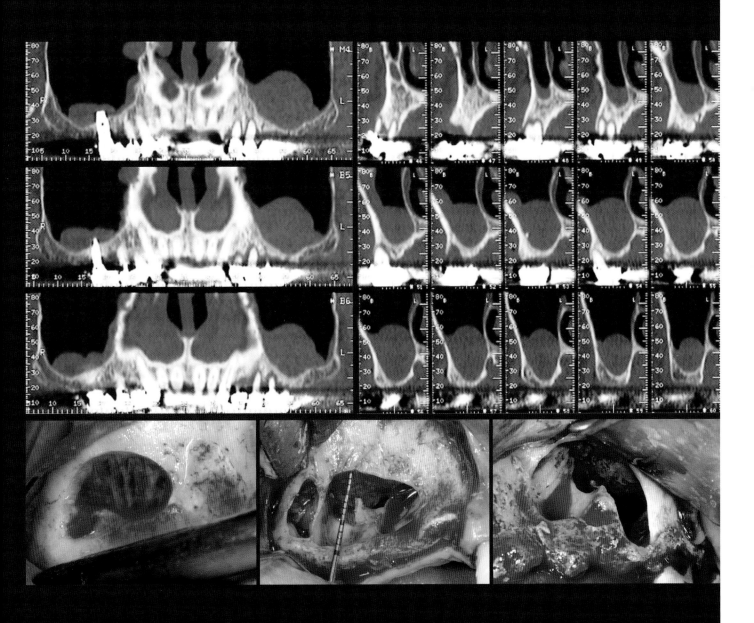

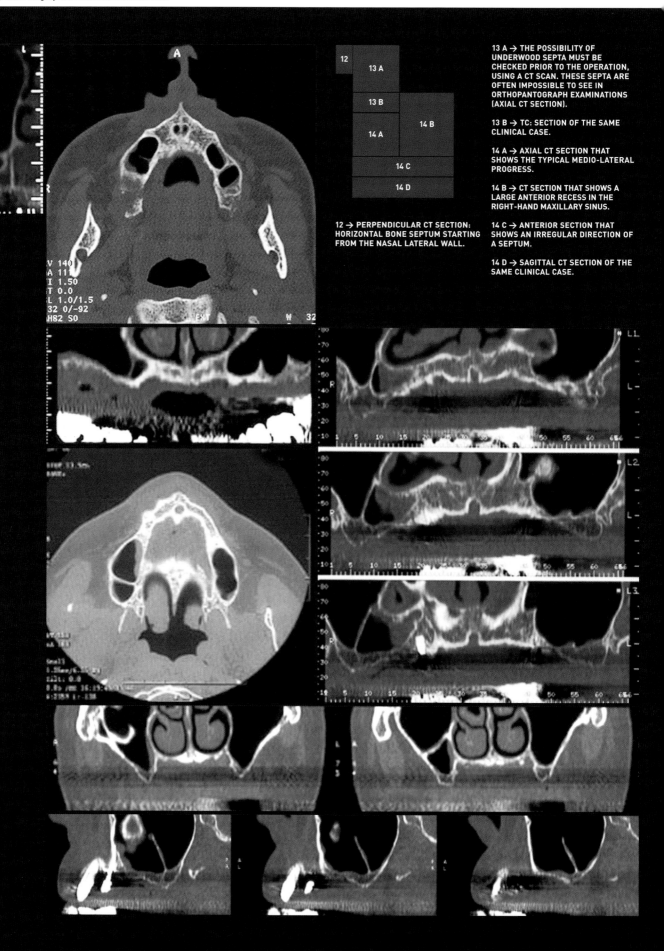

13 A → THE POSSIBILITY OF UNDERWOOD SEPTA MUST BE CHECKED PRIOR TO THE OPERATION, USING A CT SCAN. THESE SEPTA ARE OFTEN IMPOSSIBLE TO SEE IN ORTHOPANTOGRAPH EXAMINATIONS (AXIAL CT SECTION).

13 B → TC: SECTION OF THE SAME CLINICAL CASE.

14 A → AXIAL CT SECTION THAT SHOWS THE TYPICAL MEDIO-LATERAL PROGRESS.

14 B → CT SECTION THAT SHOWS A LARGE ANTERIOR RECESS IN THE RIGHT-HAND MAXILLARY SINUS.

12 → PERPENDICULAR CT SECTION: HORIZONTAL BONE SEPTUM STARTING FROM THE NASAL LATERAL WALL.

14 C → ANTERIOR SECTION THAT SHOWS AN IRREGULAR DIRECTION OF A SEPTUM.

14 D → SAGITTAL CT SECTION OF THE SAME CLINICAL CASE.

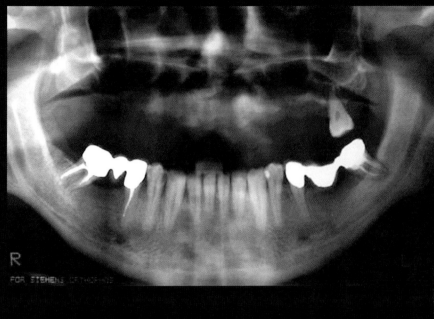

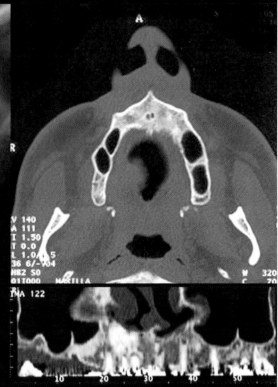

15A | 15B
| 15C

16A | 16B

15 A → EXAMPLE OF AN ORTHOPANTOGRAPH EXAMINATION WHERE SOME RADIOPAQUE AREAS CAN BE SEEN IN THE MAXILLARY SINUS.

15 B → AXIAL CT SECTION OF THE SAME CASE.

15 C → ORTHOPANTOGRAPH CT SECTION THAT SHOWS THE BILATERAL PRESENCE OF SEPTA.

16 A → AXIAL CT SECTION: MULTIPLE SEPTA.

16 B → PERPENDICULAR CT SECTIONS OF THE SAME CASE.

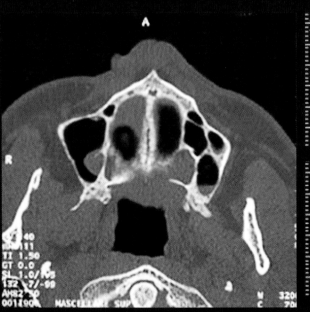

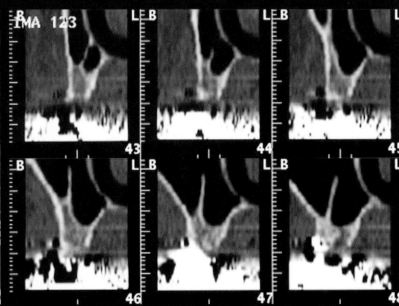

VASCULARIZATION

The maxillary vascular network is extremely large, guaranteeing a good blood supply.

The blood supply into in the maxillary sinus occurs by three arteries, all branches of the maxillary artery: 1) the infraorbital artery; 2) the medial wall supply is the posterior lateral nasal artery; 3) the posterior superior alveolar artery (branch of the internal maxillary) (Chanavaz 1990; McGowan et al. 1993; de Mol Van Otterloo 1994; Flanagan 2005).

This latter vessel often makes an intraosseous anastomosis with the infraorbital artery, starting inside the maxillary sinus lateral wall at an average distance of 19 mm from the base of the sinus **FIG. 17A**.

The intraosseous route may be seen on computer tomography in the sections that are perpendicular to the inside of the sinus lateral wall **FIG. 17B-C** (Solar et al. 1999, Elian et al. 2005).

Vascularization of the grafting material placed in sinus floor elevation procedure occurs via three routes (Solar et al. 1999):

- Extraosseous anastomosis (EA): terminal branch of the posterior superior alveolar artery (PSAA) branch of the maxillary artery (MA), with an extraosseous terminal branch of the intraorbital artery (IOA), another branch of the MA. It courses at a mean height of 23 to 26 mm from the alveolar margin. An extraosseous vestibular vascular anastomosis was observed in 44% of cases. The vessels may cause hemorrhage during flap preparation and periosteum-releasing incisions.
- Intraosseous anastomosis (IA) or alveolo-antral artery: second branch of PSAA (dental branch) with the IOA. It courses at a distance of 18.9 to 19.6 mm from the alveolar margin.
- Branches of these vessels (PSAA, IOA and IA) in the sinus membrane.

The middle portion of the Schneiderian membrane is supplied by the sphenopalatine artery, the terminal branch of the MA.

The presence of this anastomosis must be investigated to avoid hemorrhages during operations, which may occur if this artery branch is cut during the antrostomy. Severe hemorrhages during maxillary sinus grafts are rather rare, however, as the main arteries do not run inside the surgical area. Small vessels may be broken; if these are located in the exposed Schneiderian membrane, it is better to allow the hemostasis to occur naturally, perhaps helping by applying slight pressure with a gauze. An electrocoagulator may in fact cause membrane necrosis. These vessels supply both the sinus membrane and the periosteal tissues as the PSAA often has an extraosseous course. Healing and remodeling of the graft mainly depend on the vascularization branch from the sinus walls, from where the new blood vessels are created inside the graft. It is also important to preserve the blood flow to other structures involved in the surgical procedure, such as the Schneiderian membrane and the mucoperiosteal buccal flap.

The venom restorate from the maxillary sinus is by the facial vein, the sphenopalatine vein and the pterygoideus plexus. The veins may also be the route for spreading infection starting from the maxillary sinus, which may involve adjoining anatomic areas.

The loss of maxillary teeth and progessing age are causes of a marked reduction in bone vascularization. The numerical reduction of blood vessels is accompanied by a reduction in the calibre and an increase in their tortuous path. A positive link between the development of micro-vascular defects, bone atrophy and advanced age can be observed in man. Stenotic processes in the elderly reduce the blood flow to bone marrow, preventing osteoblast activity and delaying mineralization processes. Atrophy of the alveolar processes of the maxilla, an event that is only too common in the elderly, is associated

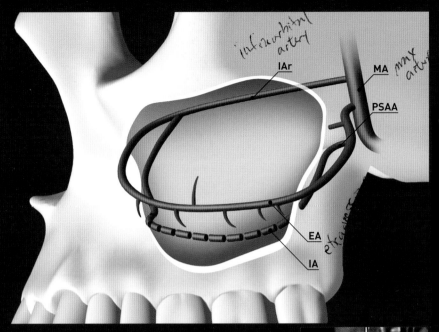

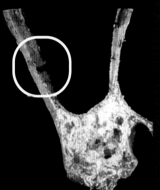

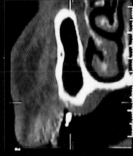

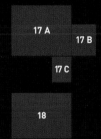

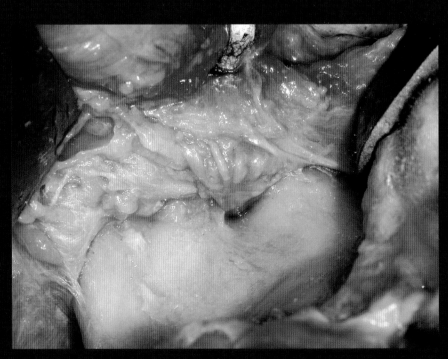

17 A → VASCULAR SYSTEM THAT INNERVATES THE MAXILLARY SINUS VESTIBULAR WALL. THE INFRAORBITAL ARTERY AND THE POSTERIOR SUPERIOR ALVEOLAR ARTERY FORM AN INTRAOSSEOUS ANASTOMOSIS (DOTTED LINE) IN ALL CASES AND AN EXTRA-OSSEOUS ANASTOMOSIS IN 40% OF CASES. (IA: INTRAOSSEOUS ANASTOMOSIS, EA: EXTRAOSSEOUS ANASTOMOSIS, IAr: INFRAORBITAL ARTERY, MA: MAXILLARY ARTERY, PSAA: POSTERIOR SUPERIOR ALVEOLAR ARTERY).

17 B → AUTOPTIC FINDING OF INTRAOSSEOUS ANASTOMOSIS ON CADAVER. THE VASCULAR FASCIA IS NOT COMPLETELY CLOSED BY BONE BUT IS ORDERED INTO A CONDUIT.

17 C → PERPENDICULAR CT SECTION. IT IS POSSIBLE TO NOTE A RADIOTRANSPARENT AREA ALONG THE MAXILLARY SINUS LATERAL WALL, WHICH CORRESPONDS TO THE ANASTOMOSIS LUMEN BETWEEN THE INFRAORBITAL ARTERY AND THE POSTERIOR SUPERIOR ALVEOLAR ARTERY.

18 → ANATOMICAL DETAIL ON CADAVER. AFTER EMERGING FROM THE INFRAORBITAL FORAMEN, THE INFRAORBITAL NERVE SPLITS INTO SMALLER BRANCHES.

with a numerical reduction of micro-circulation vessels and consequently with a drop in the blood flow to the area.

INNERVATION

Innervation of the maxillary sinus originates directly from the maxillary nerve, the second branch of the fifth cranial nerve (nervus trigeminus). With its posterior middle and superior alveolar branches, it innervates the sinus floor in the posterior area, together with the molar and premolar teeth.

The anterior superior alveolar branch, which branches from the infraorbital nerve at the infraorbital foramen, reaches the anterior sinus wall and the superior dental plexus, running below the Schneiderian membrane.

Some branches starting in the infraorbital nerve branch out from the trunk before exiting the infraorbital foramen and innervate the maxillary sinus medial wall **FIG. 18**.

Other branches involving the sinus mucosa are branches of the pterygopalatine ganglion and the sphenopalatine ganglion, with the long and short sphenopalatine nerve.

Many of the anatomic aspects examined in this chapter are important surgically when deciding which type of graft and design of lateral window to utilize.

REFERENCES

1   Blanton P.L., Biggs N.L.
    Eighteen hundred years of controversy the paranasal sinuses.
    Am. J. Anat. 1969; 124: 135-148.

2   Cawood J.I., Howell R.A.
    A classification of the edentulous jaws.
    Int. J. Oral Maxillofac. Surg. 1988; 17: 233-236.

3   Cawood J.I., Howell R.A.
    Reconstructive preprosthetic surgery. I. Anatomical considerations.
    Int. J. Oral Maxillofac. Surg. 1991; 20: 75.

4   Chanavaz M.
    Maxillary sinus: anatomy, physiology, surgery and bonegrafting related to implantology. Eleven years of surgical experience (1979-1990). J. Oral Implant. 1990; 16: 199-209.

5   de Mol Van Otterloo J.J.
    The influence of Le Fort I osteotomy on the surrounding "Midfacial" structures.
    Thesis. Amsterdam: Free University 1994; 22-24.

6   Eckert-Mobius A.
    Die Kieferhohlenentzundung im Kindersalter.
    Deutsche Stomatologie 1954; 170-177.

7   Elian N., Wallace S., Cho S.C., Jalbout Z.N., Froum S.
    Distribution of the maxillary artery as it relates to sinus floor augmentation.
    Int. J. Oral Maxillofac. Implants 2005; 20: 784-787.

8   Flanagan D.
    Arterial supply of maxillary sinus and potential for bleeding complication during lateral approach sinus elevation.
    Implant Dent. 2005; 14: 336-338.

9   Jensen O.T., Greer R.
    Immediate placement of osseointegrating implants into the maxillary sinus augmented with mineralized cancellous allograft and Gore-Tex: second-stage surgical and histologic findings. In: Laney W.R., Tolman D.E., eds. Tissue integration in oral orthopedic and maxillofacial reconstruction. Chicago: Quintessence, 1992: 321-333.

10 Kim MJ, Jung UW, Kim CS, Kim KD, Choi SH, Kim CK, Cho KS.
    Maxillary sinus septa: prevalence, height, location, and morphology. A reformatted computed tomography scan analysis.
    J Periodontol. 2006; 77(5): 903-908.

11 May M., Sobol S.M., Korzec K.
    The location of the maxillary os and its importance to the endoscopic sinus surgeon.
    Laryngoscope 1990; 100: 1037-1042.

12 McGowan D.A., Baxter P.W., James J.
    The maxillary sinus and its dental implications.
    Oxford: Wright, Butterworth-Heinemann Ltd. 1993; 1: 1-125.

13 Miles A.E.W.
    The maxillary antrum. Br. Dent. J. 1973; 134: 61-63.

14 Ritter F.N., Lee D.
    The para nasal sinuses, anatomy and surgical technique.
    St Louis: The Mosby Company 1978; 6-16.

15 Solar P., Geyerhofer U., Traxler H., Windisch A., Ulm C.W.P., Watzek G.
    Blood supply to the maxillary sinus relevant to sinus floor elevation procedure.
    Clin. Oral Implants Res. 1999; 10: 34-44.

16 Stammberger H.
    Nasal and paranasal sinus endoscopy.
    Endoscopy 1986; 18: 213-218.

17 Uchida Y., Goto M., Katsuki T., Akiyoshi T.
    A cadaveric study of maxillary sinus size and aid in bone grafting of the maxillary sinus floor.
    J. Oral Maxillofac. Surg. 1998a; 56: 1158-1163.

18 Uchida Y., Goto M., Katsuki T., Soejima Y.
    Measurement of maxillary sinus volume using computerized tomographic images.
    Int. J. Oral Maxillofac. Implants 1998b; 13: 811-818.

19 Ulm C.W.P., Solar G., Krennmair G., Matejka M., Watzek G.
    Incidence and suggested surgical management of septa in sinus lift procedures.
    Int. J. Oral Maxillofac. Implants 1995; 10: 462-465.

20 Underwood A.S.
    An inquiry into the anatomy and pathology of the maxillary sinus.
    J. Anatomical Physiol. 1910; 44: 354-369.

20 Van den Bergh J.P.A., Bruggenkate ten C.M., Disch F.J.M., Tuinzing D.B.
    Anatomical aspects of sinus floor elevations.
    Clin. Oral Implants Res. 2000; 11: 256-265.

22 Velasquez-Plata D., Hovey L.R., Peach C.C., Alder M.M.
    Maxillary Sinus septa: a 3-dimensional computerized tomographic scan analysis.
    Int. J. Oral Maxillofac. Implants 2002; 17: 854-60.

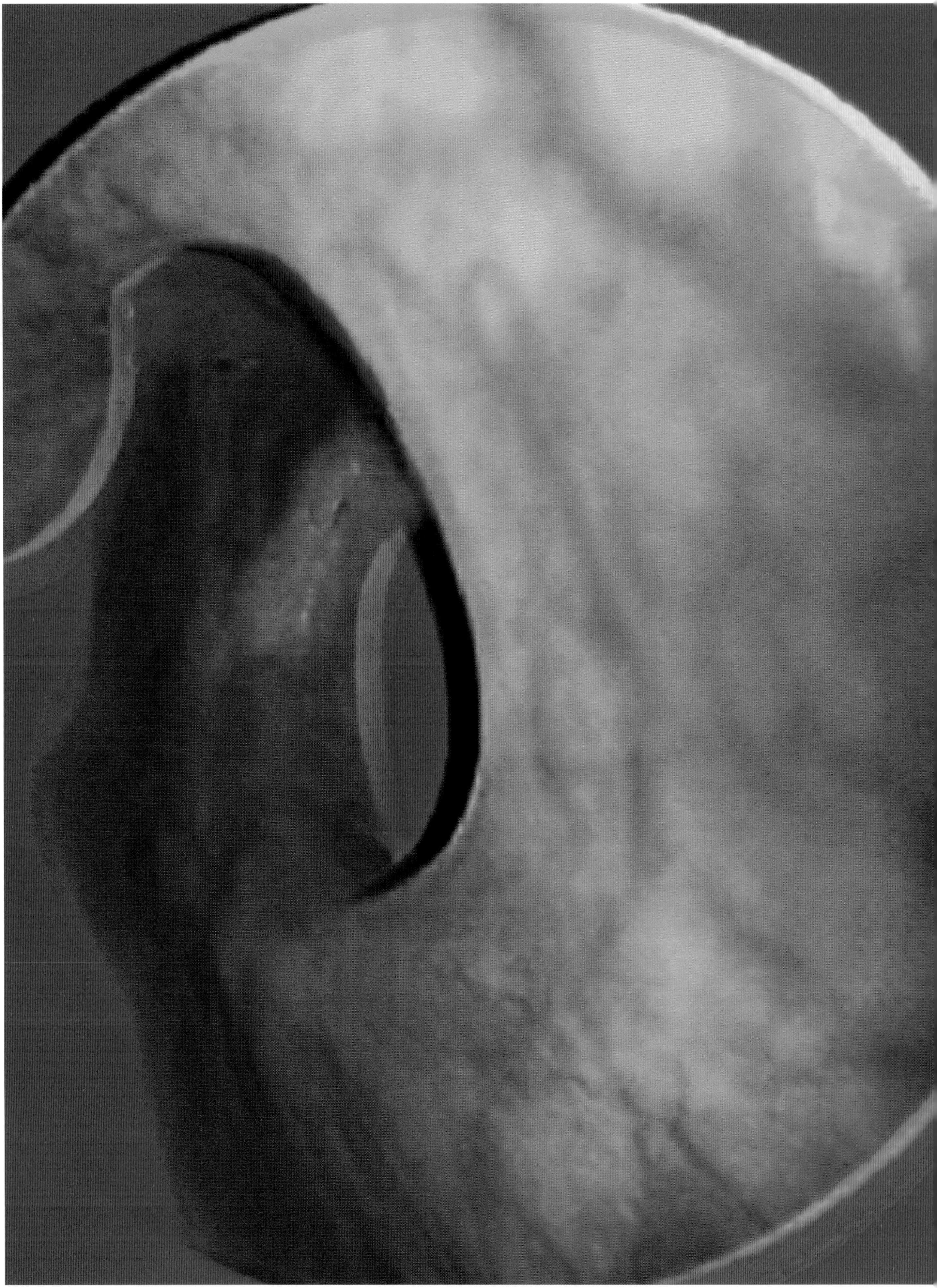

M. MANTOVANI

Otorhinolaryngological contraindications in augmentation of the maxillary sinus

03

03

Oral rehabilitation using implants has become an extremely widespread procedure, as it has a high rate of success. Even the maxillary arch, traditionally seen as a no-man's-land by implantologists, due to the presence of the maxillary sinus and the high number of the complications that may arise if it is affected, can now be rehabilitated with implants, even if there is not enough bone, thanks to the "*sinus lift*" technique. To obtain the best result, however, it is important for the clinician to be aware that carrying out a sinus lift brings about a series of anatomic alterations and interferences with sinus physiology, which should be understood to avoid complications.

The maxillary sinus, which appears to be a simple cavity full of air and lined with mucosa, is actually an anatomic formation that preserves its integrity thanks to the action of specialized micro-structures and the patency of the communication ways between the anstrum and the nasal cavities. This introduction provides us with opportunity to review the basic notions of embryology, anatomy and sinus physiology.

Of all the paranasal sinuses, the maxillary sinus is the first one to develop (around the 65th to 70th day of pregnancy). It develops in the postero-superior area above a small ridge, which is located above the lower turbinate bone

and stretches medially towards the middle turbinate bone, which is the rudiment of the unciform process [FIG. 1]. In this location, an evagination of the nasal mucosa forms. Starting from the central area of the middle meatus, the evagination stretches into the maxillary bone, forming a cavity with a larger antero-posterior axis, which is about 7 x 4 x 4 mm at birth – the outline of the maxillary sinus (Lanza et al. 1991). After birth, the maxillary sinus goes through three critical phases, corresponding to the eruption of the teeth, both deciduous and permanent: the first phase is the period between birth and 2.5 years, the second between the ages of 7 and 10, and the third between the ages of 12 and 14 (Takahashi 1984). The caudal growth of the sinus means that the sinus floor, which is located cranially compared to the nasal fossae at birth, reaches the same level at the age of 12 and then descends even more caudally, when all teeth have emerged, or further to the loss of some teeth, with a consequent resorption of the alveolar process.

The average size of the maxillary sinus, when fully developed, is 34 mm antero-posteriorly, 33 mm craniocaudally and 23 mm towards the vestibular palate; the sinus volume is on average 15 ml.

The position of the connection route between the sinus cavity and the nasal fossae, which runs from the natural ostium of the maxillary sinus and emerges in the lateral nasal wall at the middle meatus, does not change at all during lifetime, as it does not follow the "descent" of the sinus floor: this aspect means that the system cannot rely on the force of gravity for nasal draining of sinus secretions, and instead it must count on a sophisticated active transport system.

The maxillary sinus, which is usually formed by a single cavity, is lined with a pseudostratified, ciliated columnar epithelium made up of basal cells, columnar cells and "goblet cells" set against the basal membrane;

there are also serum-mucosa glands in the thin laminae directly underneath, in particular next to the ostium opening. The columnar cells have about 100 to 150 cilia per cell (Stammberger 1989) **FIG. 2A-B**.

The state of health of the maxillary sinus, like all the other paranasal sinuses, is guaranteed by the integrity of the mechanisms that work to produce and transport sinus secretions and by the oxygenation of the epithelium lining the sinus cavity. The latter needs direct gas exchange via the nasal-sinus communication routes, as the oxygen level in the blood is not sufficient.

Drainage of sinus secretions produced by the serous glands and mucosa, or mucociliary clearance, is a complex function affected by the quality and quantity of mucus produced, by the efficiency of ciliar transportation and the patency of the communication ways between the sinus and the nasal cavity.

The mucus film that covers the sinus mucosa is made up of two overlapping layers: the first serous layer is named the "sol phase", where the cilia movement takes place; the second "gel phase", which is denser, is transported by the ciliary movement, together with whatever sticks to it (e.g. dust, environmental pollutants, germs) **FIG. 2C**.

Under normal conditions, mucociliary transportation allows the antral mucus to be renewed in about 20 to 30 minutes, at a flow speed of about 1 cm/minute.

The mucus is the most important mechanism for protection of the nasal-sinus apparatus. It is made up of 96% water, 3.4% glycoprotein and also IgA-S, IgG, IgM, IgE, lysozyme, lactoferrin, prostaglandin, leukotriene and histamine. It is produced by the glands connected to the mucosa and is mainly regulated by the parasympathetic system (fibers starting from the upper salivatory center carried by the great petrosal nerve and the sphenopalatine ganglion) and the orthosympathetic system (mainly vascular function).

Some neuropeptides, including the substance P, act on the nasal-sinus mucosa, causing hypersecretion, vasodilation and plasmatic exudation. The qualitative and quantitative characteristics of mucus are also affected by hydration, environmental humidity and pharmacologic substances (e.g. atropine and atropine-like substances).

Under normal conditions, the ciliar apparatus beats 8 to 20 times per second; the temperature of the air breathed in has a direct effect on this function (optimal around 33°C. reduced under 18°C and above 40°C, absent under 12°C and above 43°C), as does the pH value (optimal between 7 and 8), oxygenation, osmotic pressure, metabolism, humidification and hydration (Watelet & Van Cauwenberge 1999) **FIG. 3**.

Observations carried out during a maxillary endoscopy reveal that penetration of the trocar through the sinus wall halts cilia movement for some minutes, probably due to a reflex phenomenon activated by the minor mucosa trauma. This allows us to predict that the raising of the Schneiderian membrane, as carried out in sinus lifting, will cause the cilia to stop beating (for a time and extent that we do not currently know due to a lack of dedicated studies) (Stammberger 1991).

Mucociliary transport occurs in a genetically predetermined pattern in the maxillary sinus. It begins in a star-like formation on the sinus floor. The mucus is transported along the anterior, medial, posterior and lateral walls, and also along the sinus roof, until it reaches the natural ostium opening. These findings were the result of careful experimental studies by Prof. Messerklinger in Graz **FIG. 4A-B**. It can be concluded that sinus secretions do not reach the respective ostiums by accidental routes, but instead follow precise paths that appear to be genetically predetermined. The bone ridges inside the sinus do not obstruct the progression of the mucus, which tends to become increasingly thick next to the upward tract.

Progression even continues in narrow points, with opposing mucosa walls, thanks to the "*bridging phenomenon*" that makes the mucus gel components progress beyond the natural ostium while the sol phase remains on the bottom. Small defects in the mucosa, for example a cut, small interruptions in the mucosa or isolated swelling of the sinus mucosa, do not interfere with mucus transportation. However, in these cases it is important for the mucus to be normal in quality, as a pathologic viscosity would make it impossible for the mucus to overcome these obstacles. One peculiar phenomenon of mucus transportation is that even if there are additional sinus-nasal openings up to 4 mm wide, mucus will still be transported towards the natural ostium without these alternative drainage routes being used. This discovery has rendered obsolete the openings that were previously made in the lower meatus in order to create spontaneous sinus drainage.

The natural ostium, the ethmoidal infundibulum and the "*hiatus semilunaris*" are the outflows for mucus towards the middle meatus of the corresponding nasal fossae: their patency is a decisive factor for maintaining normal sinus physiology.

The natural ostium of the maxillary sinus FIG. 5, which is most commonly oval in shape (7 to 11 mm long, 2 to 6 mm wide according to Lang, 1989) but which can also be circular or kidney-shaped, does not open directly onto the nasal fossae but communicates with them via a delicate, narrow "pre-chamber" formed by the ethmoid: the infundibulum, a narrow cavity in the lateral nasal wall between the unciform process medially and the orbital papyracea lamina laterally. In turn, the infundibulum opens onto the middle meatus via a two-dimensional gap, the "*hiatus semilunaris*" (bordered by the antero-inferior face of the ethmoidal bullosa posteriorly and by the free posterior edge of the unciform process anteriorly), thus allowing sinus mucus to reach the supero-medial face of the inferior turbinate and to be transported pos-

teriorly towards the rhinopharynx cavity and the underlying digestion routes.

The narrowness of the ethmoidal "prechamber" means that the opposite mucosa surfaces are close together, which, under normal conditions, allows a more efficient transportation of mucus thanks to the synergic action of the opposing cilia. The same structure also means that drainage is blocked by a minimal swelling of the mucosa, thus creating the condition for sinus pathologies, with the halting of mucus transportation (and ventilation).

Sinus ventilation, guaranteed by the patency of the same routes used by the sinus mucus transported by the cilia system across the middle meatus, allows normal clearance (mechanism function), which needs a continuous supply of oxygen to the sinus mucosa. Experimental research has revealed that 1/1000 of the sinus air content is exchanged in one breath (considering 16 breaths per minutes as normal, it would take 60 minutes for a complete exchange: however, owing to passive diffusion phenomena, it has been noted that 90% renewal of the sinus air content takes places in 5 minutes).

The delicate, complex physiologic process illustrated, involving the production of mucus, mucociliary transportation, patency of nasal drainage passages and sinus ventilation, ensures an appropriate homeostasis of the nasal-sinus system and, therefore, of the morpho-functional integrity of the latter. However, just an alteration in one of the above-mentioned physiologic processes, produced for example by: environmental noxae (micro- and macro-climatic changes, alteration in humidity of air breathed in, air pollution), systemic disorders (alteration of composition of mucus in cystic fibrosis, primary ciliary dyskinesia in Kartagener's syndrome, drug-induced ciliostatisis, dehydration or local factors lsuch as anatomic alterations of the lateral nasal wall obstructing ventilation (and drainage ways), such as hyperplasia of the unciform process, concha bullosa, stenosis of the

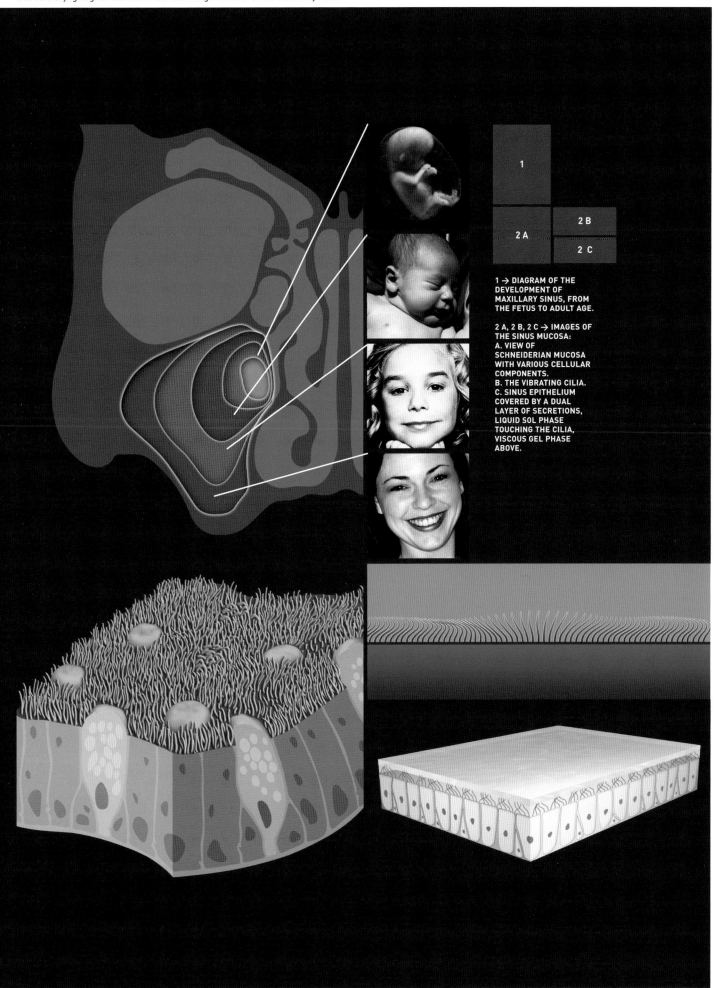

1 → DIAGRAM OF THE
DEVELOPMENT OF
MAXILLARY SINUS, FROM
THE FETUS TO ADULT AGE.

2 A, 2 B, 2 C → IMAGES OF
THE SINUS MUCOSA:
A. VIEW OF
SCHNEIDERIAN MUCOSA
WITH VARIOUS CELLULAR
COMPONENTS.
B. THE VIBRATING CILIA.
C. SINUS EPITHELIUM
COVERED BY A DUAL
LAYER OF SECRETIONS,
LIQUID SOL PHASE
TOUCHING THE CILIA,
VISCOUS GEL PHASE
ABOVE.

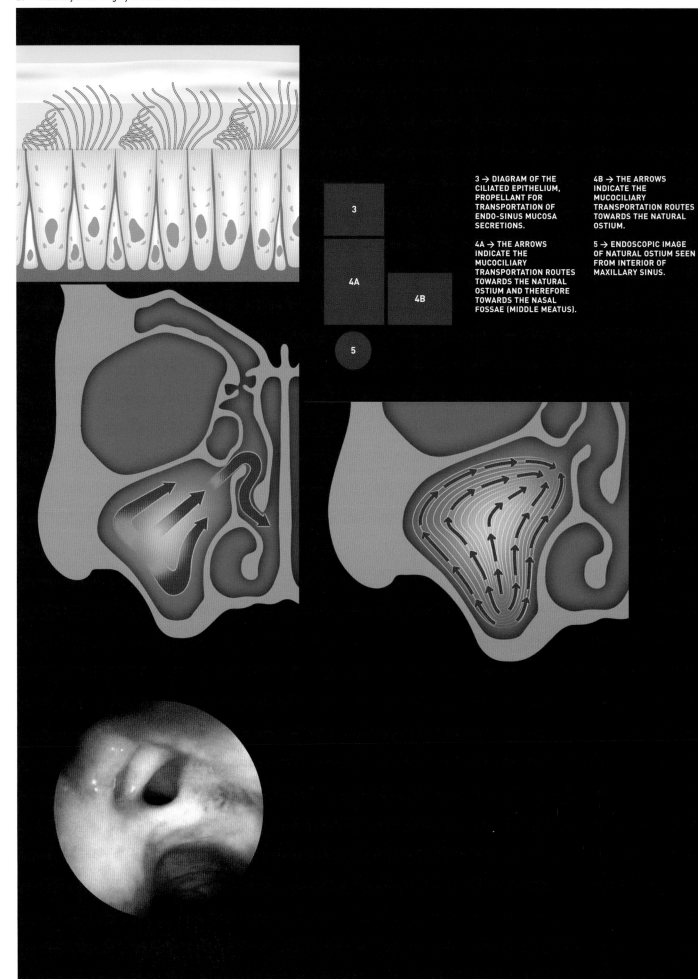

3 → DIAGRAM OF THE CILIATED EPITHELIUM, PROPELLANT FOR TRANSPORTATION OF ENDO-SINUS MUCOSA SECRETIONS.

4A → THE ARROWS INDICATE THE MUCOCILIARY TRANSPORTATION ROUTES TOWARDS THE NATURAL OSTIUM AND THEREFORE TOWARDS THE NASAL FOSSAE (MIDDLE MEATUS).

4B → THE ARROWS INDICATE THE MUCOCILIARY TRANSPORTATION ROUTES TOWARDS THE NATURAL OSTIUM.

5 → ENDOSCOPIC IMAGE OF NATURAL OSTIUM SEEN FROM INTERIOR OF MAXILLARY SINUS.

maxillary ostium, septae deviations with middle meatus contact, nasal polyps, specific and aspecific nasal hyper-reactivity, drug-induced rhinopathy and odontogenous sinus infections) can disrupt such a sophisticated system leading to sinus disease. The impairment of sinus drainage and ventilation leads to permanent damage to ciliar activity, reduction of pO_2 and increase of pCO_2 with inevitable epithelium alterations. This leads to microbial infection, which in turn causes edema and mucosae hypertrophy, and further damage to the ostiomeatal complex, jeopardizing (partly or fully, temporarily or continuously) the patency of the routes of drainage and sinus ventilation.

A typical sinus *lifting* operation involves the creation of a sub-Schneiderian membrane pocket on the maxillary sinus floor, using special separation instruments. The graft material will increase bone depth by means of an osteogenetic process. This surgical action may interfere with the normal antral physiologic processes, due to one of the following reasons:

- Inhibition of cilia activity, of variable duration and extent depending on the case (and currently not predictable as no experiments have been carried out on this matter), following a trauma produced on the mucosa while being separated from the maxillary bone.

- Alteration of the mucus composition, due to possible bacterial contamination.

- Damage to maxillary sinus natural ostium patency due to excessive elevation of the sinus floor, temporary mucosa swelling in the ostial region, or accidental penetration in the sinus lumen of fragments of filler material, through lacerations of the Schneiderian membrane (predictable in 30% of cases) (Regev et al. 1995). It should be noted that the sinus mucosa has great regeneration potential and can therefore rapidly repair the damage inflicted to its integrity by surgical action (Zimbler et al. 1998).

Considering these events, it is possible to identify two independent risk factor groups able to jeopardize the outcome of a sinus lift operation: the first, related to the operator and therefore characterized by a high inter-individual variability, is represented by the correctness of performance of the operation and, conversely, the extent of the lesions produced. The second, related to the patient, is identified in a pre-lifting sinusal anatomo-physiologyic condition named "*sinus compliance*". This term indicates the ability of the sinus to recover its homeostastasis after encountering a pathogenic noxae. With a sinus in normal conditions, both anatomical and functional, in a subject with normal local and general health, an operation that has been carried out correctly or even with accidental interruptions of the integrity of the Schneiderian membrane, there is an excellent chance of recovering its homeostasis without the development of sinusitis complications (high *compliance*). The chance of complications becomes progressively more likely as the above-mentioned risk factors increase (low *compliance*). In other words, it is possible to hypothesize the existence of a theoretical threshold for risk factors, above which the likelihood increases.

Analysing the risk factors of failure connected with the patient, we find the otorhinolaryngological contraindications for a maxillary sinus lift operation.

By introducing another variable, i.e. the criterion of the possiblity of correcting them (with *restitutio ad integrum* of the structures involved in sinus homeostasis) by suitable treatment, it is possible to split in two further sub-groups the otorhinolaryngological contraindications for the sinus lift operation: A) presumably irreversible, and B) potentially reversible.

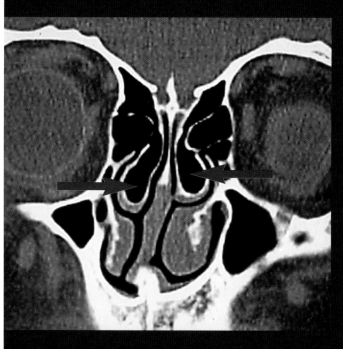

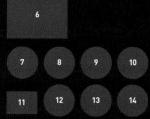

6 → DUAL CONCHA BULLOSA: CT CORONAL IMAGE. THE IRREGULAR AIR CAVITIES (INDICATED BY ARROWS) ARE VISIBLE IN THE MIDDLE TURBINATE BONES.

7 → ENDOSCOPIC VIEW OF THE ENLARGED RIGHT MIDDLE TURBINATE BONE DUE TO THE PRESENCE OF BONE PNEUMATISATION (CONCHAE BULLA).

8 → INTRA-OPERATIONAL ENDOSCOPIC VIEW DURING RESECTION OF THE LATERAL PORTION OF THE RIGHT-HAND CONCHA BULLOSA.

9 → PORTION REMOVED DURING OPERATION, INCLUDING LATERAL PORTION OF RIGHT CONCHA BULLOSA (BONE AND OVERLYING MUCOSA).

10 → ENDOSCOPIC VIEW AFTER HEALING. THE INFUNDIBULUM SPACE IS RATHER LARGE.

11 → ACUTE LEFT- MAXILLARY SINUSITIS (CORONAL CR IMAGE).

12 → ACUTE LEFT MAXILLARY SINUSITIS. THE ARROW INDICATES THE STREAM OF PURULENT MATERIAL THAT COMES OUT OF THE MAIN OSTIUM OF THE LEFT MAXILLARY SINUS. NASAL MUCOCILIARY TRANSPORTATION GUIDES IT TOWARDS THE CHOANA ALONG THE MIDDLE MEATUS.

13 → RESULTS OF A PARTIAL UNCINECTOMY (ARROW). TM, THE MIDDLE TURBINATE BONE

14 → THE NATURAL OSTIUM OF THE LEFT-MAXILLARY SINUS IS VISIBLE. PU, UNCIFORM PROCESS.

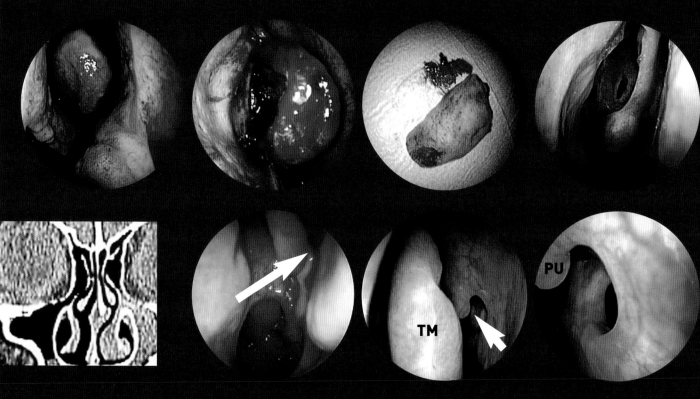

15 → THE CORONAL SECTION OF THE CT SHOWS THE MASSIVE OPACITY OF THE LEFT MAXILLARY SINUS. PARENCHYMATOUS DENSITY TISSUE PROTRUDES FROM THE LEFT SINUS OSTIUM (ARROW): ANTROCHOANAL POLYP.

16 → REMOVED ANTROCHOANAL POLYP.

17 → VIEW WITH 0° OPTICS OF LEFT MIDDLE MEATUS AND ADDITIONAL LEFT SINUS OSTIUM (ARROW) FROM WHERE THE ANTROCHOANAL POLYP EMERGED.

18 → VIEW WITH 30° OPTICS OF THE SAME ADDITIONAL SINUS OSTIUM THROUGH WHICH THE NORMAL SINUS MUCOSA CAN BE SEEN AFTER REMOVAL OF THE ANTROCHOANAL POLYP.

ENDOSCOPIC IMAGES: COURTESY OF PROF. PAOLO CASTELNUOVO, DIRECTOR, AND DR. MAURIZIO BIGNAMI, RESEARCHER, AT THE OTORHINOLARYNGOLOGICAL CLINIC, UNIVERSITY OF INSUBRIA, VARESE, ITALY

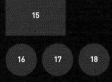

15

16 17 18

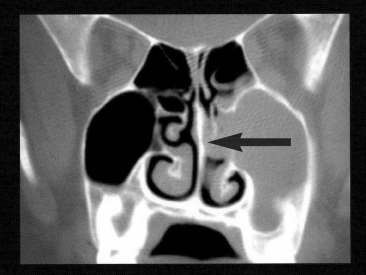

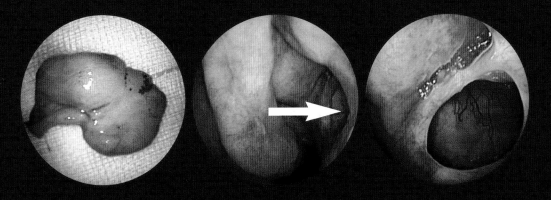

A) PRESUMABLY IRREVERSIBLE ENT CONTRAINDICATIONS

ANATOMICO-STRUCTURAL ALTERATIONS:

- Permanent and incorrigible naso-sinusal impairment, hampering antral homeostasis (e.g. posttraumatic, postsurgical and post-radiotherapy scarring on the naso-sinus walls and/or mucosal lining).

INFLAMMATORY-INFECTIVE PROCESSES

- Recurrent or chronic sinusitis, with or without polyps, which cannot undergo definitive treatment because it is associated with congenital mucociliary clearance alterations (e.g. cystic fibrosis, Kartagener's syndrome, Young's syndrome), intolerance to acetylsalicylic acid (triad: nasal polyps, asthma, intolerance to acetylsalicylic acid, ASA), immunologic deficiency (AIDS, pharmacologic immuno-suppression).

NASAL-SINUS MANIFESTATIONS OF ASPECIFIC SYSTEMIC GRANULOMATOUS DISEASES

- Wegener's granulomatosis, "*idiopathic midline granuloma*" and sarcoidosis.

TUMOR-RELATED

- Locally aggressive benign tumors (e.g. inverted papilloma, mixoma, ethmoido-maxillary fibromatosis) and naso-sinusal malignant tumors (epithelial, neuroecto-dermal, osseous, odontogenous, lymphatic, metastatic) of the maxillary sinus and/or adjacent structures that seriously interfere with naso-sinusal homeostasis both before and after treatment.

B) POTENTIALLY REVERSIBLE ENT CONTRAINDICATIONS

ANATOMICO-STRUCTURAL ALTERATIONS:

- Impairment of the drainage-ventilation ways of the maxillary sinus sustained by one or more of the following anatomic alterations: septal deviation, paradoxical bending of the middle turbinate, concha bullosa, hypertrophy of the agger nasi cells, presence of Haller cells); postsurgical scars or synechiae on the ostiomeatal complex, oro-antral fistula not associated with a wide bone flap and after a definitive surgical closure [FIG. 6-10]. Many of these alterations can today be resolved by functional endoscopic surgery: the maxillary sinus must appear to be well-ventilated before attempting a sinus lift.

INFLAMMATORY-INFECTIVE PROCESSES

- Acute viral or bacterial rhino-sinusitis [FIG. 11-14]; allergy-related rhino-sinusitis; mycotic sinusitis (non-invasive form); acute recurrent and chronic sinusitis (often sustained by one of the anatomic alterations listed above, which obstruct the sinus drainage-ventilation ways, or endo-antral foreign bodies, or nasal polyps). Functional endoscopic surgery is clearly indicated in many of these conditions.

TUMOR-RELATED

- Naso-sinusal benign tumors that impair the antral sinus ventilation drainage pathways, both before and after the *lifting* the removal of which does not hamper the mucociliary transportation system (e.g. mucosal cysts, cholesterinic granuloma, antrochoanal polyp [FIG. 15-18], all easily subject to correction by functional endoscopic surgery).

Following these preliminary remarks, it seems appropriate to underline the need for each candidate of a sinus *lift* operation to first undergo a careful clinical history investigation. This will highlight the existence of elements that may increase the risk of postoperational complications (Timmenga et al. 1997). Internal-medicine pathologies (systemic diseases that can contraindicate grafting or implants, pregnancy, *noncompensated* diabetes mellitus), recreational habits (use of cocaine, tobacco, alcohol abuse), dental pathologies (periapical pathology, untreated active periodontal disease) and otorhinolaryngological pathologies (difficulty in nasal respiration, previous naso-sinusal pathologies, chronic respiratory diseases, naso-sinusal anatomico-structural alterations) must be investigated. If necessary, suitable specialist collaboration (otorhinolaryngologist, pneumologist or immuno-internal medicine specialist) must be requested. By observing these guidelines, assuming that the operator has adequate experience and instruments, it can be concluded that, with current knowledge, the correct raising of the sinus mucosa followed by suitable grafting of the underlying cavity with appropriate material, if there are no major faults in the carrying out of the procedure and/or important reduction of the "*sinus compliance*", is a safe procedure with predictable results, i.e. an "*efficacious procedure*", as concluded unanimously during the "*Sinus Consensus Conference*" in 1996.

REFERENCES

1   **Lang J.**
    Maxillary infundibulum and the pstium of the maxillary sinus.
    Clinical anatomy of the nose, nasal cavity and paranasal sinuses. Thieme, New York, 1989.

2   **Lanza D.C., Kennedy D.W., Koltai P.J.**
    Applied nasal anatomy & embryology.
    Ear Nose Throat J. 1991; 70: 416-22.

3   **Regev E., Smith R.A., Perrott D.H., Pogrel M.A.**
    Maxillary sinus complications related to endosseous implants.
    Int. J. Oral Maxillofac. Implants 1995; 10: 451-61.

4   **Stammberger H.**
    History of rhinology: anatomy of the paranasal sinuses.
    Rhinology 1989; 27: 197-210.

5   **Stammberger H.**
    Functional Endoscopic Sinus Surgery.
    Ed. Mosby Year Book, 1991.

6   **Takahashi R.**
    The formation of the human paranasal sinuses.
    Acta Otolaryngol. Suppl. 1984; 408: 1-28.

7   **Timmenga N.M., Raghoebar G.M., Boering G., van Weissenbruch R.**
    Maxillary sinus function after sinus lifts for the insertion of dental implants.
    J. Oral Maxillofac. Surg. 1997; 55: 936-9.

8   **Watelet J.B., Van Cauwenberge P.**
    Applied anatomy and physiology of the nose and paranasal sinuses.
    Allergy 1999; 54 Suppl 57: 14-25.

9   **Zimbler M.S., Lebowitz R.A., Glickman R., Brecht L.E., Jacobs J.B.**
    Antral augmentation, osseointegration, and sinusitis: the otolaryngologist's perspective. Am. J. Rhinol. 1998; 12: 311-6.

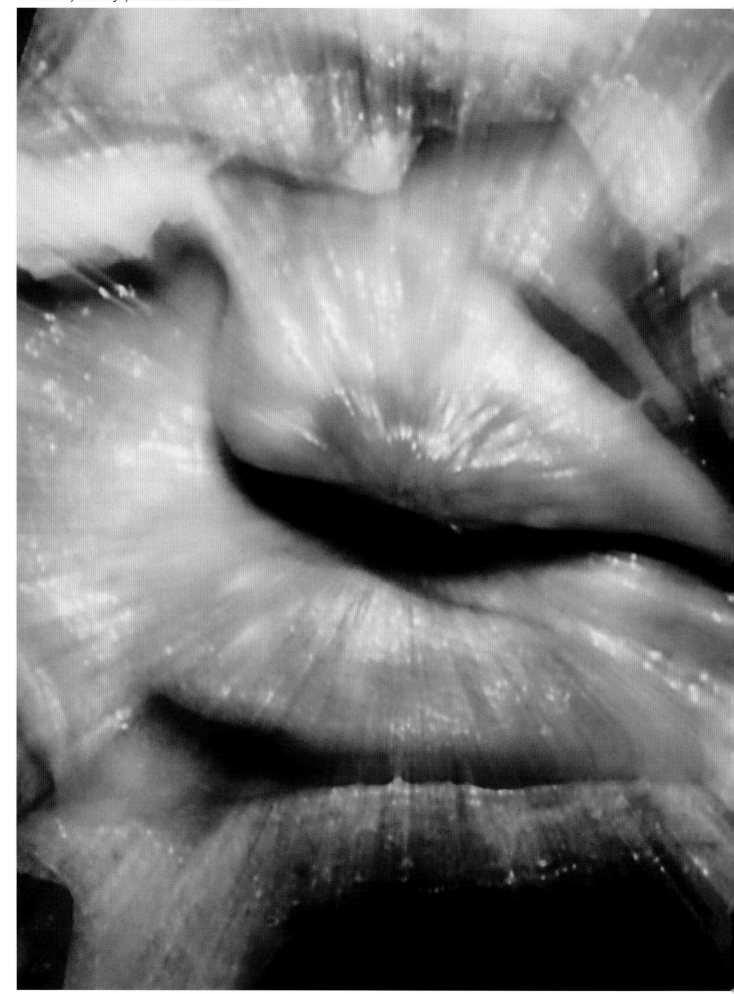

F. SANTORO
P. SALVATORI
S. TASCHIERI
T. TESTORI

The role of endoscopy in maxillary sinus augmentation. Indications for endoscopic surgery to optimize sinus functions

04

04

THE ROLE OF ENDOSCOPY IN MAXILLARY SINUS AUGMENTATION

Placing implants in the posterior area of the maxilla is frequently complicated by inadequate bone quantity and quality. Edentulism in this area is accompanied by a gradual resorption of the alveolar process craniocaudally and vestibular-orally (Atwood 1963, 1971).

The area undergoes rapid bone resorption when the functional loads on the residual crest are transformed into external loads. This brings about a reduction in the alveolar process, and also a reduction in bone trabecular density, accompanied by progressive pneumatization of the maxillary sinus (Smiler et al. 1992).

Of the surgical procedures proposed for resolving the above-stated anatomic limitations, sinus augmentation using autogenous bone or bone substitutes has proven to be a safe procedure with high predictability (Wallace & Froum 2003; Del Fabbro et al. 2004; Aghaloo 2007). This technique is also the most frequently used, especially in highly atrophic areas (Timmenga et al. 1997; Van den Bergh et al. 2000; Raghoebar et al. 1993, 2001). In minor atrophy cases (residual bone ridge height of at least 5/6 mm), a less invasive technique can be used, using a trans-alveolar approach (*osteotome technique*)

and lifting the sinus floor by using the bone collected while preparing the osteotome site (osteotome sinus floor elevation, OSFE) or using graft material (bone-added osteotome sinus floor elevation, BAOSFE) (Summers 1994).

The main complication that occurs after these types of operation is sinusitis, even though many studies base their results on criteria that are not very predictive for this type of pathology (Doud Galli et al. 2001). In fact, if an evaluation is carried out using otorhinolaryngological criteria, the appearance of chronic maxillary sinusitis after a sinus lifting operation has an incidence of 1.3% (Timmenga et al. 2001). In spite of this low percentage, these procedures bring with them a risk of damaging the maxillary sinus physiology. It has been ascertained that sinus physiology is affected by anatomic alterations.

Swelling of the sinus may also cause a reduction of ostiomeatal patency. This anatomic component plays an essential role in the appearance of sinusitis, due to interference with mucociliary drainage. If the maxillary sinus is filled, even only in part due to a hematoma or seroma, and/or ostium patency is reduced, maxillary sinusitis may occur, affecting the postoperative course of the grafting procedure (Timmenga et al. 2003a, 2003b).

The possibility of observing the ostium and sinus mucosa during the operation is therefore extremely important when assessing an individual clinical case. The use of endoscopy as a means of control has been found to be an effective technique for increasing predictability during maxillary sinus augmentation operations. Other diagnostic procedures are also facilitated: *biopsy*, *cytological smears* and *cultures*.

Moreover, when the BAOSFE technique is carried out, the endoscopic control allows checking of the integrity of the Schneiderian membrane and its elastic deformity in order to permit the maximum possible lifting of the sinus (Baumann & Ewers 1999; Nkenke 2002).

Engelke described a maxillary sinus lifting technique controlled by endoscopy (Engelke & Deckwer 1997). This technique includes the mobilization of the sinus membrane under endoscopic control, lifting via the trans-alveolar method and the simultaneous insertion of implants.

The authors proposed this technique in cases of moderate atrophy. Later, in 2003, Engelke proposed a new surgical procedure entitled "laterobasal technique". The procedure involves sinus lifting through a small cavity window for laterobasal access (Engelke et al. 2003).

It is possible to control this technique through endoscopy, which starts from the alveolar sites of the premolars and reaches the second molar. This situation allows a suitable surgical check in cases of major sinus lifting. Both procedures advise the insertion of an endoscope in the sinus lumen, through a micro-perforation made in the canine fossa. This is the most critical moment of the above-described techniques, due to its apparent traumatic nature and the targeted training that an inexperienced surgeon must complete in the otorhinolaryngological field.

Owing to this difficulty, another possibility is to simplify the endoscopic part of the surgery by making a subantral access only and avoiding micro-perforation of the maxillary sinus.

A review of literature on sinus lifting carried out using endoscopic control has shown a low occurrence of membrane lacerations, using both the ridge route (Summers 1994b; Baumann & Ewers 1999; Reiser et al. 2001; Berengo et al. 2004) and when the sinus bone floor is fractured and lifted (Nkenke 2002).

INDICATIONS FOR ENDOSCOPIC SURGERY IN OPTIMIZING SINUS FUNCTIONS

A retrospective analysis of failures and complications in maxillary sinus lifting operations places emphasis on a closer collaboration between dental surgeons and otorhinolaryngologists during the the diagnostic phase.

It is therefore the dental surgeon's task to collect clinical history data carefully, from which all the conditions that need an otorhinolaryngological evaluation can be derived, such as: difficulty in nasal breathing, previous rhino-sinus pathology, trauma and/or operations in the rhino-sinusal area or chronic and/or recurring respiratory diseases. Further important information will then be provided by radiographs.

It has already been pointed out that, of the preparatory examinations to be carried out prior to the operation, an implantology-specific CAT scan is recommended with acquisition extended to the OMC (ostiomeatal complex).

This is where vital predictive information can be found, which up to that point may be unknown, concerning negative conditions for the success of the technique, and which may result in all the anatomic alterations that cause sinus disventilation.

Endoscopy with optics will identify these alterations and will help in planning possible surgical correction. The focus point is therefore the patency of the OMC, where the natural ostium in the sinus opens through the ethmoidal *infundibulum* and where the three basic forming structures may enter into competition: the unciform process, the bulla ethmoidalis, and the agger nasi FIG. 1A–B (Takahashi 1984; Lanza et al. 1991; Levine & May 1993; Mehta 1993; Watelet & Van Cauwenberge 1999).

Competition can also arise from external interference, for example septal ridges, malformations of the middle turbinate (pneumatized by a concha bullosa bent or paradoxically bent), the existence of a large Haller cell or pathologies manifested at this level by nearby areas (such as massive ethmoidal polyposis) **FIG. 2A-D**.

Endoscopic surgery (Stammberger 1989, 1991) is in most cases – those identified as having potentially reversible contraindications – surgery extrinsic to the antrum itself (pre-chamber surgery). The aim of this type of surgery is to rehabilitate the maxillary sinus in order to allow its safe lifting. Traditional sinusotomy surgery using the Caldwell-Luc approach and involving the Schneiderian membrane disruption cannot reach the same target.

Modern endoscopic surgery, minimally invasive and functionally oriented, can be partly carried out using local anesthesia, without scarring to the oral vestibule and with healing completed within a few weeks, due to the considerable capacity of the maxillary sinus mucosa to repair itself, even after full inflammation.

The most common operating procedures are as follows:

1) UNCINECTOMY **FIG. 3A-D**

Total
(procedure following original Messerklinger technique)

Using endoscopic control with a 0° optic, the unciform process is cut, after an instru-

1A → LATERAL NASAL WALL:
  1) SUPERIOR TURBINATE
  2) MIDDLE TURBINATE
  3) INFERIOR TURBINATE

1B → LATERAL NASAL WALL:
  1) BULLA ETHMOIDALIS
  2) UNCIFORM PROCESS
  3) AGGER NASI AREA
  4) MAXILLARY SINUS' NATURAL OSTIUM

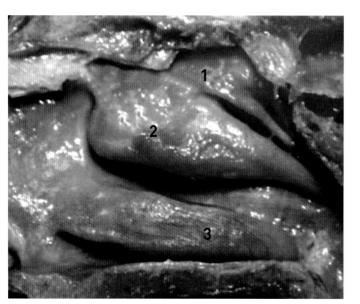

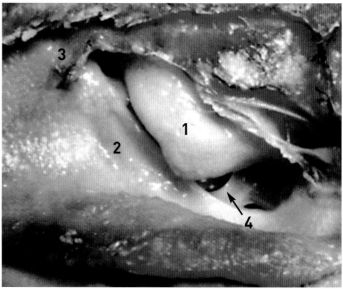

mental palpation, with a curved scalpel underneath the insertion of the middle turbinate and near to the entry point on the nasal lateral wall, in a parallel direction to avoid accidental damage to the orbital lamina papyracea. It is then moved medially, and gently removed using small Weil forceps, to open the ethmoidal infundibulum with a delicate clockwise twist of the forceps for the right nasal fossa and an anti-clockwise twist for the left one, in order to minimize damage to the lateral wall.

At this time during surgery, it is necessary to avoid large, trauma-causing, destabilizing maneuvers to the middle turbinate. In the best cases, this procedure allows the natural ostium of the maxillary sinus to be identified and provides the possibility of freeing it from obstructive pathology, by widening it.

Partial

Identification, by endoscopy with 0° optics, of the free posterior edge of the unciform process, which is later held by a retrograde clamp at the passage point between the horizontal and vertical portion of the process itself.

Section at the unciform bone, of which the lower third may be removed, carrying out the so-called *inferior uncinectomy*, or which can be brought forward delicately using the specific probe and then totally removed, using miniature cutting nasal forceps and smoothing any mucosal irregularities with a "*debrider*" **FIG. 4A-D**. This is also how a *total uncinectomy* is carried out. Sometimes these surgical procedures alone do not permit adequate removal of the infundibular obstruction and efficient sinus re-ventilation, making further ethmoidal procedures necessary that may result in the *resection of the bulla ethmoidalis and in the opening of the pneumatized agger nasi.*

2) RESECTION OF THE BULLA ETHMOIDALIS

The need to carry out a resection of the bulla depends on its pathological involvement or its growth with an antero-inferior procidence that obstructs the maxillary sinus ostium.

The bulla is opened at the safe inferomedial corner using a J-curette, and the opening completed with small Weil forceps or Strumpfel-Voss forceps, until the sinus' natural ostium is discovered.

3) OPENING OF PNEUMATIZED AGGER NASI

The agger nasi is the residue of the ascending portion of the first ethmoidal turbinate.

Marked pneumatization means that the middle turbinate is placed high and medially, narrowing the infundibular and the frontal recess, with a consequent disventilation of the maxillary sinus. This is a rare situation but it is necessary to correct it where present, opening the agger nasi cells while respecting the lateral limit towards the nearby lacrymal sac. Once this surgery has been carried out on the ethmoidal pre-chambers, the sinus' natural ostium is identified and freed from the pathology **FIG. 5A-B**.

It is then possible to proceed with plastic extension, with the anterior limit at the nasolacrymal duct and the posterior limit in the fontanelled area, with or without any additional ostium. If present they are joined to the natural ostium to avoid mucous recirculation. In this way, large endosinus mucosa cysts can be removed – using this path and suitable instruments – that are a contraindication for a maxillary sinus lifting operation. Some of the situations that condition an "*ab estrinseco*" narrowing of the infundibulum, including its prevalence, is instead a large concha bullosa on the middle turbinate.

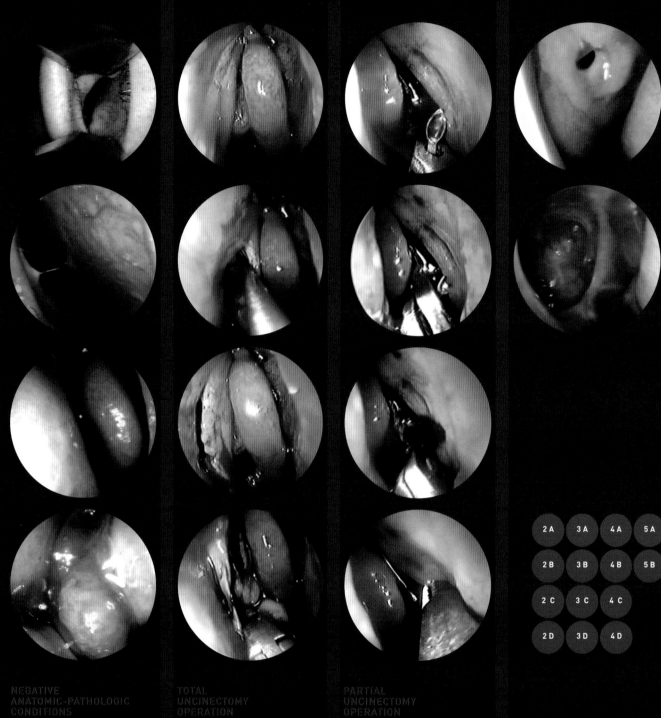

2 A	3 A	4 A	5 A
2 B	3 B	4 B	5 B
2 C	3 C	4 C	
2 D	3 D	4 D	

NEGATIVE ANATOMIC-PATHOLOGIC CONDITIONS FOR SINUS AUGMENTATION

2 A-B → RIGHT CONVEX DEVIATION OF NASAL SEPTUM.

2 C → LEFT MIDDLE TURBINATE PARADOXICALLY BENT.

2 D → LARGE LEFT ETHMOIDAL-NASAL POLYPOSIS.

TOTAL UNCINECTOMY OPERATION

3 A → UNCIFORM PROCESS.

3 B → INCISION OF UNCIFORM PROCESS.

3 C → COMPLETION OF SECTION PROCESS OF UNCIFORM.

3 D → REMOVAL OF UNCIFORM PROCESS.

PARTIAL UNCINECTOMY OPERATION

4 A → CONTACT FORCEPS WITH FREE EDGE OF LOWER THIRD OF UNCIFORM PROCESS.

4 B → ATTACHMENT OF FORCEPS TO LOWER THIRD.

4 C → COMPLETED INFERIOR UNCINECTOMY.

4 D → DEBRIDER THAT REGULATES UNCIFORM PROCESS MUCOSA.

5 A → ADDITIONAL OSTIUM.

5 B → LARGE-SCALE RIGHT ANTROSTOMY OWING TO NEED TO INCLUDE ADDITIONAL OSTIUM.

4) CONCHA BULLOSA SURGERY

Concha bullosa treatment involves the resection of the lateral lamina with a posterior extension affected by the extent of pneumatization of the middle turbinate. The upper limit will be the turbinate attachment and at the bottom the free edge will be cut to remove the lateral lamina using suitable forceps and delicate maneuvers, which do not destabilize the turbinate itself. In this way sufficient access will be obtained to the middle meatus and the infundibular area **FIG. 6A-C**.

5) COMBINED APPROACH

Endoscopic surgery allows a combined approach, when necessary, limited to the maxillary sinus cavity, via the middle meatus and the canine fossa, at a height, and with minimum bone breach (the trocar) to allow later maxillary augmentation using a standard technique.

This approach can also be used as recovery surgery for implant complications (Regev et al. 1995; Timmenga et al. 1997; Zimbler et al. 1998), such as the endosinus migration of endosseous implants **FIG. 7**.

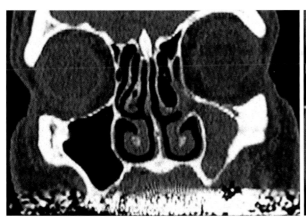
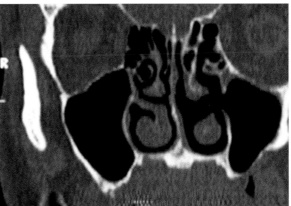
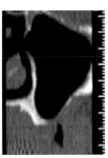

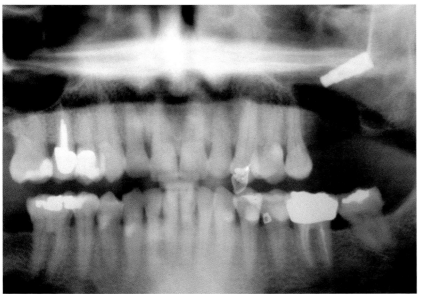

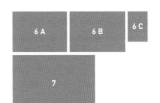

6 A → PREOPERATIONAL CT SCAN OF BULLA CONCHAE AFFECTING MAXILLARY DISVENTILATION.

6 B → POSTOPERATIVE CT SCAN.

6 C → VENTILATED SINUS AND MIDDLE ANTROSTOMY.

7 → ENDO-MAXILLARY DISLOCATION OF AN ENDOSSEOUS IMPLANT.

CONCLUSIONS

Endoscopic surgery of the sinus can treat most pathological conditions inhibiting sinus lifting, while optimizing sinus ventilation, which is an essential requisite for a correct diagnosis of sinus health.

Endoscopic surgical procedures are micro-invasive and aim to restore normal sinus physiology, allowing later implantation surgery that cannot be carried out after a sinusotomy according to the Caldwell-Luc technique.

REFERENCES

1 Atwood D.A.
Postextraction changes in the adult mandible as illustrated by microradiography of midsagittal sections and serial cephalometric roentgenograms.
J. Prosthet. Dent. 1963; 13: 810.

2 Atwood D.A.
Reduction of residual ridges: a major oral disease entity.
J. Prosthet. Dent. 1971; 26: 266.

3 Baumann A., Ewers R.
[Minimally invasive sinus lift]. Grezen und Möglichkeiten in atrophen Oberkiefer.
Mund Kiefer Gesichts Chirurgie 1999; 3: S70-S73.

4 Berengo M., Sivolella S., Majzoub Z., Cordioli G.
Endoscopic evalution of the bone-added osteotome sinus floor elevation procedure.
Int. J. Oral Maxillofac. Surg. 2004; 33: 189-94.

5 Del Fabbro M., Testori T., Francetti L., Weinstein R.L.
Systematic review of survival rates for implants placed in the grafted maxillary sinus.
J. Periodontics Restorative Dent. 2004; 24: 565-77.

6 Doud Galli S.K., Lebowitz R.A., Giacchi R.J., Glickman R., Jacobs J.B.
Chronic sinusitis complicating sinus lift surgery.
Am. J. Rhinol. 2001; 15: 181-86.

7 Engelke W., Deckwer I.
Endoscopically controlled sinus floor augmentation.
A preliminary report.
Clin Oral Implants Res. 1997; 8: 527-31.

8 Engelke W., Schwarzwaller W., Behnsen A., Jacobs H.G.
Subantroscopic laterobasal sinus floor augmentation (SALSA): an up-to-5-year clinical study.
Int. J. Oral Maxillofac. Implants 2003; 18: 135-43.

9 Lanza D.C., Kennedy D.W., Koltai P.J.
Applied nasal anatomy & embryology.
Ear Nose Throat J. 1991; 70: 416-22.

10 Levine L.H., May M.
Endoscopic Sinus Surgery.
Thieme Medical Publisher, Inc. New York 1993.

11 Mehta D.
Atlas of Endoscopic Sinunasal Surgery.
Ed. LEA & FEBIGER – Malvern, Pennsylvania, 1993.

12 Nkenke E., Schlegel A., Schiltze-Mosgau S., Neukam F.W., Wiltgang J.
The endoscopically controlled osteotome sinus floor elevation: a preliminary prospective study.
Int. J. Oral Maxillofac. Implants 2002; 17: 557-66.

13 Raghoebar G.M., Brouwer T.J., Reintsema H., Van Oort R.P.
Augmentation of the maxillary sinus floor with autogenous bone for the placement of endosseous implants: a preliminary report.
J. Oral Maxillofac. Surg. 1993; 51: 1198-203.

14 Raghoebar G.M., Timmenga N.M., Reintsema H., Stegenga B., Vissink A.
Maxillary bone grafting for insertion of endosseous implants: results after 12-124 months.
Clin. Oral Implants Res. 2001; 12: 279-86.

15 Regev E., Smith R.A., Perrott D.H., Pogrel M.A.
Maxillary sinus complications related to endosseous implants.
Jnt. J. Oral Maxillofac Impl. 1995; 10: 451-61.

16 Reiser G.M., Rabinovitz Z., Bruno J., Damoulis P.D., Griffin T.J.
Evaluation of maxillary sinus membrane response following elevation with the crestal osteotome technique in human cadavers.
Int. J. Oral Maxillofac. Imp. 2001; 16: 833-40.

17 Smiler D.G., Jonhson P.W., Lozada J.L., Misch C., Rosenlicht J.L., Tatum O.H. Jr, Wagner J.R.
Sinus lift grafts and endosseous implants.
Treatment of the atrophic posterior maxilla.
Dent. Clin. North. Am. 1992; 36: 151-86.

18 Stammberger H.
History of rhinology: anatomy of the paranasal sinuses.
Rhinology 1989; 27: 197-210.

19 Stammberger H.
Functional Endoscopic Sinus Surgery.
Ed. B. C. Decker, 1991.

20 Summers R.B.
A new concept in maxillary implant surgery: the osteotome technique. Compend. Contin. Educ. Dent. 1994a; 15-152-160.

21. Summers R.B.
The osteotome tecnique. Part 3-less invasive methods of elevating the sinus floor. Compend. Contin. Educ. Dent. 1994b; 15: 698-708.

22 Takahashi R.
The formation of the human paranasal sinuses.
Acta Otolaryngol 1984; 408: 1-28.

23 Timmenga N.M., Raghoebar G.M., Boering G., van Weissenbruch R.
Maxillary sinus function after sinus lifts for the insertion of dental implants.
J. Oral Maxillofac. Surg. 1997; 55: 936-9.

24 Timmenga N.M., Raghoebar G.M., van Weissenbruch R., Vissink A.
Maxillary sinusitis after augmentation of the maxillary sinus floor: a report of 2 cases. J. Oral Maxillofac. Surg. 2001; 59: 200-4.

25 Timmenga N.M., Raghoebar G.M., Liem R.S., van Weissenbruch R., Manson W.L., Vissink A.
Effects of maxillary sinus floor elevation surgery on maxillary sinus physiology.
Eur. J. Oral Sci. 2003a; 111: 189-97.

26 Timmenga N.M., Raghoebar G.M., van Weissenbruch R., Vissink A.
Maxillary sinus floor elevation surgery. A clinical, radiographic and histologic study.
Clin. Oral Implants Res. 2003b; 14: 322-8.

27 van den Bergh J.P., ten Bruggenkate C.M., Krekeler G., Tuinzing D.B.
Maxillary sinus floor elevation and grafting with human demineralized freeze dried bone. Clin. Oral Implants Res. 2000; 11: 487-93.

28 Wallace S.S., Froum S.J.
Effect of maxillary augmentation of survival of endosseous dental implants.
A systematic review. Ann. Periodontol. 2003; 8: 328-43.

29 Watelet J.B., Van Cauwenberge P.
Applied anatomy and physiology of the nose and paranasal sinuses. Allergy 1999; 54: 14-25.

30 Zimbler M.S., Lebowitz R.A., Glickman R., Brecht L.E., Jacobs J.B.
Antral augmentation, osseointegration, and sinusitis: the otolaryngologist's perspective.
Am. J. Rhinol. 1998; 12: 311-6.

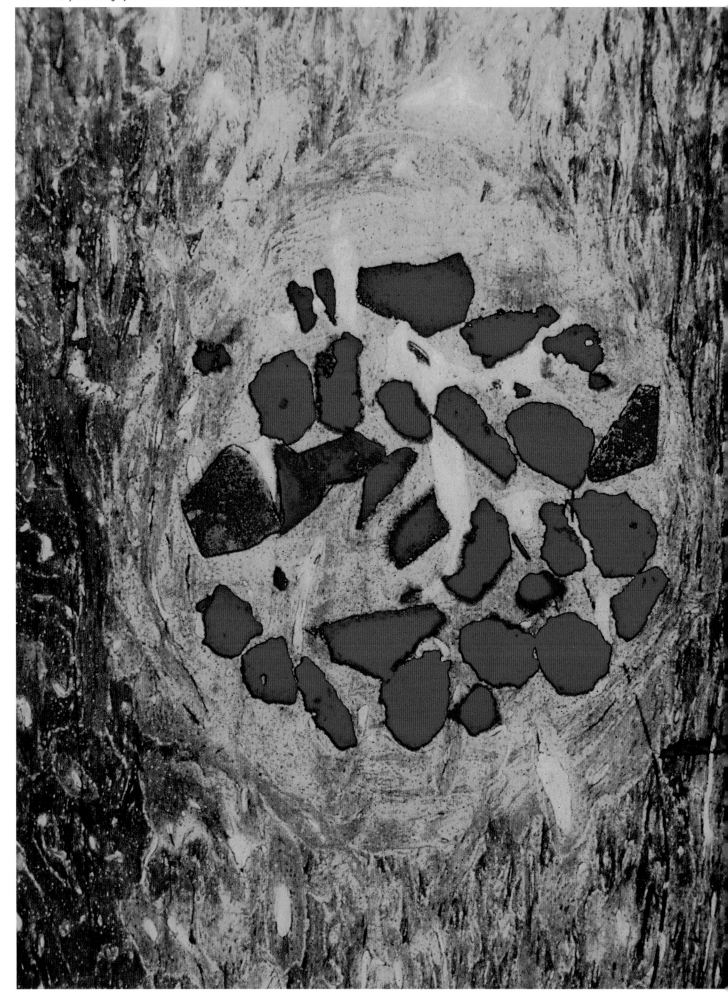

P. TRISI
G. MASSEI

Biologic and biomechanical basis of bone healing and osseointegration of implants in sinus grafts

05

05

INTRODUCTION

Specific studies on bone formation processes in sinus grafting are rare, and are usually clinically oriented towards the effects of the various graft materials and the type of implant.

Therefore, in order to understand the basic mechanisms of new bone formation inside a grafted maxillary sinus, and the later transformation of the bone under occlusal load, it is necessary to briefly mention the principles of bone repair and regeneration mechanisms and the bone response to load as they are currently understood.

MAIN PRINCIPLES OF BONE REPAIR

There are only a few basic principles involved in bone formation that must be satisfied in order to obtain successful osteogenesis (Schenk 1987):

- Sufficient blood supply: this is essential for new bone formation as the osteoblasts need high partial oxygen tension, to produce bone matrix.
  When the partial oxygen tension is low, cells produce cartilage or fiber tissue (Ham & Harris 1971) **FIG. 1**.

- Mechanical stability: this contributes to the formation of stable coagulation and thus granulation tissue that is rich in blood vessels, which ensure the blood supply to osteoprogenitor cells (Schenk 1987).

- Solid surface: osteoblasts can only deposit lamellar bone starting from a solid stable surface (Schenk 1987) **FIG. 2**.

- Size of defects: when a bone defect is overly large, i.e. more than 1 mm, it will not heal through the formation of a complete, rapid bone bridge between the walls of the defect. It will instead need several months to completely fill the defect (Johner 1972).

- Competition between cells for the most rapid proliferation: soft tissue cells that do not surround bone can proliferate much more rapidly than osteoprogenitor cells and can therefore fill the defect before the formation of new bone. Fibrous tissue is formed faster than bone tissue (Dahlin et al. 1988, 1990; Nyman et al. 1990; Seibert & Nyman 1990).

THE HEALING PROCESS OF FRACTURES

Fracture healing is an extremely complex process influenced by many different factors, such as the movement of fragments, the mobility of bone fragments with or without fixation, fragmentation and the possible exposure of the fracture site (Schenk 1992). In brief, we will consider the main histologic processes in fracture healing, which are useful for understanding the mechanisms behind implant integration or failure.

INDIRECT OR SECONDARY BONE HEALING

A fracture site can heal spontaneously thanks to the intermediate formation of a periosteal or endosteal callus **FIG. 3**, together with the formation of interfragmentary cartilage tissue and later bone remodeling. This healing process is called indirect or secondary healing

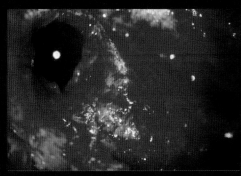

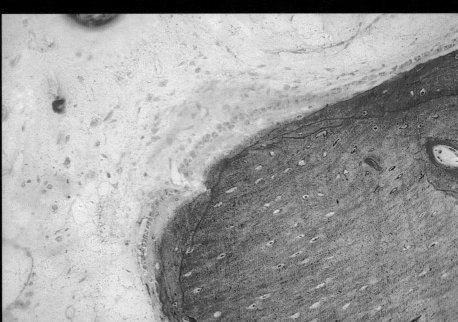

1 → A SITE THAT IS TO BE
REGENERATED MUST PRODUCE
PROFUSE BLEEDING, AS PROOF
THAT THERE IS CONSIDERABLE
BLOOD SUPPLY TO THE BONE
WOUND, AN ESSENTIAL BASIS
FOR REPAIR AND
REGENERATION.

2 → OSTEOBLASTS DEPOSIT
BONE ON A SOLID, STABLE
SURFACE, SUCH AS THAT OF
PREEXISTING BONE.

3 → AN IMPLANT PLACED IN A
RABBIT'S TIBIA CAUSED
CONSIDERABLE WEAKENING OF
THE STRUCTURAL CONTINUITY
OF BONE, BRINGING ABOUT THE
FORMATION OF A LARGE
PERIOSTEAL CALLUS COMPOSED
OF INTERWEAVED COLLAGEN
FIBER BONE.

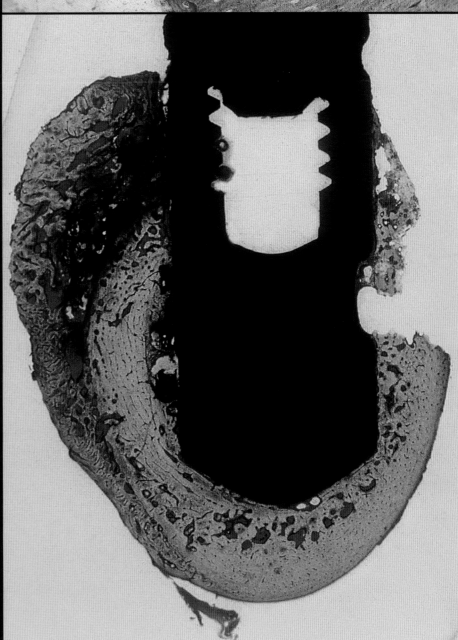

and occurs if the fractured fragments are not sufficiently stable (Schenk 1992). The intermediate formation of fibrous tissue or cartilage works to progressively reduce fragment mobility and therefore creates the stability required for bone formation (Schenk 1992).

DIRECT OR PRIMARY BONE HEALING

A check is carried out to determine when the fractured ends are perfectly reduced, are well-stabilized and proceed without the formation of periosteal callus. Initially, osteoblasts deposit new bone directly on the exposed bone surfaces within a few days and the gap can be filled completely in 4 to 6 weeks. The speed of bone filling mainly depends on the size of the defect (Schenk 1992). Small gaps in the fracture site can be filled with newly formed bone, but can also favor fragment micro-movements if they are not sufficiently stable, destroying the fragile tissue that has been newly formed for repair. This causes bone resorption (Perren et al. 1975) as the osteoclasts penetrate the fracture site, causing it to widen and the fragments to move.

CONTACT BONE HEALING

In the past, it was believed that the bone contact area between well-reduced, stabilized fracture fragments, which can be achieved using screws or plates, could prevent vascular invasion, considered to be the fundamental prerequisite for bone healing. Later it was seen that that the resorption cones of the basic multicellular unit (BMU) can cross the fracture site from one fragment to another, reforming a continuity between the ends of the fracture across the contact area.

This procedure, however, is a slow, long one, like remodeling, and is only a part of the healing process for a well-reduced, stabilized fracture. Compression of the bone matrix in the contact areas, which is achieved using compression screws or plates, does not cause bone resorption when the fracture fragments are perfectly stable and when the compact bone does not suffer necrosis due to compression when this is applied in internal fixation. Fragment compression improves fracture stability and induces healing without resorption.

The small areas of plastic deformation in the bone produced by the plate or screw are not removed by surface resorption, but by remodeling of the internal bone. Moreover, static compression applied to compact bone does not induce change in the rate of internal remodeling (Perren et al. 1975). A minimum amount of interfragmentary mobility, on the other hand, induces the formation of bone callus and the resorption of contact surfaces. In these conditions, the widening of the gap caused by resorption creates a space large enough for the invasion of osteogenetic soft tissue and therefore the new formation of bone, but this also causes a delay in the union of fractured bone parts.

HAVERSIAN REMODELING

This phenomenon is activated by any trauma in the bone, such as inflammation or alterations to the blood supply. Cortical remodeling replaces all the damaged and necrotic parts of the bone with new bone (Frost 1983a). Two or three weeks after the fracture, there is a sudden increase in the formation rate of new BMUs, a phenomenon known as regional acceleration phenomenon (RAP) that peaks at 5 to 6 weeks, with 30% of osteons active. After 8 weeks, almost 60% of the cortical osteons have been renewed and the activation rate of new BMUs begins to decline, returning to the basal level, which is about 2.5% per year in a dog's radius. The remaining 40% of cortical bone osteons will be replaced very slowly in the following months (Schenk 1992).

REPAIR OF STABLE ARTIFICIAL DEFECTS IN COMPACT BONE

- Defects of up to 100 to 200 µm in diameter made in the bone are filled concentrically with lamellar bone, and form a structure similar to a new osteon (Schenk 1992).
- Defects of 200 to 500 µm heal in 2 weeks, with the formation of a delicate woven bone network that is later reinforced by new lamellar bone and then remodeled with the formation of mature osteonic bone at a later stage (Schenk 1992) **FIG. 4**.
- Defects that are larger than 1 mm in diameter cannot be completely filled rapidly with woven bone but will take considerably longer to heal (osteogenic jump distance).
- A further increase in the size of the defect may lead to a critical diameter, which is impossible to resolve through spontaneous repair. It will instead be necessary to promote the formation of bone callus using osteoconduction, osteoinduction, osteogenetic distraction or guided bone regeneration (Johner 1972; Schmitz & Hollinger 1986; Hollinger & Kleinschmidt 1990).

REPAIR OF STABLE ARTIFICIAL DEFECTS IN SPONGY BONE

Defects produced in spongy bone in dogs' tibia, of diameter 0 to 200 µm, were consolidated by the formation of a direct woven bone bridge within one week. The woven bone trabeculae are re-inforced between the second and fourth week by new lamellar bone (lamellar compaction), which in the end covers the entire surface of the fractured trabecula (Schenk 1992). This process leads to the consolidation of cancellous bone in the gap area. In the following months, the dead trabeculae will be replaced with new lamellar bone thanks to the remodeling process that leads to the formation of new, thicker composite bone trabeculae (RAP) **FIG. 5**. Later, the remodeling processes of normal bone remodeling will replace this composite bone with new lamellar

bone (Glimcher 1987). The bone is repaired along the free surfaces of the bone marrow trabeculae, where the osteoprogenitor cells originate from the perivascular cells or from the bone marrow stromal cells.

REPAIR OF STABLE ARTIFICIAL DEFECTS IN HUMAN JAW BONES

The results of orthopedic studies previously quoted cannot be simply transferred to the human maxilla due to their peculiar biomechanical environment. The mandibular bone is subjected to heavy torque and tension and is therefore made up of compact, dense lamellar bone, as predicted by Wolff's law (Wolff 1892). The maxilla, on the other hand, does not undergo large-scale deformation and is made up of low-quality trabecular bone. Consequently, spontaneous bone regeneration conditions should be evaluated separately in human jaw bones to determine the effect of applying bone regeneration techniques. In a recent study, a new model was analysed that is useful for evaluating the biologic basis for spontaneous bone regeneration in human jaws, the bone growth device (BGD) **FIG. 6** (Trisi & Rao 1998). This device enables the simple creation and identification of a well-defined space; the sizes can always be uniform, thus allowing quantitative measurements of bone regeneration inside the space of the device itself. In ths way, we found that artificial defects in jaws, up to 2.5 mm in diameter, can heal spontaneously in about 2 months **FIG. 7** (Trisi et al. 2003a). Also, the addition of calcium phosphate resorbable ceramic graft material does not determine an increase in the amount of newly formed bone in the defect, but the density of the surrounding bone determines the density of the regenerated bone inside the defect (Trisi et al. 2003a). In 2 months, the device was filled by the newly formed bone. An analysis of larger BGD suggested that a defect of about 3.5 mm cannot heal spontaneously and com-

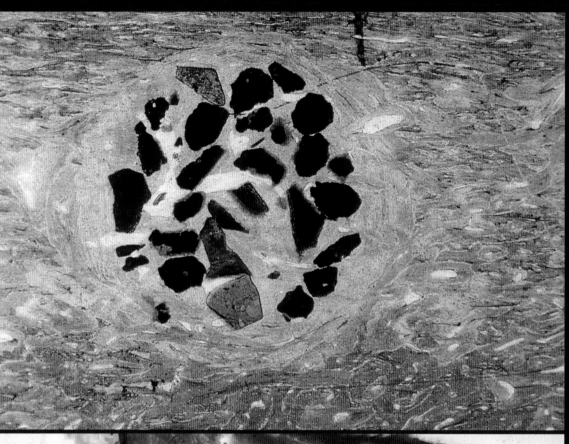

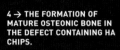

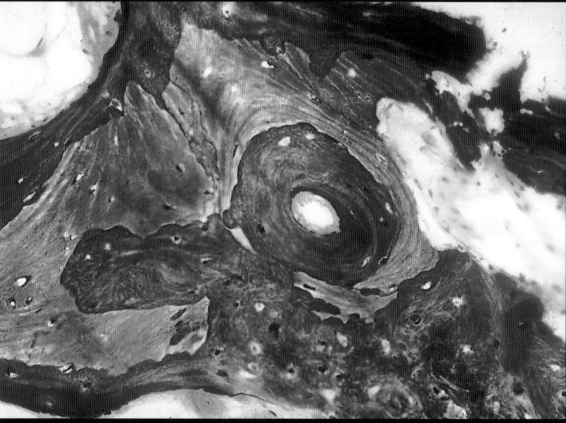

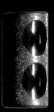

4 → THE FORMATION OF MATURE OSTEONIC BONE IN THE DEFECT CONTAINING HA CHIPS.

5 → NEW TRABECULAE FOR REPAIRING COMPOUND BONE.

6 → BGD, BONE GROWTH DEVICE.

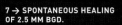

7 → SPONTANEOUS HEALING
OF 2.5 MM BGD.

8 → HISTOLOGIC SECTION OF
3.5 MM BGD THAT HAS NOT
BEEN TOTALLY FILLED WITH
BONE AFTER 6 MONTHS OF
HEALING.

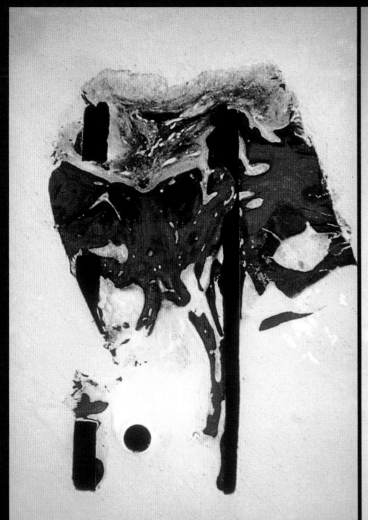
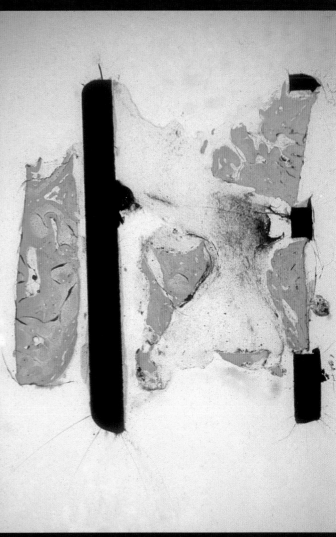

9 → HISTOLOGIC SECTION OF 3.5
MM BGD IN WHICH A
BIOMATERIAL HAS BEEN
PLACED. THE PRESENCE OF
GRAFT CHIPS HAS ALLOWED
THE COMPLETE FILLING OF THE
CRITICAL DEFECT IN ABOUT 6
MONTHS OF HEALING.

10 → FORMATION OF WOVEN
BONE IN SINUS GRAFT 12
MONTHS AFTER THE SINUS
AUGMENTATION PROCEDURE.

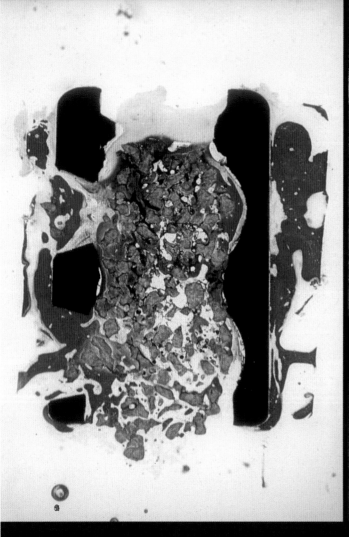

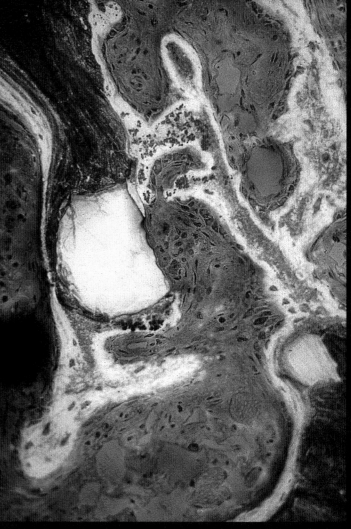

pletely in 6 months **FIG. 8**, but adding a biomaterial allows complete filling in the same time
period **FIG. 9**.

HOW IS BONE FORMED
IN THE GRAFTED SINUS?

After grafts are inserted into maxillary
sinuses, neo-osteogenesis reproduces the normal bone repair process described above.

Osteogenesis is activated by surgical
trauma, which causes the release of a large
quantity of cytokines with osteogenetic
effects (TGF-beta1, aFGF, bFGF, BMP-2 and
BMP-7) (Joyce et al. 1990a; Bolander 1992;
Bourque et al. 1993; Sandberg et al. 1993;
Bostrom et al. 1995; Onishi et al. 1998;
Sakou 1998; Trippel 1998; Tatsuyama et al.
2000; Nakajima et al. 2001; Cho et al.
2002; Rundle et al. 2002; Yu et al. 2002).
These factors start the healing process, with
the formation of new capillaries in the first
week, followed by the formation of immature
woven bone and then bone remodeling (Joyce
et al. 1990a and 1990b).

The repair reaction, with the formation of
new woven bone, originates from the bone
walls subjected to trauma, which stimulate
the osteoblast precursors, due to exposure of
the bone matrix, and act as a solid wall allowing the attachment of the osteoblasts (Boyne
& James 1980; Schenk 1987; Misch 1993).

The graft and the granulation tissue must
be mechanically stable and the neovascular
tissue must reach the entire graft, for new
bone formation to be completed.

Under the correct biologic conditions,
and having begun along the maxillary sinus
walls, osteogenesis extends progressively
towards the center and the apical area of the
graft and may continue for months after surgery (Haas et al. 2002a and 2002b) **FIG. 10**. At
this stage it is important for the biomaterial
to be extremely osteoconductive, in order to
aid the adhesion of the osteoblasts to most of
its surface, providing the highest number
possible of neo-osteogenesis nuclei. In this
way, the material physically fills the space to
be colonized on one hand, and on the other
increases the filling speed, reducing graft
consolidation times.

A gradient of osteogenesis is thus created. Maximum bone formation is obtained on
the bottom, the lateral and the medial walls,
while the most apical area has the minimum
new bone formation. The more the grafted
material is osteoinductive and osteoconductive, the faster and more complete newly
formed bone filling will be.

WHAT EFFECT DO GRAFT MATERIALS
HAVE IN THE MAXILLARY SINUS?

GENERAL PROPERTIES OF GRAFT MATERIALS

The introduction of a biomaterial into the
bone induces a complex sequence of biological
events, not only influenced by the host site's
intrinsic ability to heal, but also by the chemical,
physical and surface properties of the biomaterial itself. Endosseous biomaterials have been
classified according to the bone regeneration
mode in osteoinductives and osteoconductives.
Both bio-inert materials and bio-active materials
are considered to be osteoconductive. Osteoconduction is a biomaterial's capacity to lead
bone development above its own surface, when
placed close to bone tissue. Osteoinduction is a
specific process of the materials that have the
ability to induce the formation of new bone in
non-bone tissue (Remes & Williams 1992).
When implanted in a subcutaneous tissue,
osteoinductive materials can determine the formation of new bone, while the osteoconductive
materials induce a slight inflammatory response
and an encapsulation (Glowacki et al 1981a,
1981b; Kaban & Glowacki 1981; Mulliken et al.
1981). When implanted in bone defects, the
osteoinductive materials allow new bone to be
formed uniformly throughout the whole site, via
an endochondral or intra-membranous mecha-

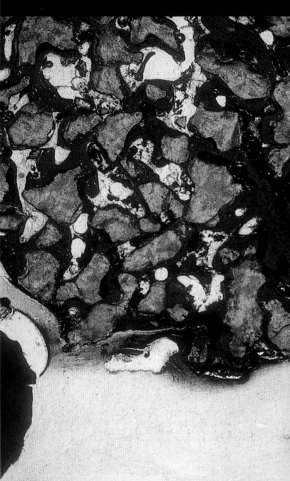

11

12

11 → BIOLOGICAL GRANULES
PARTLY FILL THE REGENERATING
SPACE, THUS HELPING TO
REDUCE THE SPACE TO BE
COLONIZED BY NEW BONE.

12 → TWO AUTOGENOUS BONE
CHIPS HAVE STARTED THE
WOVEN BONE FORMATION ON
THEIR ADJACENT SURFACES.
WHEN THE TWO EDGES MEET,
THE SPACE BETWEEN THE CHIPS
WILL BE COMPLETELY FILLED.

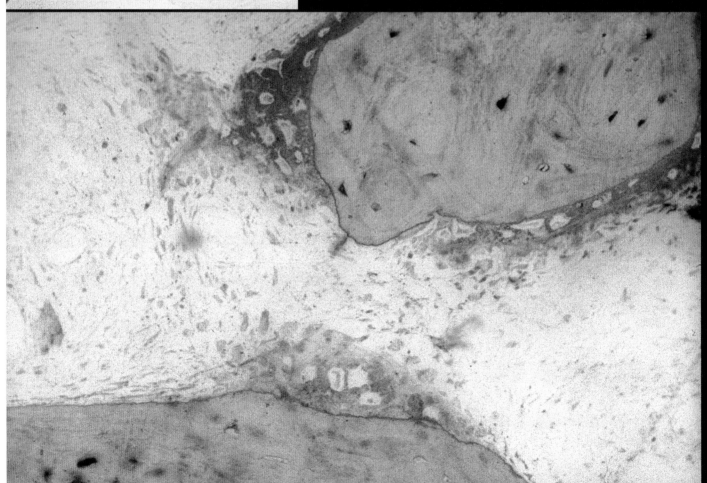

nism (Glowacki et al. 1981a; Rebaudi et al. 2003). On the other hand, osteoconductive materials implanted in bone defects support neo-osteogenesis starting from the edges of the defect, acting as scaffolding for the osteoblasts. As discussed in-depth in Chapter 9 of this book (Wallace), alloplastic materials and xenografts have varying osteoconductive properties and resorption times, while at the moment, only autogenous bone has osteoinductive capacities.

The functions that this type of material should carry out are described below:

- **Partly fill the space to be regenerated**

By using an experimental model in humans (Trisi & Rao, 1998), it was proven how, in critical jaw defects, materials can be used to fill a defect in about 6 months that was not filled in the control side **FIG. 11**. In this sense, the most obvious function that biomaterials carry out is reducing a space in the sinus cavity that must be colonized by bone, partly occupying it themselves.

- **Maintaining the volume under the sinus membrane**

The materials must play the important role of keeping the sinus membrane lifted until the new cavity is completely filled with bone. For this reason, the graft materials must be mechanically stable and must not be rapidly resorbed in the months following the grafting procedure. If resorption occurs too rapidly it would cause a loss of volume and would make the placement of suitably sized implants impossible.

- **Favor the migration of osteogenetic cells**

Osteoconduction aids and speeds up the filling of large spaces by newly formed bone, on the condition that all the prerequisites for bone regeneration are observed: suitable blood supply, mechanical stability and competition with the most rapidly proliferating tissues.

The depositing of lamellar bone begins from a solid, stable wall (Schenk 1992). The biomaterial's granules are therefore a support for the osteoblasts, from where osteogenesis can start. If all the granules are rapidly colonized by osteoblasts, there can be as many bone formation nuclei as there are granules. When the ossification fronts from the nearby granules meet and merge, the entire space will be filled by newly formed bone and granules incorporated in the newly formed bone matrix **FIG. 12**.

An alloplastic or xenogenous material's capacity to conduct bone growth determines its greater or lesser conductivity. In fact, the more the material is able to guide the cells along the whole surface, the easier and faster it will be to fill the cavity with bone. Osteo-inductive materials are those that allow the greatest rate and speed of colonization of their surfaces by newly formed bone.

- **Favoring bone formation at a certain distance from the bone walls**

Osteoblasts need a solid, stable surface where they can begin to deposit the bone matrix and then grow lamellar bone.

In 5 wall defects, with high osteogenetic potential, osteogenesis begins directly in the connective tissue, and on the traumatized bone walls, with the formation of woven bone in the initial weeks following the operation and in the areas next to the bone walls. The formation of new bone proceeds slowly in the areas furthest from the bone walls, and in the following weeks, with the deposition of lamellar bone on the newly formed woven bone trabeculae and on the graft surface (Schenk et al. 1994; Buser et al. 1998).

The quantity and quality of new bone formation depends on the osteogenetic potential of the traumatized bone site, linked to the degree of vascularization and the presence of osteogenetic cells (Schenk et al. 1994; Schmid et al. 1997; Buser et al. 1998).

13 → BIOPSY OF SINUS
LIFT WITH AUTOGENOUS BONE.
BONE FORMATION COMES FROM
THE AUTOGENOUS BONE CHIPS,
ALSO DISTANT FROM THE WALLS,
BUT THUS ACCELERATING THE
BONE-FILLING PROCESS.

14 → BIOPSY OF SINUS LIFT
WITH HUMAN DEMINERALIZED
BONE.
THERE ARE NOT ENOUGH LARGER
SPACES BETWEEN
THE PARTICLES TO ALLOW
GRANULATION TISSUE
PENETRATION.

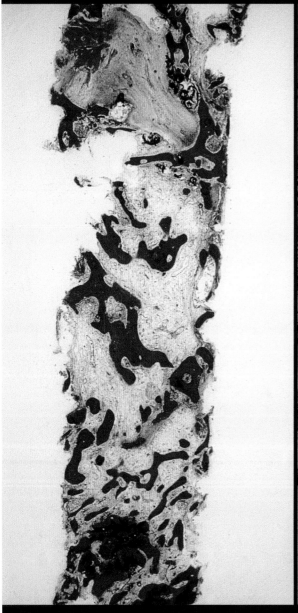

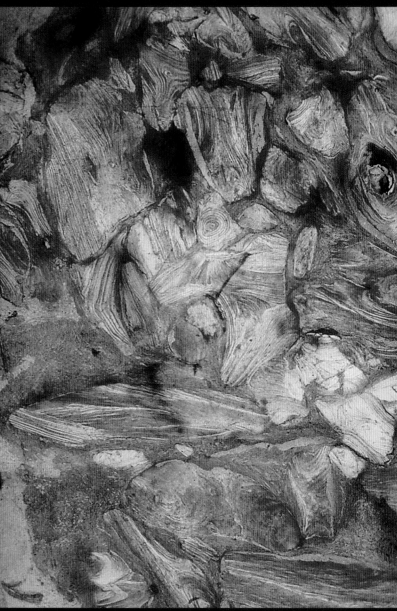

The new bone formation process will be faster and more intense near to the exposed medial and lateral walls and to the maxillary sinus floor (Boyne & James 1980; Misch 1993), while in the most central part, the quantity and speed of the new bone formation will be lower (Jensen et al. 1998).

The presence of bone grafts with osteoinductive capacities, such as cancellous autogenous bone, or *bone chips*, can alter these events, bringing cells and bone growth factors to areas that are distant from the walls and the sinus floor. In this way, neo-osteogenetic nuclei may also originate in less favorable areas, accelerating the bone growth and consolidation process. This is the reason why the addition of a certain amount of autogenous bone to alloplastic or xenogenous materials, in composite grafts, provides an improvement in the amount and speed of new bone formation inside the maxillary sinus[FIG. 13].

• **Aiding angiogenesis**

As we have already mentioned, the presence of a considerable amount of blood is essential for osteogenesis (Schmid et al. 1997), as osteoblasts need high partial oxygen pressure to produce bone matrix. It is therefore essential that a network of capillaries can penetrate to the innermost areas of the graft, furthest from the sinus walls, to achieve new bone formation.

The starting of osteogenesis from the bony walls was first described by Boyne (Boyne & James 1980) and in studies on monkeys by Misch (1993).

One important factor in this sense is the technique for compacting material in the sinus cavity. An excessively dense graft, associated with the use of granules that are too small in size or round in shape, may almost totally eliminate the residual space between one particle and another, physically preventing the rapid colonization by angiogenetic and later osteogenetic tissue[FIG. 14].

• **Allowing normal bone remodeling processes**

Another fundamental characteristic of osteoconductive materials is resorbability. The faster the material is resorbed, the faster substitution by newly formed bone will take place (Buser et al. 1998).

Resorption must occur when the material has already conducted bone growth, resulting in defect filling.

In an experimental study dealing with the defects of controlled size, Buser et al. (1998) showed that autogenous bone allows for greater defect filling in 1 month, while tricalcium phosphate (TCP), which shows the higher percentage of replacement by newly formed bone after 24 weeks, is better dissolved with the replacement by new bone. Coral hydroxyapatite and human demineralized freeze-dried bone allograft (DFDBA) provided the least favorable results in terms of quantity and quality of newly formed bone.

Similar results were obtained in humans in standardized defects histologically analyzed (Simion et al. 1994b; Trisi et al. 2003b). Resorption of the biomaterial should proceed at the same rate as new bone formation. If it is faster, the regenerative space may be reduced before the bone fills it. If, on the contrary, resorption is slower than bone formation, the newly formed bone would incorporate the graft, slowing down the possibility of removing the biomaterial. In fact, when the material is incorporated inside the newly formed bone, the phagocytic cells no longer have access to the material itself and resorption is prevented[FIG. 15]. The only possible access to the material surface will be when a remodeling process removes the bone that covers the graft, making the surface accessible to macrophages.

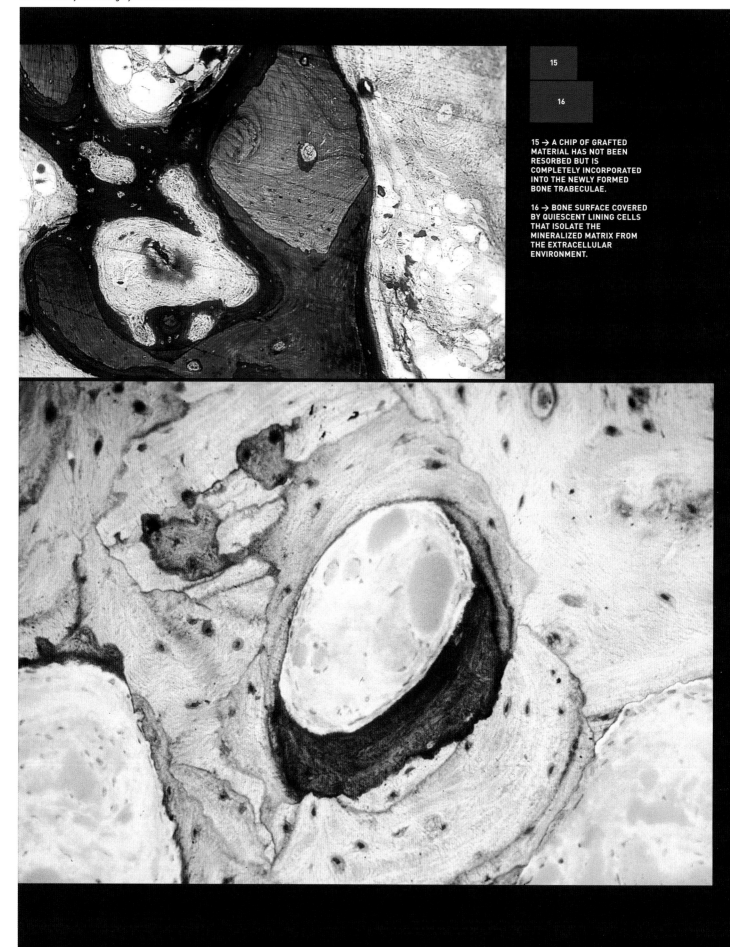

15 → A CHIP OF GRAFTED
MATERIAL HAS NOT BEEN
RESORBED BUT IS
COMPLETELY INCORPORATED
INTO THE NEWLY FORMED
BONE TRABECULAE.

16 → BONE SURFACE COVERED
BY QUIESCENT LINING CELLS
THAT ISOLATE THE
MINERALIZED MATRIX FROM
THE EXTRACELLULAR
ENVIRONMENT.

THE GOLD STANDARD - AUTOGENOUS BONE

The first studies carried out on bone grafts in the sinus used autogenous bone, which is still considered to be the best material for grafts. In fact, it has all the ideal properties: excellent biocompatibility with bone tissue, osteoconductive and osteoinductive capacities, and good mechanical properties. It can be resorbed over time and replaced with newly formed bone. However, resorbability and its mechanical properties depend on the structure of the bone, which, in turn depends on its origin (Ozaki & Buchman 1998).

The properties of autogenous bone are linked to the presence of predetermined osteogenetic cells and bone growth factors located inside the mineralized matrix (Mohan & Baylink 1991). Under normal physiologic conditions, the bone matrix is completely covered by lining cells **FIG. 16** that isolate the bone matrix from the extracellular fluids that are present in the marrow spaces, where the mesenchymal stem cells are located. After the trauma, the bone matrix is exposed to the extracellular environment, presenting the non-collagen proteins of the matrix to the cells, including the BMPs that act as bone formation promoters. This encourages cell and matrix component adhesion and stimulates the profileration of osteoblasts that will deposit osteoid during the early stages of the bone repair process (Buser et al. 1998). The next step is the beginning of the repair process, which will bring about the formation of woven bone on the exposed bone surface, until it is completely covered **FIG. 17**. When this takes place, the repair stimulus will begin to recede until the defect is completely repaired. The repair process may occur on the condition that the other prerequisites for bone formation are satisfied, such as the adequate vascularization and good mechanical stability in traumatized bone walls.

Older studies, which seemed to indicate that membranous bone grafts were superior to endochondral ones, have used grafts composed from both cortical and cancellous structures (Zins & Whitaker 1983; Kusiak et al. 1985; Dado & Izquierdo 1989). By separating these two components, it has been shown that compact bone grafts maintain their volume much better than cancellous bone grafts, whatever their origin (Hardesty & Marsh 1990; Chen et al. 1994; Ozaki & Buchman 1998). Also, no statistical difference has been found in the resorption rate between cortical grafts taken from bone of a different embryological origin. These studies clearly demonstrate that cortical bone is the best material for *onlay grafting*, regardless of its embrylogical origin. These results cast doubt on the theories that maintain that the dynamics of autogenous bone graft resorption is determined by its embryological origin.

BLOCK AUTOGENOUS BONE TRANSPLANTS

The healing of bone grafts seems to be mainly determined by the rate of vascularization achieved after the transplantation. Easier penetration of the blood vessels inside the graft also means lower mechanical resistance from the graft itself, while greater graft solidity in supporting mechanical stress also entails a more difficult revascularization and transformation into living bone (Lozano et al. 1976; Kusiak et al. 1985; Romana & Masquelet 1990; Sullivan & Szwajkun 1991a, 1991b). Years after the cortical bone graft placement, the surface or interface is the only part that can be totally revascularized and is where incorporation allowing rapid healing takes place (Lozano et al. 1976; Kusiak et al. 1985; Romana & Masquelet 1990; Sullivan & Szwajkun 1991a, 1991b).

The remaining part of the grafted cortical bone may remain non-vital for many years, while carrying out the mechanical function it is intended for (Goldberg & Stevenson 1987). The lack of vitality, however, makes the graft hypermineralized and exposed to the risk of further fractures, due to the fact that the non-vital bone

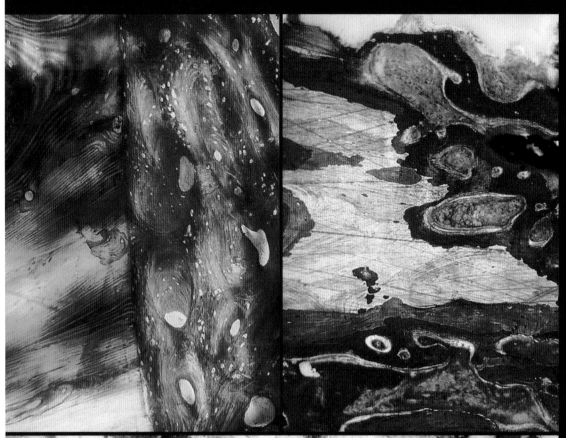

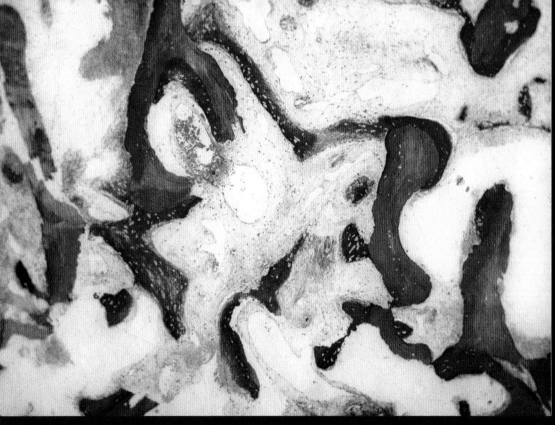

17 → POLARISED LIGHT MICROGRAPH OF AN ARTIFICIAL BONE DEFECT. AFTER 6 MONTHS, THE SECTIONED CORTICAL BONE WALL IS COMPLETELY COVERED BY NEW COMPOUND BONE.

18 → DETAIL OF AN ONLAY COMPACT BONE GRAFT FROM SYMPHYSIS. PARTIAL SUBSTITUTION OF GRAFTED BONE, 9 MONTHS AFTER INSERTION.

19 → HISTOLOGIC ASPECT OF AUTOGENOUS BONE CHIPS GRAFTED INTO THE SINUS AFTER 6 MONTHS. THE PARTICLES ARE COMPLETELY SURROUNDED AND CONNECTED TO EACH OTHER BY THE NEWLY FORMED BONE.

weakened by loading stresses has not been replaced (Enneking et al. 1980; Pelker & Friedlaender 1987). In the oral cavity, the low level of replacement with vital bone exposes the cortical *onlay graft* healed on the jaw bone to detachment when the implants are inserted. The more the graft is revascularized, the lower the risk of detachment **FIG. 18**.

AUTOGENOUS BONE TRANSPLANTS USING CHIPS

The autogenous bone chips implanted in self-contained, mechanically stable defects aid a considerable proliferation and migration of osteogenetic cells and neovascular tissue inside the defects (Wilson et al. 1985). The surface of each chip has the capacity to stimulate proliferation of osteogenetic cells, due to the availability of the BMPs contained in the exposed bone matrix. This allows the autogenous bone particles to act as a free bone wall for the deposition of new bone. After 1 week, the chips are already surrounded by new vessels and partly by new bone (Wilson et al. 1985). In critical size defects, these chips are largely covered with woven bone in 4 weeks, which connects the particles to each other and with the defect bone walls **FIG. 19** (Buser et al. 1998). The key factor for autogenous bone chip regeneration success is perfect mechanical stability of the graft. This can be easily and spontaneously achieved in self-contained defects, such as postextraction sites, but must be obtained using different means in extraalveolar regeneration, such as horizontal or vertical ridge augmentation, using membranes, grids and screws. Filling self-contained defects with autogenous bone chips may bring about an increase in the percentage of osseointegration compared to basal bone (Veis et al. 2004).

HUMAN DEMINERALIZED FREEZE-DRIED BONE ALLOGRAFT (DFDBA)

Although DFDBA is believed to be able to induce new bone formation due to its content of bone growth factors (BMP) (Urist & Strates 1970), other experimental and clinical studies have cast doubt on its osteoinduction capacity.

In some histologic studies carried out by the authors on the histologic reaction of DFDBA in humans, we observed low osteoconductivity and slow resorption during guided bone regeneration using a Gore-Tex® membrane **FIG. 20** (Simion et al. 1994a, 1994b, 1998).

DFDBA chips are resorbed very slowly and have been found in patients as long as 4 years after grafting **FIG. 21** (Simion et al. 1996). Some months after the graft, a large part of the grafted demineralized matrix is still embedded in the marrow connective tissue. The particles that are incorporated by the newly formed bone undergo the characteristic remineralization process (Simion et al. 1994a, 1994b), which takes the hydroxyapatite crystals back inside the demineralized bone, without causing replacement with vital bone. Remineralization takes place by calcification nodules that spread from the DFDBA union area with newly formed bone, or from the center of the Haversian canals, which tend to flow together, without completing transformation. The final aspect of the remineralized chip is usually granular and easily recognizable in the newly formed bone trabeculae **FIG 22**.

DFDBA has been recommended and clinically used in sinus grafts owing to its acclaimed osteoinductive characteristics, but many studies have questioned its effectiveness. Boyne (1993) used mixed autogenous bone grafts, with Bio-Oss® and DFDBA, finding only 14% of new bone in the graft area after 14 months of load. Hurzeler believes that DFDBA may have impaired new bone formation (Hurzeler et al. 1997). Several studies (Jensen & Greer 1992; Wetzel et al. 1995; Valentini & Abensur 1997; Hanisch et al. 1999; Haas et al. 2002a, 2002b) have observed negative his-

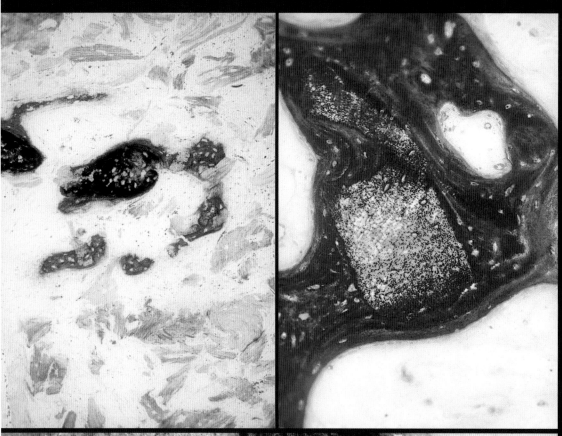

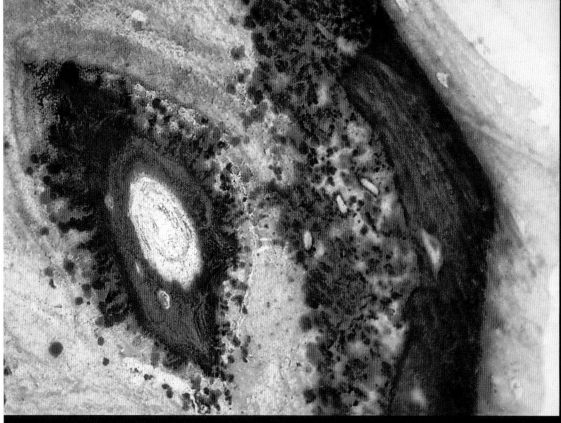

20 → DFDBA CHIPS INSERTED INTO BONE DEFECTS PROTECTED BY A GORE-TEX® MEMBRANE. MANY FRAGMENTS ARE NOT IN CONTACT WITH NEWLY FORMED BONE; THEY ARE SIMPLY SURROUNDED BY LOOSE CONNECTIVE TISSUE.

21 → 4 YEARS AFTER THE GRAFT, SOME GRAINS OF DFDBA CAN STILL BE SEEN IN THE MATURE REGENERATED BONE, WHICH HAVE NOT BEEN RESORBED AND ARE NOT FULLY REMINERALIZED.

22 → TYPICAL HISTOLOGIC ASPECT OF DFDBA WITH THE PRESENCE OF REMINERALIZATION NUCLEI INSIDE THE DEMINERALIZED MATRIX, STARTING FROM THE VASCULAR CANALS.

tologic results using DFDBA in the sinus. At the Sinus Consensus Conference (Jensen et al. 1998) it was agreed that the least positive results were found in implants inserted in sinuses grafted with DFDBA.

DFDBA use has shown worse results than autogenous bone in studies on maxillary sinuses in animals, and also worse results than negative controls. A recent analysis on human biopsies from the authors showed no signs of new bone formation using DFDBA in the maxillary sinus in a series of biopsies from patients (unpublished observation by Dr Trisi).

A COMPARATIVE EVALUATION OF VARIOUS TYPES OF GRAFTS

More than 70 biopsies originating from maxillary sinus grafts, obtained from various clinical centres and carried out after varying healing time and using different graft materials were histologically and histomorphologically analysed in our hard tissue and biomaterial research laboratory (Bio C.R.A., Pescara, Italy).

A comparative analysis of data obtained showed that the amount of newly formed vital bone increases significantly over time, regardless of the graft material used. Correlation between time and quantity of vital bone is statistically highly significant ($P < 0.002$).

Three to four months after surgery, about 20% of the volume of the regenerative space is occupied by vital bone when autogenous bone is used as graft material. Six to seven months afterwards, about 30% of the volume is occupied by vital bone, using Bio-Oss® as graft material. Nine to twelve months afterwards, the volume of vital bone increases up to about 35% in mixed grafts. After 17 months of healing, the mixed grafts show about 45% of vital bone.

We did not find statistically significant differences in the amount of newly formed bone among the various types of graft at this stage.

An important histologic study in humans by Froum showed that the volume of vital bone obtained using Osteograf N as graft material was 14.2% when used alone and 27.1% when combined with autogenous bone, after 6 to 9 months of healing (Froum et al. 1998).

WHAT FORMS AT THE IMPLANT-GRAFT INTERFACE?

IMPLANTS PLACED SIMULTANEOUS TO SINUS AUGMENTATION IS CARRIED OUT

The formation of new bone in the space below the elevated sinus membrane is a necessary, but not sufficient condition for clinical success in implantology. An implant inserted in the sinus graft at the same time as the sinus lift procedure is carried out acts biologically as a graft material. The possibility of osteoblasts colonizing its surface by depositing bone directly in contact depends on the osteoconductive properties of the implant's surface.

The formation of new bone in the sinus cavity does not necessarily mean that this bone adheres to the implant.

Experimental studies on animals (Stentz et al. 1997) and in humans (Lundgren et al. 1999) have shown that smooth titanium screws placed at the same time as regenerative therapy only reach a minimum amount of osseointegration (2.5%) at the end of the healing period.

Highly osteoconductive surfaces, such as hydroxyapatite or rough titanium, can reach high percentages of osseointegration in the same experimental conditions (Wetzel et al. 1995; Hurzeler et al. 1997; Quinones et al. 1997; Stentz et al. 1997; Haas et al. 2002c).

In a recent histologic study in humans, Trisi et al. (2002) showed that smooth titanium is one of the non-conductive materials, as it cannot make contact with the surrounding bone trabeculae in low-density bone **FIG. 23** (bone-

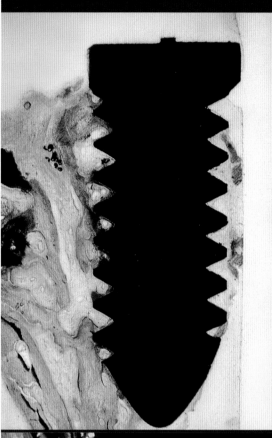

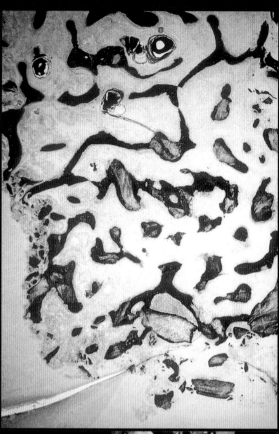

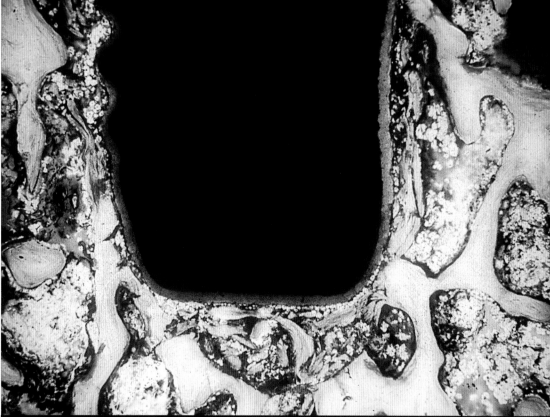

23 → EXPERIMENTAL MICRO-IMPLANT WITH DUAL SURFACE REMOVED FROM HUMAN MAXILLA. THE SMOOTH TITANIUM SURFACE PROVES NON-CONDUCTIVITY, AS IT CANNOT ACHIEVE CONTACT WITH ALL THE BONE TRABECULAE SURROUNDING IT IN LOW-TRABECULATION BONE, WHILE THE OPPOSITE ETCHED SIDE SHOWS A HIGH RATE OF OSSEOINTEGRATION.

24 → BONE BIOPSY REMOVED FROM HUMAN MAXILLARY SINUS LIFT 5 MONTHS AFTER OPERATION. THE NEWLY FORMED BONE TRABECULATION BETWEEN THE GRAFTED CHIPS IS LOW DENSITY WITH LOW MECHANICAL RESISTANCE.

25 → HISTOLOGIC EXAMINATION OF AN IMPLANT INSERTED IN FRESH BOVINE BONE AND ANALYZED IMMEDIATELY AFTER PLACEMENT. AFTER IMPLANT SITE PREPARATION, THE DELICATE TRABECULAE, BROKEN UP BY BURS, DISPERSE INTO THE ADJACENT MARROW SPACES AND ACCUMULATE AT THE APEX OF THE IMPLANT. IT IS POSSIBLE TO SEE THE PERI-IMPLANT MARROW SPACES FILLED WITH BONE DEBRIS.

implant contact < expected bone contact [BIC < EBC]) (Trisi et al. 1999, 2002, 2004). Dual acid-etched titanium surfaces (Osseotite), on the other hand, show highly conductivity, achieving a higher BIC than the EBC, both after 6 months (Trisi et al. 2002b) and after 2 months of healing (Trisi et al. 2003b).

The amount of residual basal bone, of course, can influence the percentage of primary and secondary bone-implant contact. With 5 or more millimetres of residual bone crest, bone integration with the implant neck may be sufficient to provide good primary and secondary stability, even for smooth titanium implants.

These histologic observations are also supported by clinical data (Jensen et al. 1998), that showed how 97% of plasma-sprayed titanium implants and 100% of implants with hydroxyapatite coating, but only 90% of smooth titanium surface implants achieve clinical integration in sinus grafts at the time of prosthesis insertion.

IMPLANTS INSERTED DURING A LATER SURGICAL OPERATION

Placing implants at a second surgical stage after graft healing allows a suitably sized implant site to be prepared, aiding osseointegration. In fact, the good fit of the implant is one of the essential prerequisites for obtaining osseointegration with a smooth titanium surface (Brånemark et al. 1985).

During implant site preparation in the sinus graft, the burs cut and break up the delicate trabeculae of newly formed bone and graft particles formed inside the sinus during the healing period [FIG. 24]. Many bone trabeculae are fractured and compressed laterally, while bone chips are dispersed into the peri-implant area [FIG. 25].

The bone responds to these traumatic events with a new, powerful repair process thanks to the release of several abundant growth factors in the extra-cellular fluids, which activate the osteoblasts. The release of these factors causes the formation of capillaries and woven bone inside and around the trauma site, throughout the peri-implant area, where fragments of fractured bone trabeculae can be found.

This new healing process also involves the implant surface, aiding osseointegration and new bone formation also in the most apical and distant areas from the sinus walls. The new bone repair process will follow the same biological steps that are common to all bone repair processes, with the formation of woven bone initially and later with reinforcement by lamellar bone (*lamellar compaction*) and then finally with the extremely active remodeling processes (RAP). However, in implants inserted at the same time as grafting, the bone is traumatized only in the sinus walls and floor, therefore the repair process will be limited to these graft areas. In this case, is difficult to colonize the apex of the implant with new bone, as it is too distant from the trauma areas.

The graft chips, incorporated into the newly formed bone trabeculae, may be cut by the burs while the implant site is being prepared, or may be compressed by the forced insertion of the implant, if the implant site is underprepared to allow for good primary stability. This does not disturb the osseointegration process, as the biomaterial particle maintains its osteoconductive properties and therefore enhances bone growth on its own exposed surface [FIG. 26]. If the material is excessively compressed to the interface [FIG. 27], it may prevent bone colonization of the implant surface. However, the importance of this effect is reduced by the limited size of the interface involved in this phenomenon. Also, the biomaterial walls not closely attached to the implant may be colonized by new bone, thus allowing the implant to be indirectly stabilized [FIG. 28].

Significant differences between the amount of BIC for implants inserted simultaneously or deferred in sinus grafts have also been found in experimental studies in animals (Herzeler et al. 1997).

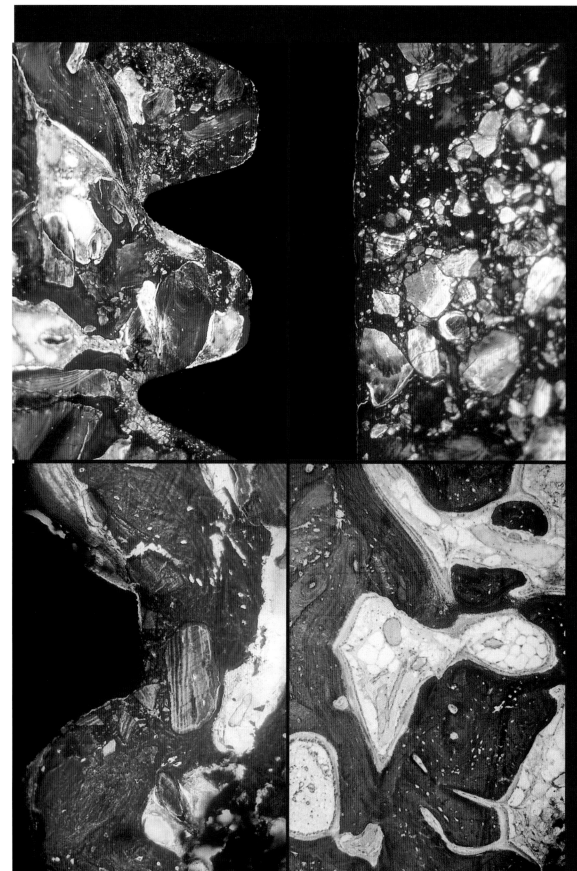

26	27
28	29

26 → DETAILS OF AN IMPLANT REMOVED BY MAJOR MAXILLARY SINUS LIFTING A FEW MONTHS AFTER PLACEMENT IN THE PREVIOUSLY GRAFTED SINUS. THE IMPLANT BIOMATERIAL SURFACE HAS BEEN CLEARLY COMPRESSED AGAINST THE BIOMATERIAL CHIPS THAT WERE GROUND BY THE PREPARATION OF THE IMPLANT SITE. THIS DOES NOT DISTURB THE OSSEOINTEGRATION PROCESS, AS THE BIOMATERIAL PARTICLES MAINTAIN THEIR OSTEOCONDUCTIVE PROPERTIES AND THEREFORE AID BONE GROWTH ON THE EXPOSED BIOMATERIAL SURFACE AND ON THE IMPLANT SURFACE.

27 → DETAILS OF APEX AREA IN AN IMPLANT INSERTED IN A PREVIOUSLY LIFTED MAXILLARY SINUS AND REMOVED AFTER 6 MONTHS OF HEALING AND 3 MONTHS OF LOAD. IN THIS CASE, THE MATERIAL WAS STRONGLY COMPRESSED TO THE IMPLANT'S APEX INTERFACE, PROBABLY DUE TO SCREWING WITHOUT PRIOR TAPPING OF THE IMPLANT SITE. IN THIS CASE, THE RESIDUAL SPACES BETWEEN THE GROUND PARTICLES DO NOT ALLOW THE FORMATION OF A NORMAL BONE MATRIX.

28 → THE BIOMATERIAL GRAINS ARE SET DIRECTLY AGAINST THE IMPLANT. HOWEVER, THE FREE PART OF THE BIOMATERIAL SURFACE HAS BEEN COLONIZED BY NEW BONE, THUS ALLOWING INDIRECT STABILIZATION OF THE IMPLANT.

29 → BONE REMODELING IS CARRIED OUT BY A POOL OF CELLS CALLED BMU, MADE UP OF OSTEOBLASTS AND OSTEOCLASTS. OSTEOCLASTS START REMODELING, BEGINNING FROM THE FREE BONE SURFACE, AFTER REMOVING THE LINING CELLS. AFTER RESORBING A BONE "PACKET", THEY LEAVE SPACE FOR THE OSTEOBLASTS, WHICH BEGIN TO SLOWLY DEPOSIT BONE AFTER A FEW DAYS ON THE SURFACE MADE BY THE OSTEOCLASTS, UNTIL THEY HAVE COMPLETELY FILLED THE CAVITY.

In a recent histologic study in human maxillae, Trisi et al. demonstrated the possibility of
obtaining about 30% osseointegration on
machined titanium implants and 70% BIC on
titanium implants with MTX surface (grit-
blasted and acid-etched; Zimmerdental),
inserted 6 to 11 months after sinus grafting
with an osseointegration period of about 6
months (Trisi et al. 2003b). The graft material
used in this study was Bio-Oss® mixed with
autogenous bone taken from the tuberosity.

Vital bone (35 to 40%) was found in the
biopsies, without significant differences in the 6
to 11 month period after grafting.

The amount of bone contact established
on completion of the healing process depends
on the quality of the regenerated bone and the
implant surface properties (Trisi et al. 2002).
The higher the bone quality and the more
osteoconductive the implant surface, the more
bone will form on the interface.

However, bone induced exclusively by the
chemical or physical osteoconductive properties
of the implant surface does not have high biomechanical qualities (Trisi et al. 1999, 2002).
Therefore, when occlusal load is initially
applied, it is advisable to adopt careful clinical
protocols such as progressive load (Misch
1993) or progressive orthodontic traction
(Misch 1993; Trisi & Rebaudi 2002).

WHAT IS THE EFFECT OF LOAD ON BONE?

REMODELING OF NORMAL BONE

Our skeleton is continuously and uniformly subjected to bone remodeling processes
that renew the bone matrix without affecting its
mechanical characteristics.

Bone remodeling is carried out by cells
known as BMU (bone multicellular units),
including osteblasts and osteoclasts **FIG. 29**. The
first phase of remodeling comprises the removal
of the predetermined bone packet by the osteoclasts, which is followed by the replacement of
new bone by osteoblasts. The same amount of
bone is resorbed and deposited in a single
remodeling cycle while the direction of the bone
lamellae and osteons may change. In cortical
bone, a new BMU initiates a new osteon, called
BSU (bone structural unit) **FIG. 30**.

Any increase or loss of bone volume is the
result of a local imbalance, during single remodeling cycles, between the depth of the osteoclast
cavity made by the osteoclasts of a single BMU
and the thickness of new bone deposited in the
cavity by the osteoblasts of the same BMU (Frost
1999).

If the amount of deposited bone increases
or the amount of bone resorbed by each BMU
decreases, the modeling is positive, with an
increase in bone mass. A reduction of the
deposited bone or an increase in the amount of
bone resorbed by the same BMU bring about a
loss of bone mass.

The speed of these changes also depends
on the frequency with which new remodeling
cycles begin (*activation frequency*) (Frost
1999). When the amount of bone resorbed and
the amount of newly formed bone by the same
BMU is the same, bone mass is maintained. In
this way, our skeleton is totally replaced every
10 years or so, with a remodeling speed of
about 5 to 10% per year (Frost 1969).

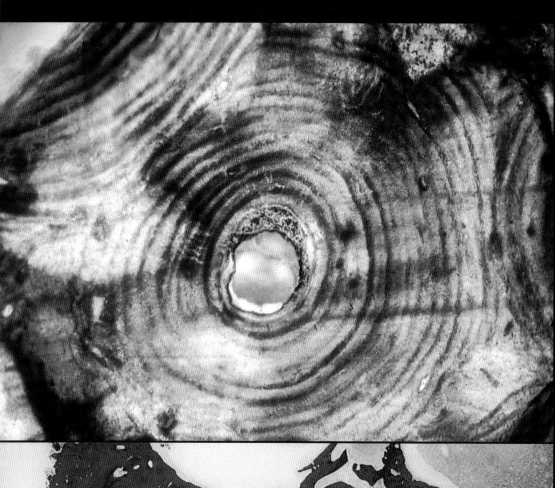

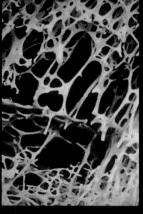

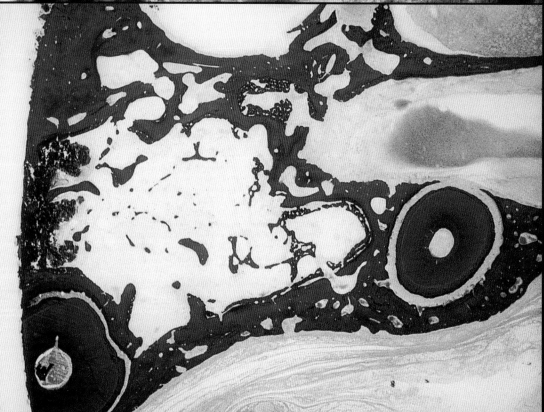

30 → IN COMPACT BONE, REMODELING TAKES PLACE VIA THE EXCAVATION OF A CYLINDRICAL TUNNEL THAT WILL THEN BE FILLED WITH CONCENTRIC LAMELLAR BONE TO FORM A NEW OSTEON. THE FUNDAMENTAL STRUCTURE OF COMPACT BONE IS TUBULAR IN APPEARANCE WITH WALL WIDTHS OF ABOUT 80 TO 100 µM, WITH THE CENTRAL HAVERSIAN CANAL THAT BRINGS NUTRITION TO ALL OSTEOCYTES CONNECTED TO THAT OSTEON. COMPLETION OF THE REMODELING PROCESS GIVES RISE TO A NEW STRUCTURAL BONE UNIT CALLED BSU.

31 → A VERY LOW DENSITY BONE STRUCTURE, LIKE THE ONE PICTURED, CAN AFFECT THE MECHANICAL INTEGRITY OF THE SKELETON AND THE INTEGRATION AND SURVIVAL OF THE IMPLANTS. (BY KIND PERMISSION OF DR. ALBERTO REBAUDI)

32 → HISTOLOGIC SECTION OF A YOUNG MAXILLA. EXCEPT FOR CORTICAL WALLS AND THE ALVEOLAR CORTEX, BONE DENSITY IS VERY LOW AND THE VOLUME IS ALMOST TOTALLY TAKEN UP BY MARROW TISSUE.

GENERAL CONCEPTS OF THE PHYSIOLOGY OF BONE REACTION TO LOAD: WOLFF'S LAW

The primary mechanical role of the skeleton is to withstand loads and moments generated during activity.

The skeleton provides rigid levers for muscular contraction and to maintain body integrity against the force of gravity. Many bones are exposed to thousands of repeated loads each day.

Bone architecture is efficient and elegant, as if its structure was designed by a sophisticated engineering project. This project is partially contained in the genetic programme of bone cells, but there is also an epigenetic component of bone design that is continually updated in response to the mechanical forces that our skeleton is subjected to during daily muscular activity.

One important principle of skeleton physiology is that bones can perceive mechanical load and modify their structure to adapt to stress changes. This principle is known as "Wolff's law".

During growth, the skeleton optimizes its architecture by adaptation to these mechanical loads. The adaptation mechanisms involve complex mechanical-transduction cellular processes such as: the conversion of mechanical forces in local mechanical signals, through fluid movement, which start up bone cell response; the transduction of the mechanical signal into a biochemical response that involves the intracellular biochemical pathways of membranes and cytoskeletons; signals between mechanical stimulus-sensitive cells (probably osteocytes and lining cells) and effector cells (osteoblasts and osteoclasts) using prostaglandins and nitric oxide as signal molecules; and the final response, bone formation or resorption, in order to induce necessary architectural changes (Turner & Pavalko 1998). These architectural changes tend to regulate and improve bone structure in relation to the mechanical environment.

According to Turner (1998), three basic phenomena regulate the biomechanical bone adaptation to load:
1. bone adaptation is led by the dynamics of the applied forces, rather than by static load;
2. only short-lasting mechanical loads can induce an adaptation response. Mechanical stimulus that lasts over time tends to reduce the adaptation response;
3. the bone cells adapt to a repetitive mechanical environment that makes them less sensitive to routine mechanical signals.

STRESS-STRAIN RATIO

Loads and moments cause deformation in bone tissue that is measured using the non-dimensional parameter called "*strain*". Deformation (*strain*) is defined as a change in the length of a object divided by its original length ($\Delta L/L$).

In biomechanical literature, the term *microstrain*, symbolized by $\mu\varepsilon$, is often used to indicate strain multiplied by one million. A strain of 0.01 (1%) coincides with 10000 *microstrains*.

If we consider the mandible of a macaque, the humerus of a tennis player, the femur of a horse, or the vertebrae of a whale, the osteoblast/osteocyte syncytium in all these situations is equally exposed to induced functional stress to the bone matrix (e.g. chewing, serving the ball, galloping or swimming).

Mechanical loads on the skeleton bring forth the hypothesis that strain induced by the former may be considered a biological signal of stimulus and adaptation for bone cells (Rubin et al. 1994). In fact, the thickness of the cortex increases in the serving humerus of the professional tennis player's arm (Jones et al. 1977) and the amount of calcium in the bone in the postcranial skeleton decreases rapidly in patients who are bedridden for long periods (Leblanc et al. 1990), or in astronauts who stay in space for long periods with no gravity (Tilton et al. 1980). These phenomena show the powerful influence of biophysical stimuli on the skeleton.

Average peaks of strain measured in a wide range of vertebrates are extremely similar in breadth, ranging from 2000 to 3500 microstrains (Rubin & Lanyon 1984). This similarity in dynamic strains among the various species suggest that skeleton morphology adapts so that functional activity induces a specific, favorable level of strain for bone tissue (Rubin & Lanyon 1984).

Forces that can induce such strain differ depending on the local mechanical properties of the bone, which vary based on the structure (cortex, cancellous bone, porosity) and the direction and frequency of load, as bone is an anisotropic, visco-elastic material. The upper level of resistance to human compact bone compression is between 160 and 210 MPa, while cancellous bone varies from 1.5 to 38 MPa (An & Draughn 2000). The elastic modulus measures 15 to 25 GPa in compact bone and 10 to 1570 MPa in cancellous bone (An & Draughn 2000).

FROST'S MECHANOSTAT THEORY AND LOAD THRESHOLDS

The increase in bone density was described by Frost in his "mechnostat theory" (Frost 1983a, 1983b, 1983c). Frost suggested that compact bone undergoes bone "hypertrophy", comprising an increase in modeling and a reduction in remodeling, when the load exceeds a certain physiologic threshold of strain. According to Burr, bone hypertrophy is caused by applying a load that can induce a strain of 2500 to 4000 microstrains (Burr et al. 1989a, 1989b).

The "mechnostat theory" also predicts the existence of other load thresholds that can determine different bone responses from the bone.

The minimum load threshold is about 200 microstrains, below which bone tissue risks atrophy, also known as disuse ostopoenia, as

happens in astronauts or long-term bedridden patients (Frost 1983a, 1983b, 1983c). The next window is that of physiologic maintenance or remodeling, ranging from 200 to 2500 microstrains, within which range bone mass and external morphology remains the same, only varying its internal structure through normal remodeling processes (Frost 1983a, 1983b, 1983c).

The threshold of 4000 microstrains indicates overload, as there is a progressive bone resorption process above this level of strain, owing to the formation of microcracks (Frost 1983a, 1983b, 1983c). Acute fractures of whole compact bone occur with deformations of 10000 to 25000 microstrains.

WHAT HAPPENS TO GRAFTS AND NEW BONE UNDER OCCLUSAL LOAD?

BIOMECHANICAL PROPERTIES OF NEWLY FORMED BONE INSIDE THE MAXILLARY SINUS

It is said that in order to obtain a long-lasting osseointegration, grafts should induce a vital bone volume of 25 to 35% (Jensen et al. 1998; Lazzara 1996). Studies on osteoporotic bone have proved that a bone volume of 10 to 16% FIG. 31 is the threshold, below which there is a large risk of losing cancellous bone mechanical integrity (Parfitt 1979; Eriksen et al. 1990). A recent study on maxillary sinus lifts indicated that when the bone volume is below 20%, the risk of implant failure is higher (Tarnow et al. 2000).

A study carried out on implants inserted in rat tibia (Brånemark et al. 1997) showed that mechanical resistance to unscrewing does not increase in the first 4 weeks of healing, but begins to increase progressively from the fifth week up to the sixteenth week. Vice versa, forced extraction load increases rapidly during the first four weeks and tprogressively increases slightly during the following 12 weeks. A histologic evaluation carried out after 0, 4, 8 and 16 weeks showed a significant correlation between the unscrewing force and the percentage of bone in contact with the implant, and between the extraction load and the thickness of the surrounding bone. These evaluations show that the increase in bone volume around the implant substantially improves the mechanical load capacity.

An in vivo biomechanical study (Haas et al. 1998) carried out on experimental cylindrical implants with titanium plasma spray inserted in sinus augmentations in sheep, showed that the force needed to extract an implant from the bone varied depending on the type of graft, and increased as time passed. Comparative tests have shown that resistance to traction after 12 weeks of healing was at a maximum when the graft material was bovine hydroxyapatite, average in sinuses grafted with autogenous bone and least in controls without grafts. The force required for implant extraction was almost double after 26 weeks of healing for test groups who had achieved similar values with each other, but in controls only a limited increase was found.

In later studies (Haas et al. 2002a, 2002b), the same authors evaluated mechanical resistance of implants inserted in human demineralized freeze-dried bone allografts (DFDBA), compared with implants inserted in non-grafted sinuses, or grafted with autogenous bone. After 12 weeks of healing, extraction force values for the implant were similar in the various groups, but after 26 weeks, the values had doubled in the group with autogenous bone but not in the control group and the group who had human DFDBA grafts. The authors concluded that time seems to be a decisive factor in increasing an implant's mechanical resistance. These conclusions are in agreement with the results of our histologic examinations that show how the quantity of vital bone increases significantly with time since the graft, regardless of the material used.

However, average pull-out resistance values obtained in these studies, from 250 to 500 N (Haas 2002b), were much lower than those obtained in native mandibular compact bone, which were about 800 N (Kraut et al. 1991).

These biomechanical data are in line with the histologic picture, which shows a low profile bone density in the grafted maxillary sinus. Therefore caution should be used when starting occlusal load on maxillary sinus implants, as even light occlusal forces may exceed the mechanical resistance threshold of newly regenerated bone.

RESPONSE OF INTERFACIAL BONE TO OCCLUSAL LOAD

In traditional conditions of delayed load, the functional stimulus takes place at the time when peri-implant bone tissue has already healed and has already undergone a first remodeling cycle. The average remodeling period (sigma) in rabbits and dogs is 2 months, while in humans it is 4 months (Frost 1969). However, during the first remodeling cycle, newly formed bone tissue is not subjected to functional masticatory stimuli. For this reason, the newly formed bone is remodeled into a hypofunctional structure that reproduces the bone morphology of the surrounding areas (Trisi et al. 2003b) **FIG. 32**, induced by the functional needs of that area, without occlusal function.

The bone quality that develops in the maxilla during the healing period is therefore rather low.

During the healing that follows long bone traumas or grafts, the bone remodeling process may take place according to various mechanisms: replacement of newly formed woven bone with new lamellar bone; maintenance of bone where strain exceeds remodeling threshold; resorption of bone devoid of mechanical function; repairing of microcracks. All these stresses are regulated by strains induced locally (Frost 1999). The same processes must also take place inside the bone that forms in the sinus grafts.

According to the mechanostat theory, Frost (1999) hypothesizes that small strains of about

500 to 1000 microstrains in maxillary sinus grafts may improve bone quality during the healing period. However, as the mechanical strength of newly formed bone, which is extremely spongy, is very low, these loads should be about 1% of normal masticatory forces, as greater forces may place graft healing at risk.

We know that modeling induced by function may cause bone hypertrophy as a functional response to the increase in mechanical load on the peri-implant bone. The graft itself cannot react to the load, but deformation of the vital bone matrix surrounding the implants and the graft can initiate a positive biological response.

Unfortunately, the study of these processes is complicated by the fact that real clinical conditions cannot be reproduced reliably in experimental *in vitro* studies. Van Oosterwyck stated that it is important to set up *in vivo* studies with loaded implants that exactly reproduce clinical reality (Van Oosterwyck et al. 1998). To date, only a few studies have been published on the adaptation of bone around dental implants in animals (Barbier & Schepers 1997; Quinones et al. 1997).

An increase in bone density was seen in a series of cases we analyzed, on implants placed in maxillary sinus augmentations in voluntary patients loaded for differing time periods, using the progressive load protocol (Misch 1993).

CORTICALIZATION AND BIC

We were able to observe how the speed of new bone formation undergoes a sharp acceleration at the beginning of loading, by using tetracycline labeling. After 12 months of healing on unloaded implants, the percentage of bone remodeling was 36% per year, while after 3 months of loading, the percentage of bone sites with active bone formation increased to 676% per year. This demonstrates that occlusal load on implants plays an important role in stimulating bone remodeling, which

allows a remodeling of the peri-implant bone structure. This phenomenon was also seen in studies on animals and humans (Roberts et al. 1984; Garetto et al. 1995), and is expected according to the mechanostat theory.

The final effect of remodeling depends on the balance between the amount of newly deposited bone, the amount of bone resorbed by each BMU, and the number of BMUs activated in the time unit.

After unloaded healing periods of 6 to 18 months, we found bone formation adhering to the implant with varying percentages of osseointegration depending on the implant surface. The density of newly formed vital bone varied from 20 to 50%, and a thin layer of bone, about 50 μm thick, covered a large part of the implant surface **FIG. 33**. The percentage of bone contact with the implant surfaces was already high at the end of the healing period and showed no significant increase with the increasing occlusal load periods. In an experimental study in animals, Quinones et al. found an increase in the percentage of bone contact after 6 months of occlusal load compared with non-loaded implants (Quinones et al. 1997).

In our case, 3 months of load caused an increase in the thickness of the bone layer covering the implant. Whereas after 12 months of healing without any load, the bone trabeculae adhering to the implant surface was about 50 μm thick, it increased to 150-200 μm after 3 months of functioning. After about 60 to 80 months it reached 300 to 350 μm **FIG. 34**. Statistical analysis shows a significant correlation between the loading time and the thickness of the peri-implant bone trabeculae. The functional bone adaptation to occlusal load was limited to the layer of bone that adheres directly to the implant surface, up to a distance of about 0.5 mm from the latter. The total bone volume showed significant differences among the various load times.

These observations show us how activation of the BMU leads to positive remodeling aimed at an increase in peri-implant bone density, especially located in the 500 µm nearest to the implant interface.

In this way, a cortical bone layer is formed around the implant, similar to the alveolar cortex that surrounds the roots of natural teeth. This process begins immediately after starting functional load and is almost complete after 3 months.

PERI-IMPLANT BONE REACTION TO OCCLUSAL OVERLOAD

At the same time as peri-implant cortex was formed, a deep infra-osseous pocket also formed in some of the samples examined **FIG. 35**. This defect was narrow and deep, covered by a junctional epithelial, that stopped about 300 to 400 µm from the first bone contact point and did not shown signs of inflammatory cell infiltration in the sub-epithelial connective tissue or in the thickness of the epithelium **FIG. 36**.

Moreover, the bone surrounding the implant neck was found to have greater tetracycline labeling. These observations allow the hypothesis that the infraosseous defect that develops without inflammation, and in the presence of a high bone turnover, is linked to an overload in the implant neck. In fact, we know that the maximum concentration of stress under load is found at the implant neck (Van Oosterwyck et al. 1998) **FIG. 37**.

If an implant is subjected to excessive load, it is more likely for the physiologic bone load threshold to be exceeded at this level. This may activate bone resorption, not mediated by inflammation, as would have been the case in the presence of peri-implantitis caused by bacterial plaque, but by the onset of microcracks **FIG. 38** (Hoshaw et al. 1994). The implants used in our study on sinus grafts were small in diameter (3.25 mm) and in length (7 mm), in order to be able to retrieve them, leaving the minimum defect possible in the residual bone.

However, in the posterior maxilla, where these implants were placed, the occlusal load is up to eight times more than in the anterior areas of the oral cavity. It is therefore possible that small implants with high occlusal stresses, such as those in the posterior maxillae, may have been subject to overloading conditions.

If we also consider that the maximum concentration of stress is located at the implant neck, it may be expected to find bone resorption caused by overload in this area. It has been shown that areas undergoing overload and bone resorption due to microcracks react by forming woven bone, as an attempt to rapidly react to overloaded (Nunamaker et al. 1990; Turner et al. 1994).

In our observations, new woven bone developed in the crest area where infrabony pockets were found **FIG. 39**, supporting the hypothesis of overload origin.

CONCLUSIONS

To conclude, all the experimental data taken from animal studies and from patients allowed us to state that the peri-implant bone reaction to occlusal load reflects the general theories of bone response to load, described in orthopedic literature. The lack of occlusal load brings about the formation of an atrophic peri-implant bone, adhering to the implant, but with low mechanical and structural strength. A few months of load can stimulate positive bone modeling processes that induce an increase in bone density in the implant interfacial area. An excessive occlusal load causes bone resorption in the implant neck area and on the bone crest, which can deeply penetrate the implant interface by creating a cycle that may lead to implant failure.

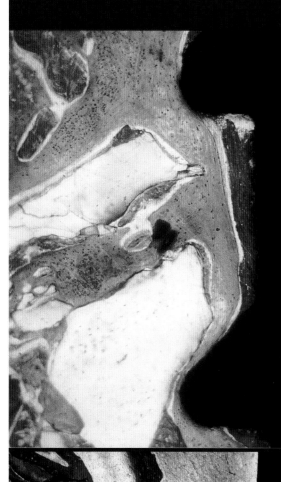

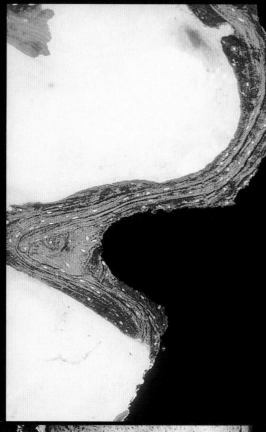

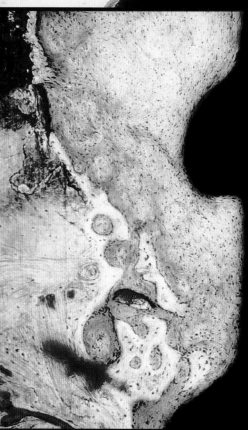

33 → HISTOLOGIC SECTION OF IMPLANT TAKEN AFTER 12 MONTHS OF HEALING IN THE GRAFTED UNLOADED MAXILLARY SINUS. IT IS POSSIBLE TO SEE A THIN BONE STRUCTURE ADHERING TO THE IMPLANT SURFACE, BUT THIS IS EXTREMELY WEAK.

34 → HISTOLOGIC SECTION OF AN IMPLANT TAKEN AFTER 6 MONTHS OF HEALING AND 3 MONTHS OF LOAD IN THE GRAFTED MAXILLARY SINUS. IT IS POSSIBLE TO SEE THE THICKENING OF THE BONE LAYER THAT COVERS THE IMPLANT SURFACE THAT WILL REACH A FEW HUNDRED MICRONS AFTER A FEW YEARS.

35 → HISTOLOGIC SECTION OF AN IMPLANT TAKEN AFTER 6 MONTHS OF HEALING AND 12 MONTHS OF LOAD IN THE GRAFTED MAXILLARY SINUS. THE INFRAOSSEOUS POCKET IN THIS CASE HAS A DEEP, NARROW MORPHOLOGY AND NO INFLAMMATORY CELL INFILTRATIONS CAN BE SEEN.

36 → HISTOLOGIC SECTION OF AN IMPLANT TAKEN AFTER 6 MONTHS OF HEALING AND 9 MONTHS OF LOAD IN THE GRAFTED MAXILLARY SINUS. THERE IS A MONO-STRATIFIED EPITHELIUM IN THE POCKET ADHERING TO THE IMPLANT SURFACE, WHICH STOPS AT 300 TO 400 μM ABOVE FIRST BONE CONTACT. THERE ARE NO SIGNIFICANT INFLAMMATORY CELL INFILTRATIONS.

37 **38**

39

37 → IMPLANT INSERTED IN PHOTOELASTIC RESIN AND STRAINED BY LATERAL LOAD. IT IS POSSIBLE TO SEE HOW THE MAXIMUM CONCENTRATION OF STRESS IS PRESENT AT THE IMPLANT NECK.

38 → HISTOLOGIC SECTION OF AN IMPLANT TAKEN AFTER 6 MONTHS OF HEALING AND 12 MONTHS OF LOAD IN THE GRAFTED MAXILLARY SINUS. MICROCRACKS CAN BE SEEN AT THE TOP OF THE THREADS, PROBABLY CAUSED BY AN OCCLUSAL OVERLOAD.

39 → HISTOLOGIC SECTION OF AN IMPLANT TAKEN AFTER 6 MONTHS OF HEALING AND 8 MONTHS OF LOAD IN THE GRAFTED MAXILLARY SINUS. A CERTAIN AMOUNT OF NEWLY FORMED WOVEN BONE IS PRESENT IN THE INFRAOSSEOUS POCKET, USUALLY ONLY PRESENT DURING THE INITIAL PHASES OF THE HEALING PROCESS. THIS OBSERVATION SUPPORTS THE HYPOTHESIS OF THE EXISTENCE OF A FUNCTIONAL OVERLOAD IN THE IMPLANT NECK AREA.

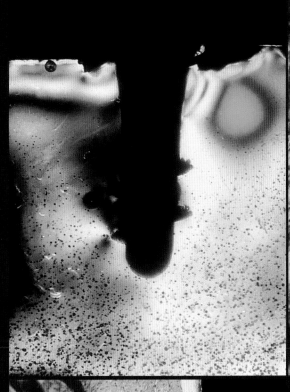

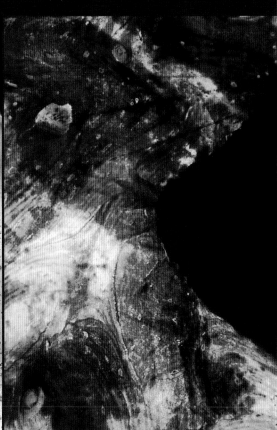

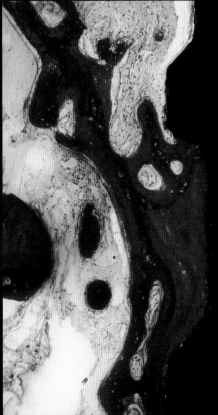

REFERENCES

1   An Y.H., Draughn R.A.
    Mechanical testing of bone and the bone-implant-interface.
    CRC Press, Boca Raton. 2000.

2   Barbier L., Schepers E.
    *Adaptive bone remodeling around oral implants under axial
    and nonaxial loading conditions in the dog mandible.*
    Int. J. Oral Maxillofac. Implants. 1997; 12: 215-223.

3   Bolander M.E.
    Regulation of fracture repair by growth factors.
    Proc. Soc. Exp. Biol. Med. 1992; 200: 165-170.

4   Bostrom M.P., Lane J.M., Berberian W.S., Missri A.A., Tomin E.,
    Weiland A., Doty S.B., Glaser D., Rosen V.M.
    *Immunolocalization and expression of bone morphogenetic
    proteins 2 and 4 in fracture healing.*
    J. Orthop. Res. 1995; 13: 357-367.

5   Bourque W.T., Gross M., Hall B.K.
    Expression of four growth factors during fracture repair.
    Int. J. Dev. Biol. 1993; 37: 573-579.

6   Boyne P.J.
    *Analysis of performance of root-form endosseous implants
    placed in the maxillary sinus.*
    J. Long. Term. Eff. Med. Implants. 1993; 3: 143-159.

7   Boyne PJ., James R.A.
    *Grafting of the maxillary sinus floor with autogenous marrow
    and bone 10.* J. Oral Surg. 1980; 38: 613-616.

8   Brånemark R., Ohrnell L.O., Nilsson P., Thomsen P.
    *Biomechanical characterization of osseointegration during
    healing: an experimental* in vivo *study in the rat.*
    Biomaterials 1997; 18: 969-978.

9   Burr D.B., Schaffler M.B., Yang K.H., Wu D.D., Lukoschek M.,
    Kandzari D., Sivaneri N., Blaha J.D., Radin E.L.
    The effects of altered strain environments on bone tissue kinetics.
    Bone 1989b; 10: 215-221.

10 Burr D.B., Schaffler M.B., Yang K.H., Lukoschek M., Sivaneri
    N., Blaha J.D., Radin E.L.
    *Skeletal change in response to altered strain environments: is
    woven bone a response to elevated strain?*
    Bone 1989a; 10: 223-233.

11 Buser D., Hoffmann B., Bernard J.P., Lussi A., Mettler D.,
    Schenk R.K.
    *Evaluation of filling materials in membrane-protected bone
    defects. A comparative histomorphometric study in the
    mandible of miniature pigs.*
    Clin. Oral Implants Res., 1998; 9: 137-150.

12 Chen N.T., Glowacki J., Bucky L.P., Hong H.Z., Kim W.K.,
    Yaremchuk M.J.
    *The roles of revascularization and resorption on endurance of
    craniofacial onlay bone grafts in the rabbit.*
    Plast. Reconstr. Surg. 1994; 93: 714-722.

13 Cho T.J., Gerstenfeld L.C., Einhorn T.A.
    *Differential temporal expression of members of the
    transforming growth factor beta superfamily during murine
    fracture healing.*
    J. Bone Miner. Res. 2002; 17: 513-520.

14 Dado D.V., Izquierdo R.
    *Absorption of onlay bone grafts in immature rabbits: mem-
    branous versus enchondral bone and bone struts versus paste.*
    Ann. Plast. Surg. 1989; 23: 39-48.

15 Dahlin C., Linde A., Gottlow J., Nyman S.
    Healing of bone defects by guided tissue regeneration.
    Plast. Reconstr. Surg. 1988; 81: 672-676.

16 Dahlin C., Gottlow J., Linde A., Nyman S.
    *Healing of maxillary and mandibular bone defects using a
    membrane technique. An experimental study in monkeys.*
    Scand. J. Plast. Reconstr. Surg. 1990; 24: 13-19.

17 Enneking W.F., Eady J.L., Burchardt H.
    *Autogenous cortical bone grafts in the reconstruction of
    segmental skeletal defects.*
    J. Bone Joint Surg. Am. 1980; 62: 1039-1058.

18 Eriksen E.F., Hodgson S.F., Eastell R., Cedel S.L.,
    O'Fallon W.M., Riggs B.L.
    *Cancellous bone remodeling in type I (postmenopausal)
    osteoporosis: quantitative assessment of rates of formation,
    resorption, and bone loss at tissue and cellular levels.*
    J. Bone Miner. Res. 1990; 5: 311-319.

19 Frost H.M.
    Tetracycline-based histological analysis of bone remodeling.
    Calcif. Tissue Res. 1969; 3: 211-237.

20 Frost H.M.
    The regional acceleratory phenomenon: a review.
    Henry Ford Hosp. Med J. 1983a; 31: 3-9.

21 Frost H.M.
    *A determinant of bone architecture. The minimum effective
    strain.* Clin. Orthop. 1983b; 286-292.

22 Frost H.M.
    The skeletal intermediary organization.
    Metab. Bone Dis. Relat. Res. 1983c; 4: 281-290.

23 Frost H.M.
    Vital biomechanics of the bone-grafted dental implants.
    In The sinus bone graft. O.T. Jensen, editor. Quintessence,
    Chicago, Carol Stream. 1999; 17-29.

24 Froum S.J., Tarnow D.P., Wallace S.S., Rohrer M.D., Cho S.C.
    *Sinus floor elevation using anorganic bovine bone matrix
    (OsteoGraf/N) with and without autogenous bone: a clinical,
    histologic, radiographic, and histomorphometric analysis-Part
    2 of an ongoing prospective study.*
    Int. J. Periodontics Restorative Dent. 1998; 18: 528-543.

25 Garetto L.P., Chen J., Parr J.A., Roberts W.E.
    *Remodeling dynamics of bone supporting rigidly fixed titanium
    implants: a histomorphometric comparison in four species
    including humans.*
    Implant Dent. 1995; 4: 235-243.

26 Glimcher M.J.
    *Chemistry, structure, and organization of bone and their
    influence on bone healing. In Fracture healing.*
    Lane J.M., editor. Churchill Livingstone, New York,
    Edinburgh, London, Melbourne 1987; 39-48.

27 Glowacki J., Altobelli D., Mulliken J.B.
    *Fate of mineralized and demineralized osseous implants in
    cranial defects.*
    Calcif. Tissue Int. 1981a; 33: 71-76.

28 Glowacki J., Kaban L.B., Murray J.E., Folkman J., Mulliken J.B.
    *Application of the biological principle of induced osteogenesis
    for craniofacial defects.*
    Lancet 1981b; 1: 959-962.

29 Goldberg V.M., Stevenson S.
    Natural history of autografts and allografts.
    Clin. Orthop. 1987; 7-16.

30 Haas R., Haidvogl D., Donath K., Watzek G.
Freeze-dried homogeneous and heterogeneous bone for sinus augmentation in sheep. Part I: histological findings.
Clin. Oral Implants. Res. 2002a; 13: 396-404.

31 Haas R., Haidvogl D., Donath K., Watzek G.
Freeze-dried homogeneous and heterogeneous bone for sinus augmentation in sheep. Part II: biomechanical findings.
Clin. Oral Implants. Res. 2002b; 13: 581-586.

32 Haas R., Mailath G., Dortbudak O., Watzek G.
Bovine hydroxyapatite for maxillary sinus augmentation: analysis of interfacial bond strength of dental implants using pull-out tests.
Clin. Oral Implants. Res. 1998; 9: 117-122.

33 Haas R., Baron M., Donath K., Zechner W., Watzek G.
Porous hydroxyapatite for grafting the maxillary sinus: a comparative histomorphometric study in sheep.
Int. J. Oral Maxillofac. Implants 2002; 17: 337-346.

34 Ham A.W., Harris W.R.
Repair and transplantation of bone. In The biochemistry and physiology of bone. Development and growth.
G.H. Bourne, editor. Academic Press, New York, NY. 1971; 337-399.

35 Hanisch O., Lozada J.L., Holmes R.E., Calhoun C.J., Kan J.Y., Spiekermann H.
Maxillary sinus augmentation prior to placement of endosseous implants: a histomorphometric analysis.
Int. J. Oral Maxillofac. Implants 1999; 14: 329-336.

36 Hardesty R.A., Marsh J.L.
Craniofacial onlay bone grafting: a prospective evaluation of graft morphology, orientation, and embryonic origin.
Plast. Reconstr. Surg. 1990; 85: 5-14.

37 Hollinger J.O., Kleinschmidt J.C.
The critical size defect as an experimental model to test bone repair materials. J. Craniofac. Surg. 1990; 1: 60-68.

38 Hoshaw S.J., Brunski J.B., Cochran G.V.B.
Mechanical loading of Branemark implants affects interfacial bone modeling and remodeling.
Int. J. Oral Maxillofac. Implants 1994; 9: 345-360.

39 Hurzeler M.B., Quinones C.R., Kirsch A., Gloker C., Schupbach P., Strub J.R., Caffesse R.G.
Maxillary sinus augmentation using different grafting materials and dental implants in monkeys.
Part I. Evaluation of anorganic bovine-derived bone matrix.
Clin. Oral Implants Res. 1997; 8: 476-486.

40 Jensen O.T., Greer R.O.
Immediate implant placement of osseointegrating implants into the maxillary sinus augmented with mineralized cancellous allograft and Gore-Tex®: second-stage surgical and histological findings. In Tissue integration in oral, orthopedic, and maxillofacial reconstruction.
Laney W.R., Tolman D.E., editors. Quintessence, Chicago. 1992; 321-333.

41 Jensen O.T., Shulman L.B., Block M.S., Iacono V.J.
Report of the Sinus Consensus Conference of 1996.
Int. J. Oral Maxillofac. Implants. 1998; 13: 11-45.

42 Johner R.
Dependence of bone healing on defect size.
Helv. Chir. Acta 1972; 39: 409-411.

43 Jones H.H., Priest J.D., Hayes W.C., Tichenor C.C., Nagel D.A.
Humeral hypertrophy in response to exercise.
J. Bone Joint Surg. Am. 1977; 59: 204-208.

44 Joyce M.E., Roberts A.B., Sporn M.B., Bolander M.E.
Transforming growth factor-beta and the initiation of chondrogenesis and osteogenesis in the rat femur.
J. Cell Biol. 1990a; 110: 2195-2207.

45 Joyce M.E., Jingushi S., Bolander M.E.
Transforming growth factor-beta in the regulation of fracture repair.
Orthop. Clin. North Am. 1990b; 21: 199-209.

46 Kaban L.B., Glowacki J.
Induced osteogenesis in the repair of experimental mandibular defects in rats.
J. Dent. Res. 1981; 60: 1356-1364.

47 Kraut R.A., Dootson J., McCullen A.
Biomechanical analysis of osseointegration of IMZ implants in goat mandibles and maxillae.
Int. J. Oral Maxillofac. Implants. 1991; 6: 187-194

48 Kusiak J.F., Zins J.E., Whitaker L.A.
The early revascularization of membranous bone.
Plast. Reconstr. Surg. 1985; 76: 510-516.

49 Lazzara R.J.
The sinus elevation procedure in endosseous implant therapy.
Curr. Opin. Periodontol. 1996; 3: 178-183.

50 Leblanc A.D., Schneider V.S., Evans H.J., Engelbretson D.A., Krebs J.M.
Bone mineral loss and recovery after 17 weeks of bed rest.
J. Bone Miner. Res. 1990; 5: 843-850.

51 Lozano A.J., Cestero H.J. Jr., Salyer K.E.
The early vascularization of onlay bone grafts.
Plast. Reconstr. Surg. 1976; 58: 302-305.

52 Lundgren S., Rasmusson L., Sjostrom M., Sennerby L.
Simultaneous or delayed placement of titanium implants in free autogenous iliac bone grafts. Histological analysis of the bone graft- titanium interface in 10 consecutive patients.
Int. J. Oral Maxillofac. Surg. 1999; 28: 31-37.

53 Misch C.E.
Contemporary Implant Dentistry. Mosby, St. Louis. 1993.

54 Mohan S., Baylink D.J.
Bone growth factors. Clin. Orthop. 1991; 30-48.

55 Mulliken J.B., Glowacki J., Kaban L.B., Folkman J., Murray J.E.
Use of demineralized allogeneic bone implants for the correction of maxillocraniofacial deformities 2.
Ann. Surg. 1981; 194: 366-372.

56 Nakajima A., Nakajima F., Shimizu S., Ogasawara A., Wanaka A., Moriya H., Einhorn T.A., Yamazaki M.
Spatial and temporal gene expression for fibroblast growth factor type I receptor (FGFR1) during fracture healing in the rat.
Bone. 2001; 29: 458-466.

57 Nunamaker D.M., Butterweck D.M., Provost M.T.
Fatigue fractures in thoroughbred racehorses: relationships with age, peak bone strain, and training.
J. Orthop. Res. 1990; 8: 604-611.

58 Nyman S., Lang N.P., Buser D., Bragger U.
Bone regeneration adjacent to titanium dental implants using guided tissue regeneration: a report of two cases.
Int. J. Oral Maxillofac. Implants. 1990; 5: 9-14.

59 Onishi T., Ishidou Y., Nagamine T., Yone K., Imamura T., Kato M., Sampath T.K., ten Dijke P., Sakou T.
Distinct and overlapping patterns of localization of bone morphogenetic protein (BMP) family members and a BMP type II receptor during fracture healing in rats.
Bone 1998; 22: 605-612.

60 Ozaki W., Buchman S.R.
    Volume maintenance of onlay bone grafts in the craniofacial skeleton: micro-architecture versus embryologic origin.
    Plast. Reconstr. Surg. 1998, 102: 291-299.

61 Parfitt A.M.
    Quantum concept of bone remodeling and turnover: implications for the pathogenesis of osteoporosis.
    Calcif. Tissue Int. 1979; 28: 1-5.

62 Pelker R.R., Friedlaender G.E.
    Biomechanical aspects of bone autografts and allografts.
    Orthop. Clin. North Am. 1987; 18: 235-239.

63 Perren S.M., Rahn B., Cordey J.
    Mechanics and biology of fracture healing.
    Fortschr. Kiefer Gesichtschir. 1975; 19: 33-37.

64 Quinones C.R., Hurzeler M.B., Schupbach P., Arnold D.R., Strub J.R., Caffesse R.G.
    Maxillary sinus augmentation using different grafting materials and dental implants in monkeys. Part IV. Evaluation of hydroxyapatite-coated implants.
    Clin. Oral Implants Res. 1997; 8: 497-505.

65 Rebaudi A., Silvetrini P., Trisi P.
    Use of a Resorbable Hydroxyapatite-Collagen Chondroitin Sulfate Material on Immediate Postextraction Sites: A Clinical and Histologic Study.
    Int. J. Periodont. Rest. Dent. 2003; 23: 371-379.

66 Remes A., Williams D.F.
    Immune response in biocompatibility.
    Biomaterials 1992; 13: 731-743.

67 Roberts W.E., Smith R.K., Zilberman Y., Mozsary P.G., Smith R.S.
    Osseous adaptation to continuous loading of rigid endosseous implants. Am. J. Orthod. 1984; 86: 95-111.

68 Romana M.C., Masquelet A.C.
    Vascularized periosteum associated with cancellous bone graft: an experimental study.
    Plast. Reconstr. Surg. 1990; 85: 587-592.

69 Rubin C.T., Lanyon L.E.
    Dynamic strain similarity in vertebrates; an alternative to allometric limb bone scaling.
    J. Theor. Biol. 1984; 107: 321-327.

70 Rubin C., Gross T., Donahue H., Guilak F., McLeod K.
    Physical and environmental influences on bone formation. In Bone Formation and Repair.
    Brighton C.T, Friedlaender G.E and Lane J.M, editors.
    American Academy of Orthopaedic Surgeons, Rosemont, U.S. 1994; 61-78.

71 Rundle C.H., Miyakoshi N., Ramirez E., Wergedal J.E., Lau K.H., Baylink D.J.
    Expression of the fibroblast growth factor receptor genes in fracture repair.
    Clin. Orthop. 2002; 253-263.

72 Sakou T.
    Bone morphogenetic proteins: from basic studies to clinical approaches.
    Bone 1998; 22: 591-603.

73 Sandberg M.M., Aro H.T., Vuorio E.I.
    Gene expression during bone repair.
    Clin. Orthop. 1993; 292-312.

74 Schenk R.K.
    Cytodinamics and histodynamics of primary bone repair. In Fracture Healing.
    Lane J.M., editor. Churchill Livingstone, New York, Edinburgh, London, Melbourne. 1987; 23-32.

75 Schenk R.K.
    Biology of fracture repair. In Skeletal Trauma.
    Browner B.D., Jupiter J.B., Levine A.M. and Trafton P.G., editors. W.B. Saunders Co., Philadelphia. 1992; 31-76.

76 Schenk R.K., Buser D., Hardwick W.R. and Dahlin C.
    Healing pattern of bone regeneration in membrane-protected defects: a histologic study in the canine mandible.
    Int. J. Oral Maxillofac. 1994; Implants 9: 13-29.

77 Schmid J., Wallkamm B., Hammerle C.H., Gogolewski S., Lang N.P.
    The significance of angiogenesis in guided bone regeneration. A case report of a rabbit experiment.
    Clin. Oral Implants. Res. 1997; 8: 244-248.

78 Schmitz J.P. and Hollinger J.O.
    The critical size defect as an experimental model for craniomandibulofacial nonunions.
    Clin. Orthop. 1986; 299-308.

79 Seibert J., and Nyman S.
    Localized ridge augmentation in dogs: a pilot study using membranes and hydroxyapatite.
    J. Periodontol. 1990; 61: 157-165.

80 Simion M., Dahlin C., Trisi P. and Piattelli A.
    Qualitative and quantitative comparative study on different filling materials used in bone tissue regeneration: a controlled clinical study.
    Int. J. Periodontics Restorative Dent. 1994a; 14: 198-215.

81 Simion M., Trisi P. and Piattelli A.
    Vertical ridge augmentation using a membrane technique associated with osseointegrated implants.
    Int. J. Periodontics Restorative Dent. 1994b; 14: 496-511.

82 Simion M., Trisi P., Piattelli A.
    GBR with an e-PTFE membrane associated with DFDBA: histologic and histochemical analysis in a human implant retrieved after 4 years of loading.
    Int. J. Periodontics Restorative Dent. 1996; 16: 338-347.

83 Simion M., Jovanovic S.A., Trisi P., Scarano A., Piattelli A.
    Vertical ridge augmentation around dental implants using a membrane technique and autogenous bone or allografts in humans.
    Int. J. Periodontics Restorative Dent. 1998; 18: 8-23.

84 Stentz W.C., Mealey B.L., Gunsolley J.C., Waldrop T.C.
    Effects of guided bone regeneration around commercially pure titanium and hydroxyapatite-coated dental implants. II. Histologic analysis.
    J. Periodontol. 1997; 68: 933-949.

85 Sullivan W.G., Szwajkun P.R.
    Revascularization of cranial versus iliac crest bone grafts in the rat.
    Plast. Reconstr. Surg. 1991b; 87: 1105-1109.

86 Sullivan W.G., Szwajkun P.
    Membranous versus endochondral bone.
    Plast. Reconstr. Surg. 1991a; 87: 1145.

87 Tarnow D.P., Wallace S.S., Froum S.J., Rohrer M.D., Cho S.C.
    Histologic and clinical comparison of bilateral sinus floor elevations with and without barrier membrane placement in 12 patients: part 3 of an ongoing prospective study.
    Int. J. Periodontics Restorative Dent. 2000; 20: 117-125.

88 Tatsuyama K., Maezawa Y., Baba H., Imamura Y., Fukuda M.
Expression of various growth factors for cell proliferation and cytodifferentiation during fracture repair of bone.
Eur. J. Histochem. 2000; 44: 269-278.

89 Tilton F.E., Degioanni J.J., Schneider V.S.
Long-term follow-up of Skylab bone demineralization.
Aviat. Space Environ. Med. 1980; 51: 1209-1213.

90 Trippel S.B.
Potential role of insulinlike growth factors in fracture healing.
Clin. Orthop. Relat. Res. 1998; S301-S313.

91 Trisi P., Rebaudi A.
Progressive bone adaptation of titanium implants during and after orthodontic load in humans.
Int. J. Periodontics Restorative Dent. 2002; 22: 345-353.

92 Trisi P., Rao W.
The bone growing chamber: a new model to investigate spontaneous and guided bone regeneration in human artificial jaw bone defects.
Int. J. Periodontics Restorative Dent. 1998; 18: 151-159.

93 Trisi P., Marcato C., Todisco M.
Bone-to-implant apposition with machined and mtx® microtextured implant surfaces in human sinus grafts.
Int. J. Periodontics Restorative Dent. 2003b; 23: 427-437.

94 Trisi P., Lazzara R.J., Rebaudi A., Rao W., Testori T.
Bone-implant contact on machined and Osseotite dual acid etched surfaces after 2 months of healing in the human maxilla.
J. Periodontol. 2004. 74: 945-956

95 Trisi P., Lazzara R., Rao W., Rebaudi A.
Bone-implant contact and bone quality: evaluation of expected and actual bone contact on machined and osseotite implant surfaces.
Int. J. Periodontics Restorative Dent. 2002; 22: 535-545.

96 Trisi P., Rao W., Rebaudi A., Fiore P.
Histologic effect of pure-phase beta-tricalcium phosphate on bone regeneration in human artificial jawbone defects.
Int. J. Periodontics. Restorative. Dent. 2003a; 23: 69-77.

97 Trisi P., Rao W., Rebaudi A.
A histometric comparison of smooth and rough titanium implants in human low-density jawbone.
Int. J. Oral Maxillofac. Implants. 1999; 14: 689-698.

98 Turner C.H.
Three rules for bone adaptation to mechanical stimuli.
Bone 1998; 23: 399-407.

99 Turner C.H., Pavalko F.M.
Mechanotransduction and functional response of the skeleton to physical stress: the mechanisms and mechanics of bone adaptation.
J. Orthop. Sci. 1998; 3: 346-355.

100 Turner C.H., Forwood M.R., Rho J.Y., Yoshikawa T.
Mechanical loading thresholds for lamellar and woven bone formation.
J. Bone Miner. Res. 1994; 9: 87-97.

101 Urist M.R., Strates B.S.
Bone formation in implants of partially and wholly demineralized bone matrix. Including observations on acetone-fixed intra and extracellular proteins.
Clin. Orthop. 1970; 71: 271-278.

102 Valentini P., Abensur D.
Maxillary sinus floor elevation for implant placement with demineralized freeze-dried bone and bovine bone (Bio-Oss): a clinical study of 20 patients.
Int. J. Periodontics Restorative Dent. 1997; 17: 232-241.

103 Van Oosterwyck H., Duyck J., Vander S.J., van der P.G., De Cooman M., Lievens S., Puers R., Naert I.
The influence of bone mechanical properties and implant fixation upon bone loading around oral implants.
Clin. Oral Implants. Res 1998; 9: 407-418.

104 Veis A.A., Trisi P., Papadimitriou S., Tsirlis A.T., Parisis N.A., Desiris A.K., Lazzara R.J.
Osseointegration of osseotite and machined titanium implants in autogenous bone graft. A histologic and histomorphometric study in dogs.
Clin. Oral Implants Res. 2004; 15: 54-61.

105 Wetzel A.C., Stich H., Caffesse R.G.
Bone apposition onto oral implants in the sinus area filled with different grafting materials. A histological study in beagle dogs.
Clin. Oral Implants. Res. 1995; 6: 155-163.

106 Wilson J.W., Rhinelander F.W., Stewart C.L.
Vascularization of cancellous chip bone grafts.
Am. J. Vet. Res. 1985; 46: 1691-1699.

107 Wolff J.
Das Gesetz der Transformation der Knochen.
Verlag von August Hirschwald, Berlin. 1892.

108 Yu Y., Yang J.L., Chapman-Sheath P.J., Walsh W.R.
TGF-beta, BMPS, and their signal transducing mediators, Smads, in rat fracture healing.
J. Biomed. Mater. Res. 2002; 60: 392-397.

109 Zins J.E., Whitaker L.A.
Membranous versus endochondral bone: implications for craniofacial reconstruction.
Plast. Reconstr. Surg. 1983; 72: 778-785.

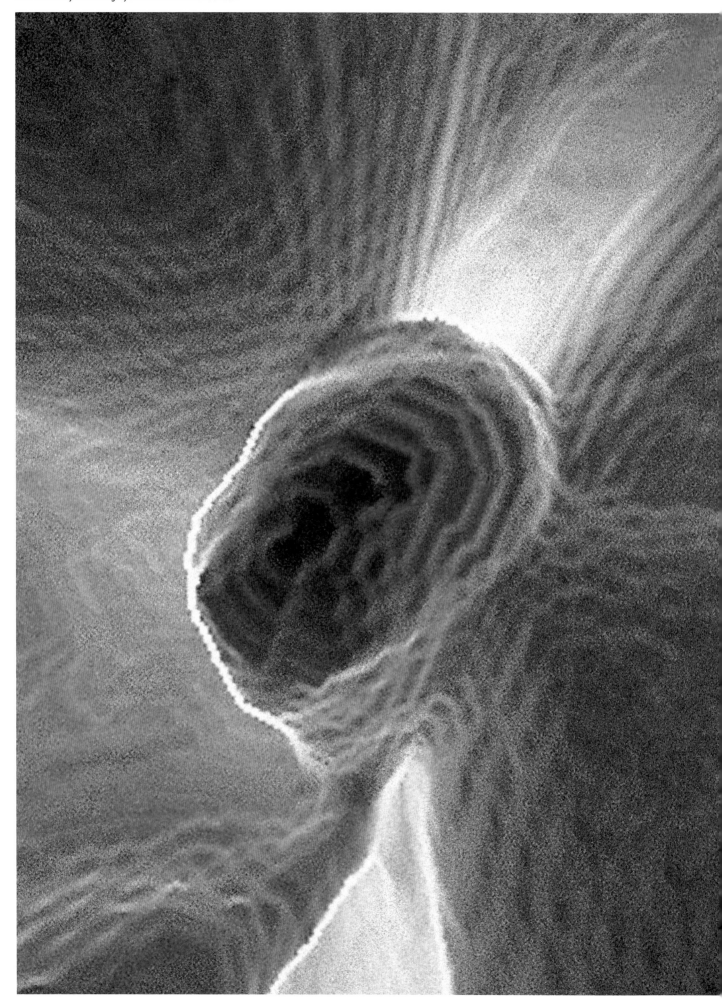

G. BELLONI

The role of CT scans in maxillary sinus augmentation surgery

06

06

INTRODUCTION

Modern implantology, by allowing new possibilities for the functional rehabilitation of edentulism, has stimulated the creation and perfection of increasingly sophisticated and accurate diagnostic methods. Dental and maxillofacial surgeons are offered more precise information about implant site evaluation, thus allowing correct, detailed prosthodontic treatment.

Diagnostic imaging has a primary role in presurgical planning. Computerized tomography (CT) has become standard for assessing the feasibility of implant surgery (Besimo et al. 1995; Bolin & Eliasson 1995; Testori et al. 1993).

Three-dimensional diagnostic assessments have a decisive value in presurgical treatment planning, especially in situations in which the alveolar process has pronounced resorption, and therefore insufficient bone volume for placing endosseous implants. These situations, which once limited the placement of implants in the posterior maxilla, can now be overcome via maxillary sinus augmentation procedures.

In these cases, diagnostic imaging, in particular using CT scans, plays a vital role, providing reliable and necessary information (Dula et al. 1994; Dula & Buser 1996; Seipel et al. 1995).

COMPUTERIZED TOMOGRAPHY

The use of spiral CT equipment in diagnostic imaging together with reconstruction programs has revolutionized the use of this method of imaging in dental applications. Volumetric acquisitions and multi-level, 3D reconstructions have provided a new overview of the problems linked to the dental apparatus, both in diagnostics of lesions and in orthodontic and implantology therapy.

Progress in diagnostics is due to the new multislice CT systems that allow for even better precision and the possibility of sub-millimeter acquisitions (acquisitions with collimation up to 0.6 mm and interpolar reconstructions up to 0.3 mm) (Dula et al. 1994; Dula & Buser 1996).

CT ADVANTAGES AND LIMITS

CT undoubtedly offers considerable advantages compared with traditional diagnostics (orthopantography, intraoral x-rays), overcoming the limit of two-dimensionality and insuring 3D information on the implant site.

Information on bone densitometry **FIG. 1A-B**, on bone cortical walls and on bone resorption in the alveolar processes **FIG. 2** is important for correct planning of prosthetic treatment, either from a functional or an esthetic point of view (Dula & Buser 1996).

Information on associated orosinus pathologies is also important **FIG. 3A-B**. In complex dental operations, CT must be considered as an essential presurgical diagnostic method **FIG. 4** (Schom et al. 1996; Testori et al. 1993; Seipel et al. 1995).

Limits that are still impossible to overcome are the items linked to the presence of metal restoration that cause a scatter effect, which interferes with diagnostic imaging.

RADIATION DOSE

Spiral CT exposes patients to an absorbed radiation dose with a higher absolute value compared with traditional x-ray methods.

Modern CT equipment, however, is equipped with effective collimation of the radiation beam, inducing radiation levels to structures near the scanning levels (thyroid) to a reduced dose, similar to that of traditional methods.

Compared with conventional CT equipment, the use of spiral CT results in a lower absorbed dose **TAB. 1**. This is due to the new solid state stability and performance of the monitor, and the possibility of rotation in less than one second (0.5 seconds).

Finally, the dose optimization systems included in the most recent CT equipment allow further reduction (up to 20%) of radiation dose (Clark et al. 1990; Diederichs et al. 1996; Belloni et al. 1999; Hassfeld et al. 1998; Hidajat et al. 1998).

CT IN SINUS AUGMENTATION PLANNING

What questions do the dental surgeon and the maxillofacial surgeon ask the radiologist when planning maxillary sinus augmentation operations?

The first information required from diagnostic procedures is linked to the volume of the maxillary sinus, especially the area of remaining bone.

Anatomic information, the presence of septa and the presence of alterations in mucosa caused by ongoing orosinus pathologies are important. Correct identification of the position and patency of the maxillary sinus ostium, together with the presence of any additional foramen are required.

- CT allows accurate calculations of the recipient site and possibly also the donor site volume in the event of maxillary sinus lifting, or augmentation of the mandibular alveolar ridge.

Analysis of the values of radiation dose absorbed with a spiral CT compared with a conventional CT

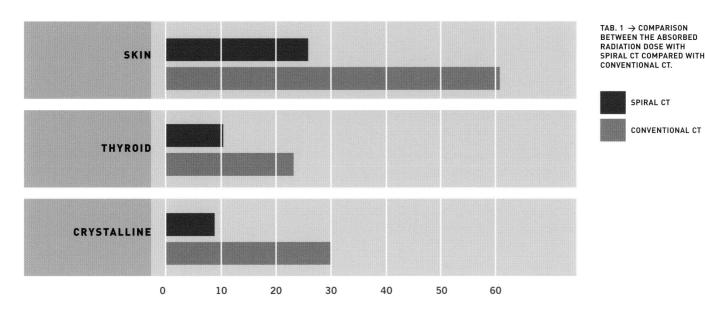

TAB. 1 → COMPARISON BETWEEN THE ABSORBED RADIATION DOSE WITH SPIRAL CT COMPARED WITH CONVENTIONAL CT.

SPIRAL CT

CONVENTIONAL CT

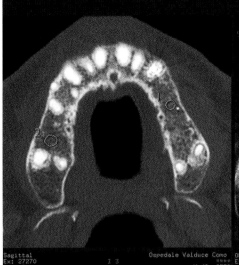

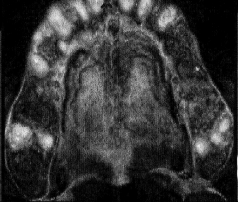

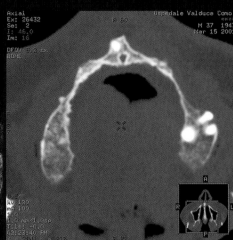

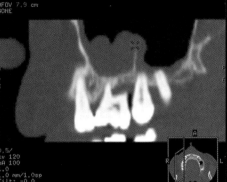

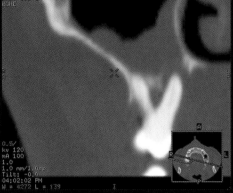

1 A	1 B	2
3 A	3 B	
	4	

**1 A - B → POSSIBILITY OF
DENSITOMETRIC MONITORING IN BONE
DENSITY AREAS OF INTEREST, AND 3D
RECONSTRUCTION WITH VOLUME
RENDERING TECHNIQUE.**

**2 → EVALUATION OF BONE RESORPTION
IN ALVEOLAR RIDGES.**

**3 A - B → ASSOCIATED OROSINUS
PATHOLOGIES: BOTH PRIMARY SINUSITIS
AND OF DENTAL ORIGIN WITH PRESENCE
OF OROSINUS FISTULA.**

**4 → IN COMPLEX SURGERY, 3D
RECONSTRUCTIONS PROVIDE DIAGNOSTIC
SYNTHESIS IMAGES.**

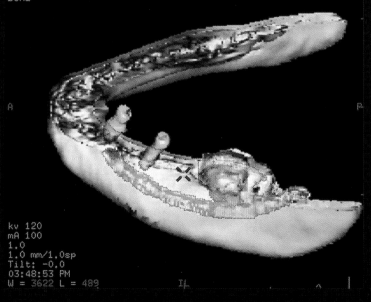

Three-dimensional reconstructions are an accurate and reliable method for calculating the amount of bone tissue needed to obtain adequate reconstruction of the alveolar process, in order to permit the placement of dental implants **FIG. 5A-B**.
In cases where bone graft is taken from an intraoral site, CT allows calculation of the amount of tissue that can be removed without running into anatomical problems caused by inadequate bone availability. The need for bone from distant sites such as the iliac crest or the tibia can also be assessed if insufficient intraoral bone is available for harvesting.

• CT has considerably improved diagnostic assessment of the local situation. Axial images, with sub-millimeter thickness thanks to the latest-generation of equipment, are very important in locoregional diagnostic capacities. A morpho-volumetric analysis of the planned surgical site becomes relatively simple, and the densitometric information available for areas of interest ensures much higher diagnostic confidence compared with conventional radiologic investigation. The substantial inclusion of information technology in the diagnostic field has made electronic reconstructions possible. These are now available in various rendering modes that represent "synthesis images" of an enormous amount of information, contained in hundreds of axial images produced. In addition to being immediate and diagnostically exhaustive, these images are easy to interpret for the operators **FIG. 6**.
One important advantage of spiral CT over other methods is the possibility of reconstructing images in multiple projections from just one acquisition, with an undoubted reduction in the dose absorbed by the patient.
Three-dimensional reconstructions using *volume rendering* images have today reached

much higher diagnostic levels than early 3D reconstructions, which used the *surface* technique, and are now obsolete **FIG. 7A-B**.
In particular cases, such as the analysis of maxillary sinus lumen morphology, it may be useful to use virtual endoscopy, which can simulate and help the planning of sinoscopy operations **FIG. 8A-B**.

• The identification of the maxillary sinus ostium, in particular the integrity of the anatomic structure, known as the ostiomeatal complex, is a key role in planning sinus augmentation. This is the morpho-functional unit used for drainage and aeration of the anterior ethmoidal cells, the maxillary sinuses and the frontal sinuses. CT allows precise evaluation of its numerous components, showing up any irregularities in development (e.g. concha bullae, septum deviation, presence of inflammation that involves the maxillary sinus ostium). It is important to determine the position of the ostium and its patency when planning sinus elevation operations. Respecting this structure is essential for a successful operation **FIG. 9**.

STUDY TECHNIQUE

In the otorhinolaryngological field, when evaluation of paranasal sinuses is needed, axial and coronal projections are carried out (that are reformatted from the volume acquired) with 3.5-mm collimation, proportional to the extension of the region being examined. Some authors suggest thin scanning, 1 to 2 mm thick, for the evaluation of the ostiomeatal region.

In contrast, when planning sinus elevations, a collimation of 1 mm or less is preferred in the maxillary sinus in an axial projection, proportional to the more limited region involved. This is due to the undeniable advantage of better precision in locoregional evaluations and the possibility of 1:1 scale monitoring.

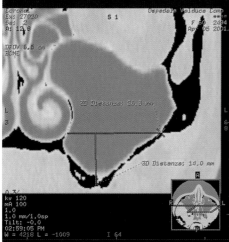

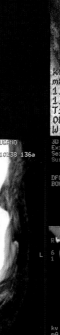

5 A - B → EXAMPLE OF CALCULATION OF BONE QUANTITY VOLUME REQUIRED FOR SINUS AUGMENTATION.

6 → WEALTH OF DIAGNOSTIC DETAILS IN A 3D CONSTRUCTION.

7 A - B → DIFFERENCE IN WEALTH OF DIAGNOSTIC INFORMATION BETWEEN A VOLUME RENDERING RECONSTRUCTION AND A SURFACE RECONSTRUCTION.

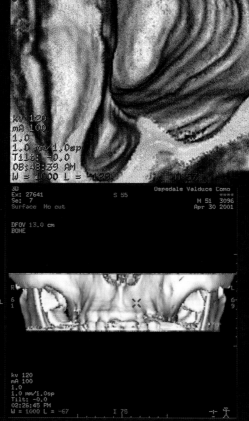

POSTOPERATIONAL CONTROLS

A CT scan, especially if it can be compared with a presurgical investigation, provides an effective confirmation of correct grafting of the maxillary sinus **FIG. 10A-B**.

Densitometric evaluation provides information on graft mineralization. Monitoring of the position of implants and any sinus complications is also possible. It must be remembered, however, that information on dental implant osseointegration cannot be obtained, except via the histologic analysis of a biopsy sample.

NEW DIAGNOSTIC PROSPECTS: MAGNETIC RESONANCE (MR)

The possibility of using an imaging method that is less harmful biologically and does not use ionizing radiation has aroused interest in its use for implantology.

Magnetic resonance is based on electromagnetic fields and radiofrequencies. Hydrogen atoms are stimulated, owing to their high diffusion in biologic organisms and the characteristics of their nuclei.

The hydrogen nuclei, placed in a magnetic field and stimulated by a radiofrequency, first absorb and then give out energy as an electrical signal, which is transformed into digital information and is translated by a computer into grayscale, forming a digital image. White corresponds to a high-intensity signal, gray to an intermediate-intensity signal and black to a low-intensity signal.

Tissue response varies depending on the type of sequence used. Weighted T1, T2 and proton density sequences (PD) exist.

Magnetic resonance is mostly used in diagnostics in the study of the central nervous system, where it has proved to have a decisive superiority compared with CT.

Modern equipment, owing to higher magnetic fields, allows this imaging method to be used in a wide variety of fields, configuring a range of use for MR that is comparable with that of CT.

Using MR in dental surgery is not new: it is now an essential method in studying temporomandibular joints, especially in evaluating the joint meniscus.

The investigation is carried out using PD, T1 and T2 sequences with an echo gradient and good spatial resolution using a dedicated coil. This allows good differentiation between the bone and the joint meniscus. The multi-level nature of the MR provides sagittal and coronal-oblique sequences with the mouth closed. Evaluation with dynamic sagittal oblique sequences allows assessment of the condyle, and it can be checked whether the meniscus is recaptured during the opening-closing of the joint or whether it remains dislocated.

The diagnostic improvement in assessing the temporomandibular joint, using this method, has been decisive, thus making MR the first-choice examination method.

MR IN THE STUDY OF MAXILLARY SINUSES

Magnetic resonance has been found to have greater sensitivity than CT when identifying the presence of inflammatory pathologies in the maxillary sinuses, which is important when planning sinus augmentation surgery.

Magnetic resonance offers the advantage of identifying the presence of acute, ongoing inflammation immediately, showing a hyperintense signal of mucosa thickening in the maxillary sinus.

The importance of this method, however, lies in its capacity to make a differential diagnosis between the stagnation of mucus and the presence of polyps or cystic retention in the maxillary sinuses.

Magnetic resonance is as effective as CT in the study of the ostiomeatal complex and canal pathologies that support or accompany sinus alterations.

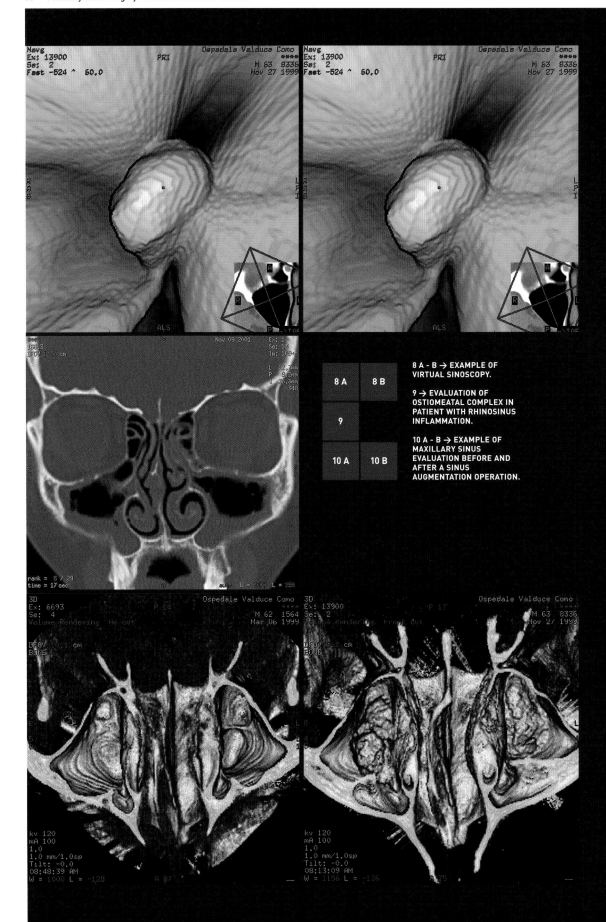

8 A - B → EXAMPLE OF VIRTUAL SINOSCOPY.

9 → EVALUATION OF OSTIOMEATAL COMPLEX IN PATIENT WITH RHINOSINUS INFLAMMATION.

10 A - B → EXAMPLE OF MAXILLARY SINUS EVALUATION BEFORE AND AFTER A SINUS AUGMENTATION OPERATION.

MR IN IMPLANTOLOGY

New studies and experiences are moving efforts towards the evaluation of using MR instead of CT for dental implantology applications.

Currently, MR allows sequences according to favorable scanning levels for the study of the maxilla and mandible: oblique, parallel to horizontal branches, coronal, and perpendicular.

This is possible for limited areas, and the use of weighted T1 and T2 scans provides valid diagnostic images for the study of implant sites or for sinus augmentation therapy. It is still difficult to obtain images on a 1:1 reconstruction scale. Reconstructions can be carried out using dental programs with 3D acquisitions in weighted T1 sequences, although practically speaking, results show a lower spatial resolution than a CT scan.

Limits to the potential use of this method are that it cannot be used for patients with pacemakers, endocranial surgical clips and all iron-magnetic prostheses in the sequence field or surrounding area. Dental therapy using ferrous materials may create artefacts in the acquired images (Gray et al 2003).

CONCLUSIONS

CT in sinus augmentation is an essential tool for correct diagnosis and for precise treatment planning.

The multiple uses and the possibility of reconstructing images means that close collaboration between dental surgeons and radiologists is necessary in order to exploit fully the diagnostic potential.

MR has a promising role in imaging diagnostics, although currently DentaScan reconstructions have a lower spatial resolution than CT.

At present, this equipment is mainly limited to neuro and osteo-articular investigations. Development of MR will be an interesting test for dental surgery in the near future, especially using dedicated coils and low intensity mag-

netic field equipment, used for both planning and for the follow up of complex operations.

REFERENCES

1 **Belloni G.M., Testori T., Francetti L., Bianchi F.**
TC spirale in implantologia. Valutazione della dose radiante assorbita. Dental Cadmos 1999; 2: 55-8.

2 **Besimo C., Lambrecht J.T., Nidecker A.**
Dental implant treatment planning with reformatted computed tomography. Dentomaxillofac. Radiol. 1995; 24: 264-7.

3 **Bolin A., Eliasson S.**
Panoramic and tomographic dimensional determinations for maxillary osseointegrated implants. Comparison of the morphologic information potential of two and three dimensional radiographic systems.
Swed. Dent. J. 1995; 19: 65-71.

4 **Clark D.E., Danforth R.A., Barnes R.W., Burtch M.L.**
Radiation absorbed from dental implant radiography: a comparison of linear tomography, CT scan, and panoramic and intra-oral techniques. J. Oral Implantol. 1990; 16: 156-64.

5 **Diederichs C.G., Engelke W.G., Richter B., Hermann K.P., Oestmann J.W.**
Must radiation dose for CT of the maxilla and mandible be higher than that for conventional panoramic radiography? AJNR Am. J. Neuroradiol. 1996; 17: 1758-60.

6 **Dula K., Buser D., Porcellini B., Berthold H., Schwarz M.**
Computed tomography/oral implantology (I). Dental CT: a program for the computed tomographic imaging of the jaws: the principles and exposure technic. Schweiz Monatsschr Zahnmed. 1994; 104: 450-9.

7 **Dula K., Buser D.**
Computed tomography/oral implantology. Dental-CT: a program for the computed tomographic imaging of the jaws. The indications for preimplantological clarification. Schweiz Monatsschr Zahnmed. 1996; 106: 550-63.

8 **Gray C.F., Redpath T.W., Smith F.W., Staff R.T.**
Advanced imaging: Magnetic resonance imaging in implant dentistry. Clin. Oral Implants Res. 2003; 14: 18-27.

9 **Hassfeld S., Streib S., Sahl H., Stratmann U., Fehrentz D., Zoller J.**
Low-dose computerized tomography of the jaw bone in pre-implantation diagnosis. Limits of dose reduction and accuracy of distance measurements.
Mund Kiefer Gesichtschir. 1998; 2: 188-93.

10 **Hidajat N., Schroder R.J., Vogl T., Maurer J., Steger W., Felix R.**
Dose distribution in conventional CT and spiral CT and on the topic of dose reduction with spiral CT.
Radiologe 1998; 38: 438-43.

11 **Schom C., Engelke W., Kopka L., Fischer U., Grabbe E.**
Indications for dental-CT. Case reports.
Aktuelle Radiol. 1996; 6: 317-24.

12 **Seipel S., Wagner I.V., Koch S., Schneider W.**
A virtual reality environment for enhanced oral implantology.
Medinfo 1995; 8 Pt 2: 1710.

13 **Testori T., Sacerdoti S., Barenghi A. et al.**
La tomografia assiale computerizzata nella moderna implantologia: reali vantaggi per una corretta programmazione chirurgico-protesica; dose assorbita dal paziente.
Ital J. Osseointegrataion 1993; 1: 19-28.

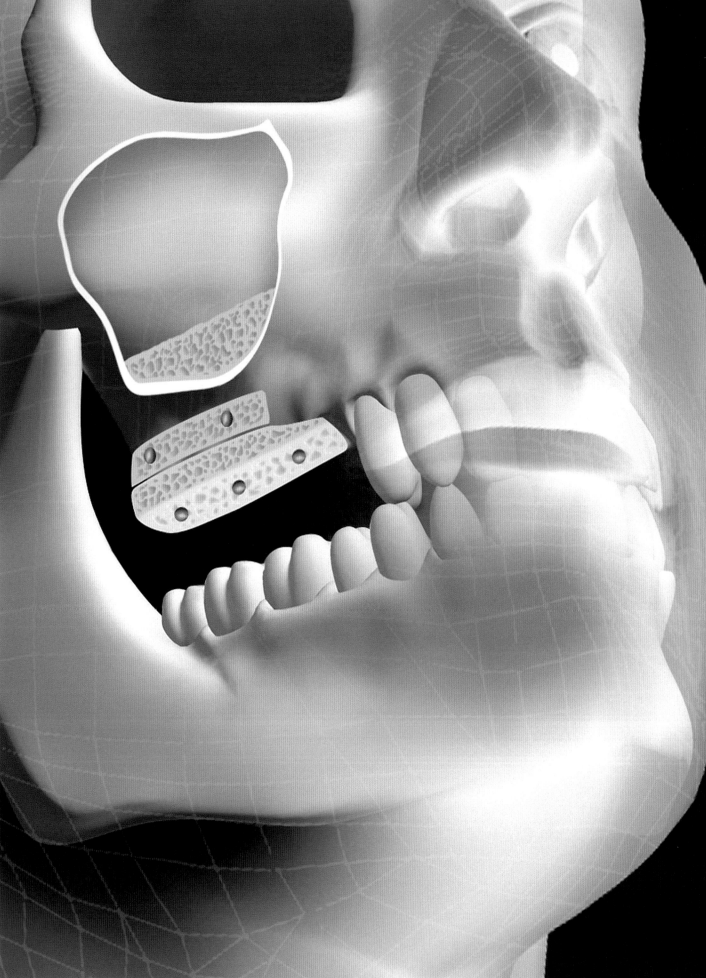

A.B. GIANNÌ
R. MONTEVERDI
A. BAJ
F. CARLINO
O. TOMIC

Maxillary atrophy: classification and surgical protocols

07

07

Tetsch 1991; Brusati et al. 1997; Carlino et al. 1998). However, it is commonly found that when teeth are lost, the alveolar bone is resorbed at varying rates, owing to the lack of mechanical stimulus transmitted by the roots. Resorption first begins on the horizontal level, and then later affects the height of the alveolar bone, which decreases progressively, in some cases reaching as far as the basal bone.

In addition to the physiologic bone resorption of edentulous ridges, mechanical trauma caused by removable prostheses often occurs, and it causes further progressive resorption of the edentulous ridges (Cawood & Howell 1988; Bianchi 1999; Romeo et al. 2003).

Moreover, it is necessary to have adequate shape and volume of the ridges and a normal maxillo-mandibular skeleton relationship on the three planes in order to achieve satisfactory long-term results of fixed implant prostheses.

On the sagittal plane, a Class III skeletal relationship is often found in patients with total maxillary edentulism, as the loss of teeth

INTRODUCTION

An optimal esthetic and functional prosthesis can be achieved when the maxillary bone has precise morphologic requisites: the height and thickness of edentulous bone must be at least 5 mm, and there must be a sufficient quantity of keratinized tissue and an adequate depth of the vestibular fornix (Cawood & Howell 1988; Van Steenberghe 1988; Sailer 1989; Hirsch & Ericsson 1991;

1 A → ATROPHY OF THE MAXILLA WITH FLATTENING OF THE NASOLABIAL ANGLE AND LOSS OF UPPER LIP SUPPORT.

1 B → ANTI-CLOCKWISE MANDIBULAR ROTATION DUE TO THE LOSS OF MAXILLARY VERTICAL DIMENSION AND SUBSEQUENT PSEUDO-PROGNATHISM.

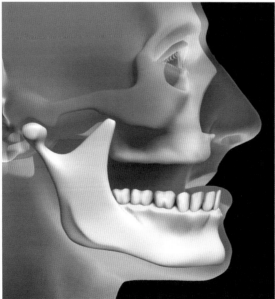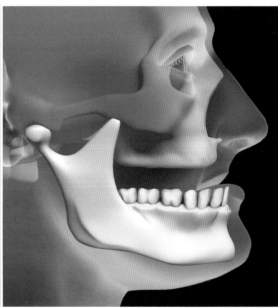

and subsequent alveolar atrophy cause a reduction of the anterior facial height with a consequent counter-clockwise mandibular rotation and the appearance of a prognathic profile **FIG. 1**.

On the sagittal plane, a correct relationship, compatible with skeletal Class I (ANB angle 2° ± 2°), should be maintained although small discrepancies may be compensated for by the future prosthesis.

On the vertical plane, on the other hand, the distance between the alveolar ridge and the ideal occlusion plane must be greater than or equal to 5 mm, with a vertical maxillomandibular distance of at least 1 cm. The maximum limit of the vertical height, especially regarding the maxilla, is connected to a normal labiodental relationship and an esthetically acceptable length of the prosthetic crowns.

Finally, on the horizontal plane, it is necessary to make sure that the opposing ridges allow for the construction of a prosthesis with a correct interocclusal relationship (Carlino et al. 1998; Chiapasco & Rossi 2003).

Since these requirements are not found in all patients who undergo implant prosthesis rehabilitation, it is often necessary to perform reconstructive surgery, with the aim of restoring ideal conditions for the future implant rehabilitation.

ATROPHY OF THE MAXILLA

The most commonly found maxillary atrophies that represent contraindications for implant treatment are vertical and/or horizontal alveolar atrophy and/or a total reduction in the sagittal and/or vertical size of the maxilla (Isaksson et al. 1993; Brusati et al. 1997; Chiapasco & Rossi 2003).

The first contraindication is represented by a reduced distance between the alveolar ridge and the nasal fossae and the maxillary sinuses, which are often pneumatised after molar and premolar loss. In the event of horizontal resorption, there is often inadequate thickness for the diameters of the most commonly used implants and it may be difficult to achieve the correct interarch relationship on the horizontal plane.

In some cases, maxillary bone atrophy can also be associated with a vertical or sagittal discrepancy in the maxillomandibular relationship, which could be corrected by maxillary and/or mandibular osteotomies used in orthognathic surgery. The loss of maxillary teeth often worsens or even creates a class III maxillomandibular relationship, due to the aforementioned counterclockwise mandibular rotation following the loss of the vertical maxillary dimension **FIG. 1**.

There are extreme cases in which, in addition to the total loss of alveolar ridge, there is also resorption of the basal bone, making bone reconstruction extremely complex, not only due to the amount of bone needed for an optimal reconstruction, but, above all, due to the extreme difficulty in covering the graft in the immediate postoperative phase. In severe atrophies, complex reconstruction techniques can be used, which are derived from post-oncological reconstructive surgery, like the use of microvascular bone flaps (Hayter & Cawood 1996).

Lips and perioral tissue must also be considered. Patients with severe anterior maxillary atrophy have an aged appearance owing to the loss of anterior vertical height and a lack of support from the teeth and the maxillary bone. The lack of support can only be partly corrected by the prosthetic rehabilitation and therefore secondary correction with plastic facial surgery such as lipofilling and liposculpture is required (Coleman 1991, 1997).

Several classifications have been proposed for maxillary and/or mandibular bone defects that, although precise and localized, are limited to the exclusive classification of the shape and size of the alveolar ridge. To achieve an esthetic and functional result it is necessary to make an accurate preliminary evaluation of the perioral and facial soft tisssue in relation to the bony structures.

A proposal for a comprehensive classification of maxillary atrophies and the reconstructive surgery options are adressed in this chapter.

The essential prerequisite for success of an implant rehabilitation is the preoperative study of the case, obtained by clinical examination and instrumental assessments, such as orthopantograph, cephalometric radiograph, CT scan and study casts. Only a correct diagnosis of the type of defect will lead to clinical success, with a long-term result of the prosthetic rehabilitation.

The following diagnostic protocol in patients with partial or total edentulism of the maxilla is suggested.

Clinical examination: The clinical examination must entail an intraoral examination and an extraoral examination;

- an objective intraoral examination to assess the volume of the edentulous ridges, the quality and quantity of the keratinized tissue, the vertical, sagittal and horizontal interarch distances;

- an objective examination of the face with detailed examination of the interlabial relationships, the exposure of the maxillary incisors, if present, the length and support of the lips and soft tissue and a careful evaluation of any discrepancy in the condylar centric position and maximum intercuspidation. The following characteristics become more or less evident in a patient with maxillary edentulism and consequent bone atrophy: a reduction in facial length (loss of anterior face height), the disappearance of the labiomental angle, retrusion of the upper lip, a prognathic chin, deepening of nasolabial grooves, and increase in nasolabial angle **FIG 2-3**.

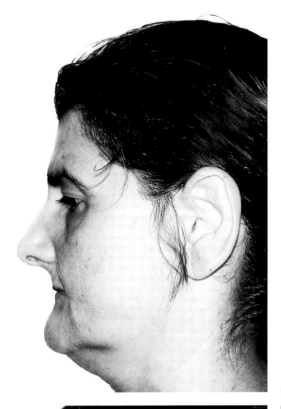

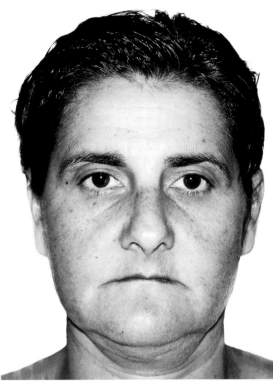

2 A-B → SAGITTAL PROFILE
AND FRONTAL VIEW OF
EDENTULOUS PATIENT WITH
PSEUDOPROGNATHISM AND
LACK OF PERIORAL SOFT
TISSUE SUPPORT.

3 A-B → SAGITTAL PROFILE
AND FRONTAL VIEW OF
PATIENT ON COMPLETION OF
IMPLANT PROSTHETIC
REHABILITATION
TREATMENT.
THE RESTORATION OF
PERIORAL SOFT TISSUE
SUPPORT CAN BE NOTED.

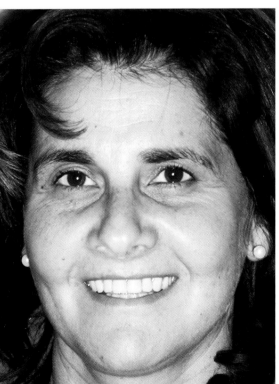

Instrumental examinations: Orthopantograph and cephalometric radiographs are always necessary to exclude the existence of bone pathologies, such as cysts and osteitis, to evaluate the alveolar ridge height, the maxillary sinus pneumatization and the maxillomandibular relationship on the vertical and sagittal planes.

The use of maxillary CT is necessary only when the clinical and/or instrumental examinations show an initial height and/or thickness of the alveolar ridge (lower than or equal to 10 mm and 5 mm respectively) for the insertion of implants of at least 10 mm in height and 3.75 mm in thickness, or when an accurate evaluation of the maxillary sinus and/or nasal fossae is necessary for planning future sinus augmentation procedures or a maxillary osteotomy with an interposed bone graft.

Articulated study casts evaluate the morphology of the edentulous arches, with an articulator of the facial arch in order to measure the three-dimensional relationship of the arches and to quantify the extent and the site of bone grafts, or the direction of osteotomic movement of the maxilla prior to surgery.

GRAFT MATERIAL

Autogenous bone is still the gold-standard material in reconstructive pre-implant surgery: it is safe, economic and above all is currently the only graft material that contains all three healing modes of the alveolar bone: osteogenesis, osteoinduction and osteoconduction.

Healing has three phases:

1) Osteogenesis: the surviving vital cells in the grafted bone stimulate the formation of new bone with maximum activity in the first 4 weeks. This mechanism only takes place in fresh bone grafts, especially autogenous ones, and cancellous bone grafts are richer in vital cells than cortical bone grafts.

2) Osteoinduction: from the second week to the sixth month, with peak activity at the sixth week, the release of bone morphogenetic proteins (BMP) from dead cells induces the osteoinductive phase, which is the differentiation of mesenchymal cells into chondrogenic and osteogenetic cells. The formation of new bone comes almost exclusively from the creeping substitution, i.e. the process in which the mesenchymal vessels and cells in the receiving bed invade the graft, resorb the bone component and replace it with new bone. Graft incorporation is therefore a process in which the receiving bed will have revascularized the graft area and will have replaced the graft bone with new bone.

3) Osteoconduction: the inorganic material acts as a guide for the osteoconductive phase from the second to the twenty-fourth month.

With regards to the embryologic origin of the donor site, some studies have shown that intra-membranous origin grafts, such as calvaria bone, are more stable and resorb less than intrachondral bone grafts, such as iliac bone. Other authors, however, have shown that the graft's behavior has less to do with its embryologic origin and more to do with the three-dimensional bone structure of the transposed bone and the prevalence of cancellous or cortical tissue (Hardesty & Marsh 1992; Isaksson et al. 1993; Triplett et al. 1996).

SURGICAL TECHNIQUES

Two reconstructive techniques are traditionally described in cases of severe maxillary atrophies: onlay or appositional bone grafts and inlay or interpositional bone grafts.

From a technical point of view, the first bone grafts are performed by the insertion of autogenous bone above the bone surface that is to be increased and the graft is then stabilized as firmly as possible and covered by mucosa to avoid any contamination from the external environment **FIG. 4**. The second involves the use of full maxillary or alveolar ridge osteotomies and therefore the interposition of the graft between two pedunculated bony surfaces that are vascularized. Grafts are revascularized in the first 4 to 8 weeks after insertion, via a process known as "*creeping substitution*", i.e. the progressive resorption and apposition of new bone (Hardesty & Marsh 1992).

Inlay grafts have an intuitive biologic advantage compared with onlay grafts: the graft can receive a blood supply from two vital bone surfaces, so revascularization will be quicker and there will be less bone resorption during the healing phases **FIG. 5**.

The possibility of "lengthening" the bone using osteodistraction and, in some cases, microvascular flaps, has recently been advocated as a therapeutic option.

Bone distraction is a surgical procedure that uses a biologic process for new bone formation between the edges of ostetomised bone segments, when they are separated by growing traction. After carrying out an osteotomy in the area to be increased, the bone is lengthened by about 1 mm per day, using a specific instrument called a distractor. After about 65 days, mature bone will have grown in the gap. This method is mostly used for the mandibular bone (Chin & Toth 1996) **FIG. 6**.

The second technique, which is more technically complex and riskier in terms of morbidity, involves a donor site extremely distant from the oral cavity, such as the fibula, which may be associated with skin and muscle, together with its own vascular peduncle that is isolated and sectioned beforehand **FIG. 7**. The bone flap is transposed to the site that must be reconstructed, and is modeled and fixed as necessary.

At this point, microvascular anastomosis is carried out between the flap peduncle and the vessels in the areas to be reconstructed (mostly facial artery and vein for maxillary bone and thyroid artery and outer jugular vein for mandibular bone) that will keep the transposed bone vital. Unlike a graft, the bone here is vital and therefore is not resorbed in the first 2 months, as it does not heal with the creeping substitution mechanism, and if it becomes infected, antibiotics can be used to sterilize the part. A rigid bond already exists after 7 weeks, while in bone grafts at 7 weeks there is only fibrous tissue in the host graft-site interface. Immediate revascularization allows all the flap cells to survive, and the regenerative capacity of a microvascular flap is equal to that of the bone, with a healing process that is similar to that of a fracture, i.e. without creeping substitution and therefore without resorption (Hidalgo 1989; Hayter & Cawood 1996).

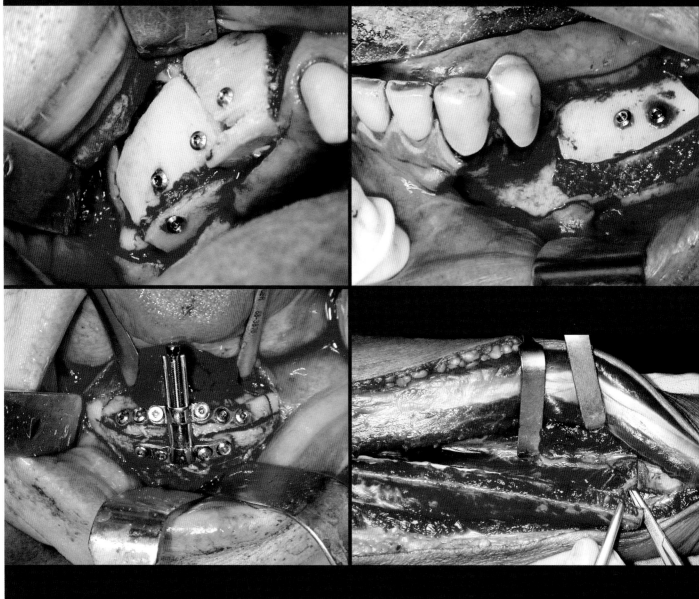

4 → EXAMPLE OF ONLAY
MAXILLARY BONE GRAFT.

5 → EXAMPLE OF INLAY
MANDIBULAR BONE GRAFT.

6 → MANDIBULAR
DISTRACTOR APPLIED TO
THE SYMPHYSIS.

7 → MICROVASCULAR
FIBULA.

VESTIBULAR PLASTIC SURGERY

An adequate depth of the vestibular fornix is an essential requirement for the stability of removable prostheses. The placement of two implants in the mandible or four implants in the maxilla usually guarantees prosthesis stability.

It is, however, essential for most authors to obtain good fornix depth, in addition to 2 to 3 mm of peri-implant keratinized tissue that favors correct oral hygiene procedures, in order to avoid the risk of reccurring peri-implantitis (Van Steenberghe 1988; Tetsch 1991).

To obtain fornix depth, the classical vestibular plastic surgery may be used together with a mucosal graft or a skin graft. The skin graft, however, especially in the anterior areas, cannot provide an esthetic result owing to the obvious dischromy.

It is preferable to use a partial thickness flap for apical transposition of the mucosa, which is no longer stabilized at the periostium but with screws fixed to the bone (Triaca & Carlino 1996) **FIG. 8-15**.

Once healing by secondary re-epithelization, and therefore fornix depth, has been obtained, small peri-implant keratinized grafts can be performed.

CLASSIFICATION OF MAXILLARY ATROPHIES

As already mentioned, the parameters taken into consideration in classifying single maxillary bone atrophies do not only concern the shape and size of the alveolar bone, but also the 3D relationship between the jaws and the state of oral and facial soft tissue. Once the diagnostic process is completed, patients needing pre-implant surgery in the maxilla are divided according to the classification below.

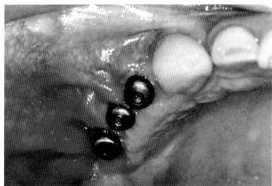
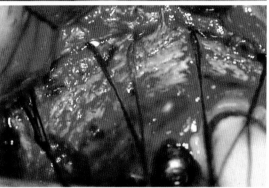
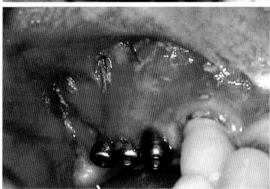

8-9-10 → RE-ESTABLISHMENT OF CORRECT FORNIX DEPTH, VIA VESTIBULAR PLASTIC SURGERY WITH PARTIAL THICKNESS FLAP.

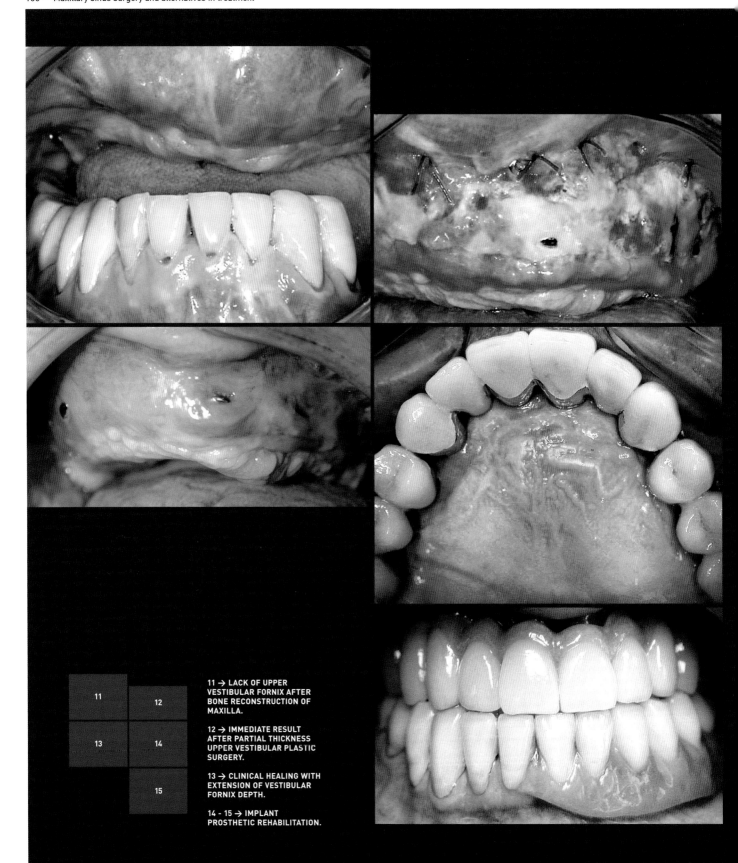

11 → LACK OF UPPER VESTIBULAR FORNIX AFTER BONE RECONSTRUCTION OF MAXILLA.

12 → IMMEDIATE RESULT AFTER PARTIAL THICKNESS UPPER VESTIBULAR PLASTIC SURGERY.

13 → CLINICAL HEALING WITH EXTENSION OF VESTIBULAR FORNIX DEPTH.

14 - 15 → IMPLANT PROSTHETIC REHABILITATION.

SURGICAL PROTOCOL IN MAXILLARY BONE ATROPHIES

The correct taxonomic placement of the patient in one of these categories therefore allows the most suitable reconstructive treatment to be chosen, after considering the cost-benefit ratio of each surgical intervention.

1) POSTERIOR SECTORIAL ATROPHY

HYPERPNEUMATIZATION OF THE MAXILLARY SINUS TYPE A

The ideal surgical intervention in patients with sinus hyperpneumatization is sinus augmentation with autogenous bone graft FIG. 16-17. In the event of a monolateral operation, surgery can be carried out under local anesthetic by an expert, with the removal of intraoral bone from the symphysis or the ascending ramus. For a bilateral sinus augmentation, it is advisable to use general anesthesia, which allows a sufficient amount of bone to be taken from the iliac crest or the calvaria bone. In selected cases (e.g. patients with health problems) it may be necessary to carry out bilateral sinus lift under local anesthesia or under sedation, preferably in the operating theatre. This is performed in one or two sessions, using autogenous bone grafts taken from intraoral sites or from the iliac crest with a trephine bur. Before carrying out a sinus augmentation, as anticipated, it is mandatory to check that the

SECTORIAL BONE ATROPHIES

1) POSTERIOR SECTORS (PREMOLAR AND MOLAR REGIONS)
A) HYPERPNEUMATIZATION OF SINUS
B) HORIZONTAL DEFICIENCY
C) VERTICAL DEFICIENCY
D) COMBINED DEFICIENCY

2) ANTERIOR SECTORS (INTER-CANINE AREA)
A) HORIZONTAL (OR SAGITTAL) DEFICIENCY
B) VERTICAL DEFICIENCY
C) COMBINED DEFICIENCY

MULTI-SECTORIAL OR SEVERE BONE ATROPHIES

3) WITH NORMAL MAXILLOMANDIBULAR RELATIONSHIP
A) HORIZONTAL DEFICIENCY
B) VERTICAL DEFICIENCY
C) COMBINED DEFICIENCY

4) WITH ALTERED MAXILLOMANDIBULAR RELATIONSHIP

EXTREME BONE ATROPHIES

5) TOTAL RESORPTION OF ALVEOLAR BONE AND BASAL BONE

SECTORIAL BONE ATROPHIES

1) POSTERIOR

TYPE A: HYPERPNEUMATIZATION OF SINUS

Normal interarch distance.
Ridge height ≤ 5-8 mm
Ridge thickness ≥ 6 mm

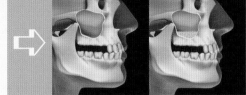

Sinus lift with surgery.

TYPE B: HORIZONTAL DEFICIENCY

Normal interarch distance.
Ridge height between 5 and 8 mm
Ridge thickness ≤ 6 mm

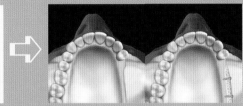

Sinus lift with bone graft.

TYPE C: VERTICAL DEFICIENCY

Increased interarch distance.
Ridge height < 5 mm
Ridge thickness ≥ 6 mm

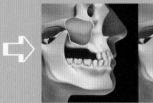

Vertical onlay bone graft
+/– sinus lift.

TYPE D: COMBINED DEFICIENCY

Increased interarch distance.
Ridge height < 5 mm
Ridge thickness ≤ 6 mm

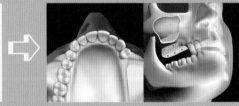

Vertical and transverse onlay bone
graft +/– sinus lift
with autogenous bone graft.
Vestibular plastic surgery at 3
months with mucosal graft.

2) ANTERIOR

TYPE A: HORIZONTAL DEFICIENCY

Normal interarch distance.
Ridge height < 10 mm
Ridge thickness < 6 mm

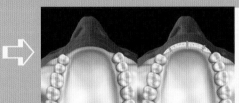

Horizontal onlay bone graft.

TYPE B: VERTICAL DEFICIENCY

Increased interarch distance.
Ridge height < 10 mm
Ridge thickness ≥ 6 mm

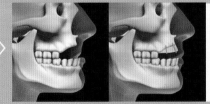

Vertical onlay graft.

TYPE C: COMBINED DEFICIENCY

Increased interarch distance.
Ridge height < 10 mm
Ridge thickness < 6 mm

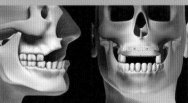

Vertical and horizontal
bone onlay graft.

MULTI-SECTORIAL OR SEVERE BONE ATROPHIES

3) WITH NORMAL MAXILLOMANDIBULAR RELATIONSHIP

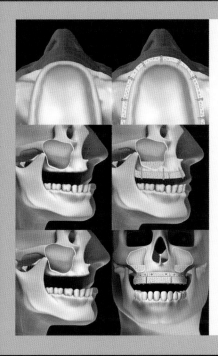

The diagnostic parameters of three identified deficiencies:

horizontal (type a)

vertical (type b)

and combined (type c).

4) WITH ALTERED MAXILLOMANDIBULAR RELATIONSHIP

Altered maxillomandibular
three-dimensional relationship.
Increased interarch distance.
Variable thickness of ridge.

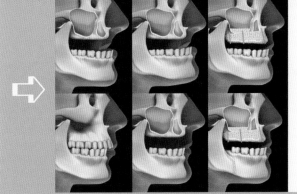

Le Fort I Osteotomy
with interposition bone graft
+/– onlay bone grafts
+/– mandibular osteotomy.

EXTREME BONE ATROPHIES

5) TOTAL RESORPTION OF ALVEOLAR BONE AND BASAL BONE

Extreme atrophy with serious
resorption also of basal bone.
Increased interarch distance.

 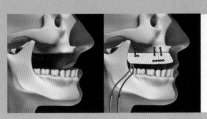

Microvascular bone flap.

maxillary sinus is normally ventilated and that there are no pathologic conditions (see previous chapter) that are contraindications to the operation. It must be remembered that the presence of a mucosal cyst in the maxillary sinus, a frequent and totally asymptomatic event, is not a contraindication for the performance of a sinus lift. On the contrary, during the surgery the surgeon can remove it or aspirate it through a small bone operculum placed above the usual antrostomy used for a sinus augmentation procedure.

HORIZONTAL DEFICIENCY TYPE B

The horizontal bone deficiency is corrected either by a vestibular onlay graft **FIG. 18-19** or, if the ridge is at least 3 to 4 mm thick, by splitting the ridge and placing an interposition bone graft. As already mentioned, in patients with sinus hyperpneumatization, surgery can be carried out under local anesthesia, even for affixation onlay grafts, if the horizontal bone deficiency does not exceed 3 to 4 mm and above all if two to three implant sites are involved. In other cases, considering the amount of necessary autogengous bone operative time, it is advisable to carry out the procedure under general anesthesia **FIG. 20-23**.

For ideal bone graft healing, the following factors should be considered:
- Firm stabilization of the graft with titanium plates and/or screws **FIG. 21** to avoid any microtrauma that could hamper the neo-angiogenesis process.
- Coverage of the graft with a tension-free, suture, to avoid any exposure and thus infection of the graft. For this purpose, the flaps must be carefully mobilized, with periosteal incisions. Even partial graft exposure, especially of cortical bone, usually leads to total graft removal.
- Careful filling of any residual gap between the graft and maxillary bone with bone chips, possibly associated with a membrane, in order to avoid interposition of

16 → MAXILLARY SINUS HYPERPNEUMATIZATION.

17 → SURGICAL CORRECTION WITH MAXILLARY SINUS AUGMENTATION PROCEDURE.

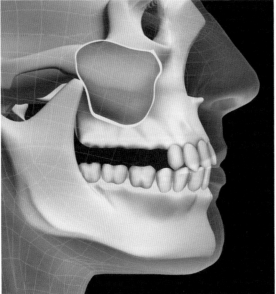
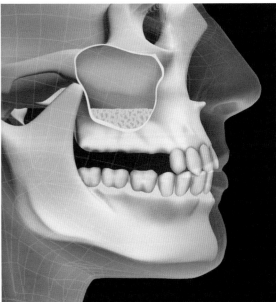

connective tissue during the healing process. The formation of connective tissue between the grafted bone and the maxillary bone makes bone integration with the maxilla precarious and prevents later osseointegration of the implants placed in the reconstructed maxilla.

During implant placement, it is recommended that the fixation screws are not removed, to avoid mobilization of the graft from the host site. When implants are being uncovered, the fixation screws are removed, and reconstruction of peri-implant tissue may also be carried out at the same time.

In the authors' experience it has been found that it is advisable to place implants at a later date, from 3 months (iliac bone), to 4 to 5 months (calvaria and intraoral bone), to avoid excessive bone graft resorption.

Whenever it is possible to carry out a sagittal osteotomy including a horizontal expansion, day surgery can be performed for up to five implants, as the amount of bone to be placed is less than the amount of bone required to carry out an onlay graft. Under normal conditions, this technique does not lead to the use of intraosseous fixation devices, as the osteotomized section is not completely fractured at the alveolar ridge base, as a greenstick fracture is later performed, and it maintains the horizontal expansion achieved owing to the perfect balance between expansion forces (interposed bone graft) and retaining forces represented by sutured flaps. However, this technique, if not carried out by expert surgeons, may easily cause a full fracture of the external alveolar ridge with a consequent need for stabilization by osteosynthesis.

With regard to implants, especially in day surgery, preference is given to the immediate implant placement that will only obtain primary stability if placed at least 5 mm in a non-osteotomized maxillary bone.

If, however, alveolar *splitting* involves more than 4 mm of the ridge height, it is preferable to postpone placement for 3 to 4

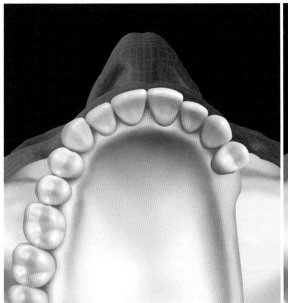 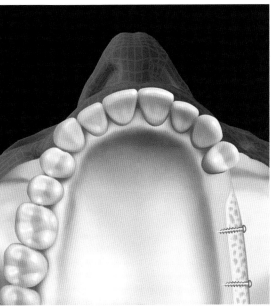

18 → POSTERIOR HORIZONTAL BONE ATROPHY OF THE MAXILLA.

19 → SURGICAL CORRECTION WITH HORIZONTAL APPOSITIONAL BONE GRAFT.

months. In this case, 2 to 3 months after implant placement, peri-implant tissue reconstruction can be carried out where necessary, in particular of the adherent gum using a palatal mucosal graft.

VERTICAL DEFICIENCY
TYPE C

In patients with a posterior vertical height deficiency, with an increase in the interarch distance, a vertical onlay graft of autogenous bone is recommended; it can be stabilized by titanium screws and/or plates with or without membranes **FIG. 24-25**. This type of surgery can often be carried out under local anesthesia in a day surgery setting if the vertical deficiency is not severe. In cases of more severe deficiency, intraoral harvesting is not a sufficient source of bone graft, and bone substitutes are still not the

graft material of choice for large reconstructions.

If the maxillary sinus is hyperpneumatized with excessive increase of the vertical interarch distance, it is advisable to carry out the sinus lift and an onlay graft at the same time.

Placement of implants can only be performed at the same time as grafting if the residual crestal bone can guarantee sufficient primary stability for the implants; in all other cases, it is preferable to postpone implant placement after 3 months in cases reconstructed with iliac bone, and no later than 4 to 5 months for calvaria bone or intraoral bone, to avoid excessive resorption of the grafts.

In the event of delayed implant placement, the fixation screws will be removed, and the fornix and the keratinized tissue will be reconstructed with a palatal mucosal graft during the same surgical session.

20 → INTRAORAL VIEW OF MAXILLARY POSTERIOR HORIZONTAL TRANSVERSE BONE DEFICIENCY.

21 → INTRA-OPERATIVE CLINICAL VIEW OF BONE RECONSTRUCTION WITH ILIAC BONE GRAFT.

22 → POST-SURGICAL ORTHOPANTOGRAPH.

23 → CLINICAL VIEW OF HEALING AT 2 MONTHS.

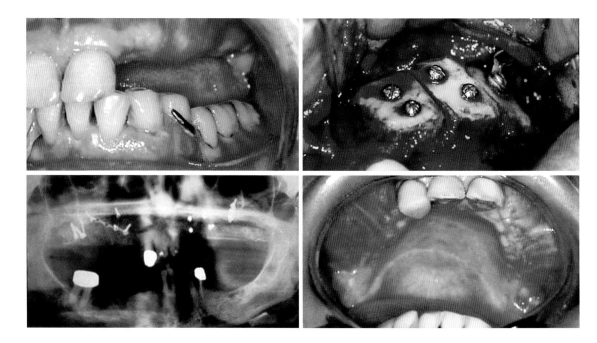

**COMBINED DEFICIENCY
TYPE D**

In patients with both vertical and horizontal ridge bone deficiency, the reconstructive procedures described for patients in groups 1B and 1C will be carried out at the same time **FIG. 26-28**.

Of course, the longer surgical time and the increase in the amount of autogenous extraoral bone required do not allow this surgery to be performed in a day surgery setting **FIG. 29-33**.

2) ANTERIOR SECTORIAL ATROPHIES

**HORIZONTAL DEFICIENCY
TYPE A**

Similar to posterior atrophy, when alveolar ridge height in the anterior sections is less than 5 to 6 mm, it is advisable to use vestibular onlay bone grafts **FIG. 34-35** or *splitting* of the ridge.

The anterior area has important esthetic implications: the bone volume, the inclination and position of the prosthetic incisors can affect labiodental exposure and the smile line. It is mandatory to use articulated study casts in order to optimise the esthetic and the functional results, and to assess preoperatively the soft tissue support, especially the thickness and length of the upper lip and labial competence. These clinical data will dictate bone

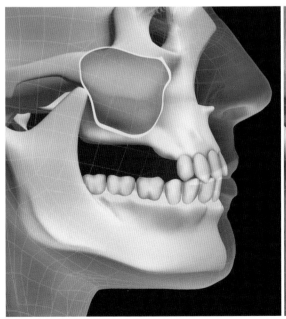
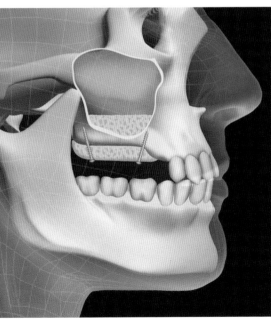

24 → POSTERIOR VERTICAL BONE ATROPHY AND SUBSEQUENT INCREASE IN INTERARCH DISTANCE.

25 → SURGICAL CORRECTION WITH MAXILLARY SINUS AUGMENTATION PROCEDURE AND VERTICAL ONLAY GRAFT.

reconstruction, which will allow for the placement of adequate sized implants. On the other hand, the size of the upper lip must not be altered, creating labial incompetence or a reduction of the nasolabial angle.

Patients with a class III skeletal relationship and vestibular-lingual discrepancies of less than 7 to 8 mm can be compensated with a fixed hybrid prosthesis in the mandible, and a removable meso and supra-structure in the maxilla, to re-establish corect soft tissue support, smile line, type of occlusion and access for maintenance maneuvers.

Discrepancies of more than 7 to 8 mm require maxillofacial intervention if a fixed prosthesis is required **FIG. 36-40**.

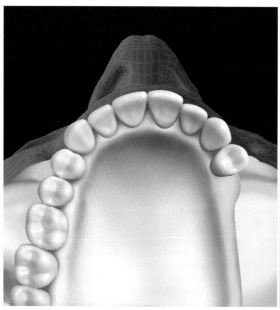

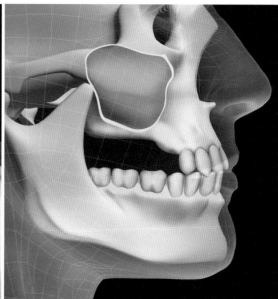

26 TO 28 → MAXILLARY
POSTERIOR HORIZONTAL BONE
ATROPHY.

SURGICAL CORRECTION WITH
MAXILLARY SINUS
AUGMENTATION PROCEDURE
WITH VERTICAL AND HORIZONTAL
ONLAY GRAFT.

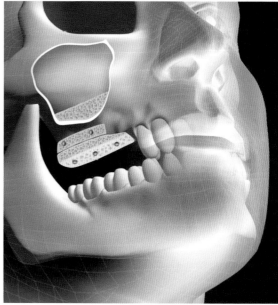

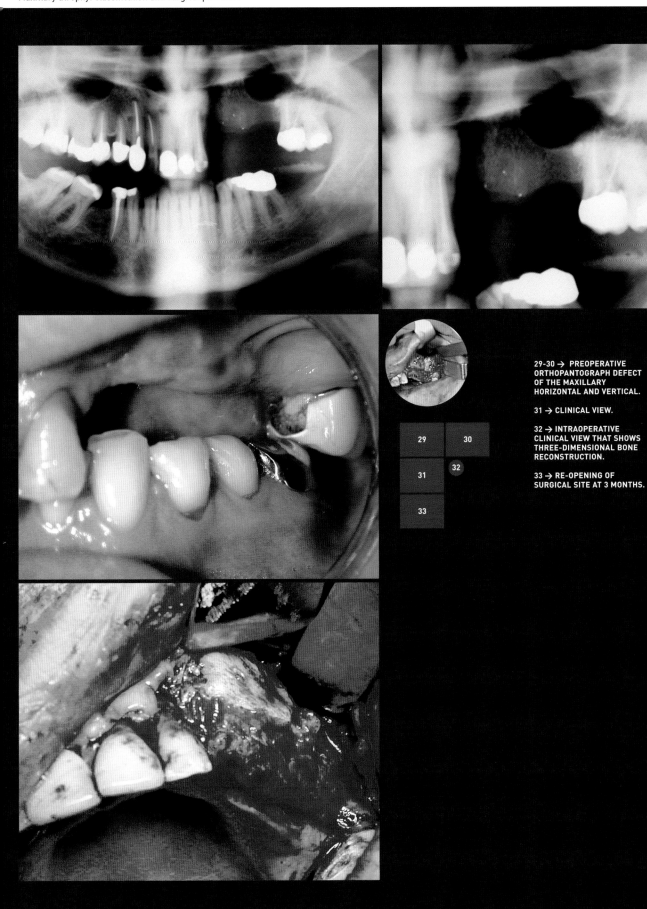

29-30 → PREOPERATIVE ORTHOPANTOGRAPH DEFECT OF THE MAXILLARY HORIZONTAL AND VERTICAL.

31 → CLINICAL VIEW.

32 → INTRAOPERATIVE CLINICAL VIEW THAT SHOWS THREE-DIMENSIONAL BONE RECONSTRUCTION.

33 → RE-OPENING OF SURGICAL SITE AT 3 MONTHS.

29	30
31	32
33	

VERTICAL DEFICIENCY
TYPE B

The increase in the interarch distance dictates the vertical bone reconstruction with grafting procedures from the iliac crest or the calvaria**FIG. 41-42**. The exact size and location of the graft must be planned carefully prior to the surgery from the clinical and instrumental information gathered. The lips are clinically analyzed, with particular reference to the length, aiming for a labiodental exposure of 2 to 3 mm at the incisor margin, after prosthetic treatment. In addition to using orthopantograph and computerized tomography (CT), lateral cephalometric radiographs will also be taken to assess the interarch distance and the relationship between the maxillary bone and the upper lip. Finally, the articulated study casts will allow assessment of the vertical size of the bony reconstruction to achieve correct occlusion and an ideal implant–crown ratio.

The loss of the fornix, which is caused by the apical repositioning of the flap to cover the graft, must be treated after 3 months with a palatal gingival graft.

In some cases, at the end of treatment there may still be some deficiency associated with deficiencies of the lip in the perinasal area, which may be treated with a liposculpture intervention (see below).

COMBINED DEFICIENCY
TYPE D

In cases with both vertical and horizontal deficiency of the anterior area, a three-dimensional bone reconstruction will be carried out with grafts from the iliac and/or calvaria bone

34 → MAXILLARY HORIZONTAL
BONE ATROPHY IN THE
ANTERIOR REGION.

35 → SURGICAL CORRECTION
WITH HORIZONTAL
APPOSITIONAL BONE GRAFT.

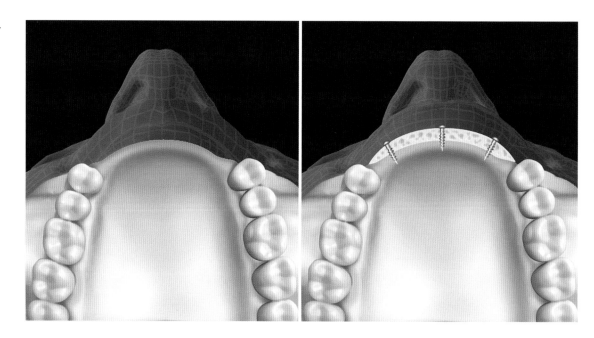

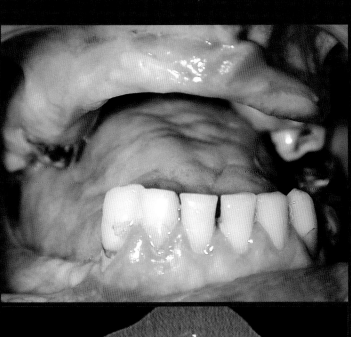

36	
37	38
39	40

36-37-38 → CLINICAL CASE OF MAXILLARY ANTERIOR HORIZONTAL BONE DEFICIENCY OF THE MAXILLA. AXIAL CT AND LATERAL CEPHALOMETRIC RADIOGRAPH.

39-40 → HARVESTING AND RECONSTRUCTION WITH CALVARIA.

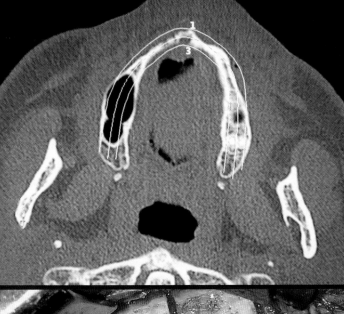

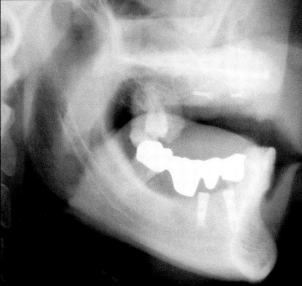

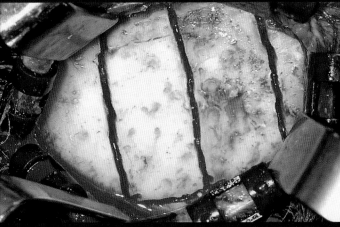

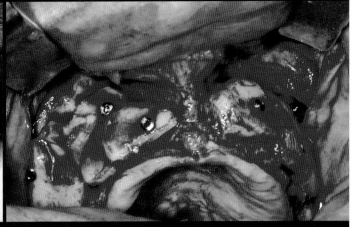

FIG. 43-45. The diagnostic and surgical problems are those discussed in previous sections **FIG. 46-51**.

Before systematically treating multisectorial bone atrophies, it must be pointed out that it is not unusual to find extruded dental elements **FIG. 52-53**. In these cases, the interarch distance may seem normal. The extrusion of natural teeth may be pronounced depending on several factors, the most important of which is the duration of edentulism. If not corrected, extrusion of the dentoaveolar segment will make it impossible to fabricate a correct prosthesis, due to lack of maxillomandibular space. In these cases, bone reconstruction should be carried out together with a dentoalveolar osteotomy to reposition the extruded segment, which is technically faster and safer than orthodontic treatment **FIG. 52–62**.

3) SEVERE ATROPHIES WITH NORMAL MAXILLOMANDIBULAR RELATIONSHIP

The therapeutic strategies are a combination of different surgical approaches used in sectorial atrophies **FIG. 63-69**. The only change is the need to restore the fornix depth and soft tissues in two separate sessions, which could be achieved at implant placement or uncovering **FIG. 70-81**.

41 → VERTICAL BONE ATROPHY OF ANTERIOR MAXILLA, WITH LOSS OF UPPER LIP SUPPORT.

42 → SURGICAL CORRECTION USING VERTICAL APPOSITIONAL BONE GRAFT AND SUBSEQUENT NORMALIZATION OF SOFT TISSUE PROFILE.

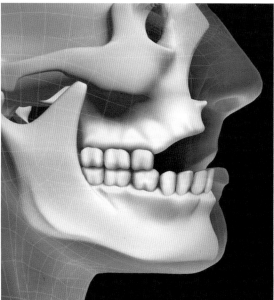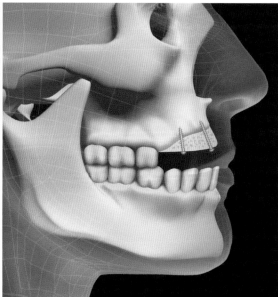

4) SEVERE ATROPHIES WITH ALTERED THREE-DIMENSIONAL RELATIONSHIP

When bone atrophy is associated with an altered maxillary–mandibular relationship, it is necessary not only to reconstruct the alveolar ridges, but also to establish the normal maxillo-mandibular three-dimensional relationship. In cases of full maxillary edentulism, especially if the condition has existed for several years, it is not unusual to find a Class III skeletal relationship, caused by maxillary retrusion after the resorption of the basal bone FIG. 82-86. If the patient had a Class III skeletal relationship before losing his teeth, the situation will deteriorate even further after losing the anterior maxillary teeth, due to both the lack of lip support and the subsequent

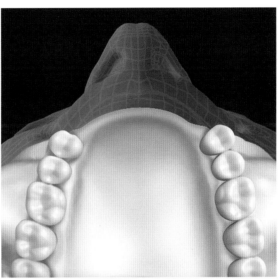

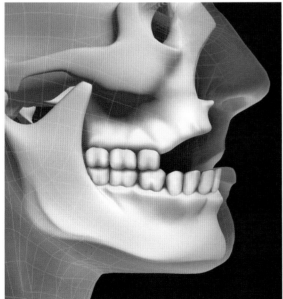

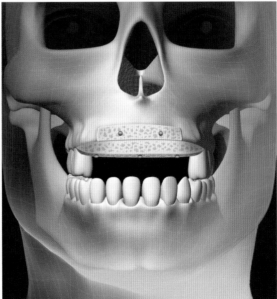

43-44 → MAXILLARY VERTICAL AND HORIZONTAL BONE ATROPHY IN THE ANTERIOR REGION.

45 → SURGICAL CORRECTION WITH VERTICAL AND HORIZONTAL APPOSITION OF BONE GRAFT.

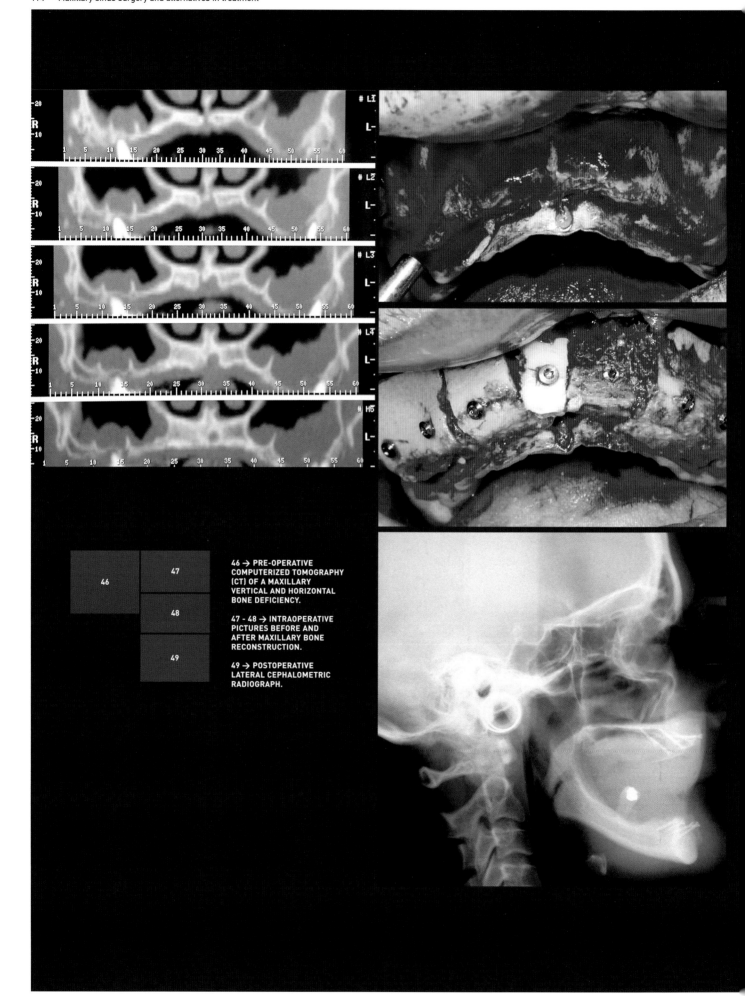

46 → PRE-OPERATIVE COMPUTERIZED TOMOGRAPHY (CT) OF A MAXILLARY VERTICAL AND HORIZONTAL BONE DEFICIENCY.

47 - 48 → INTRAOPERATIVE PICTURES BEFORE AND AFTER MAXILLARY BONE RECONSTRUCTION.

49 → POSTOPERATIVE LATERAL CEPHALOMETRIC RADIOGRAPH.

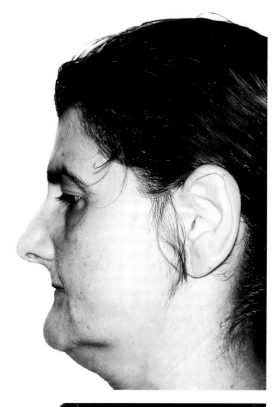
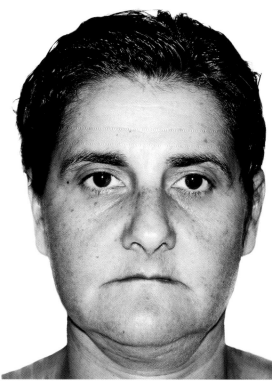
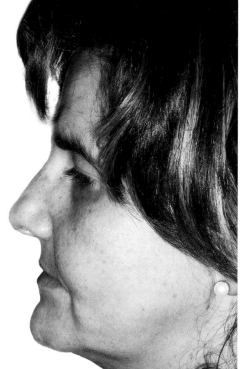
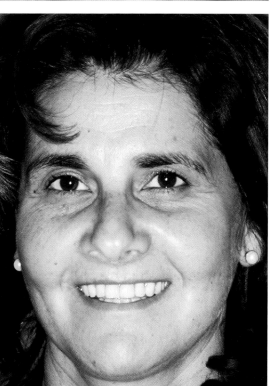

50 A-B → SAGITTAL AND FRONTAL VIEW OF PATIENT BEFORE TREATMENT. NOTE THE LACK OF PERIORAL SOFT TISSUE SUPPORT.

51 A-B →SAGITTAL AND FRONTAL VIEW OF PATIENT AFTER THE REHABILITATION TREATMENT. THE RESTORATION OF PERIORAL SOFT TISSUE SUPPORT CAN BE NOTED.

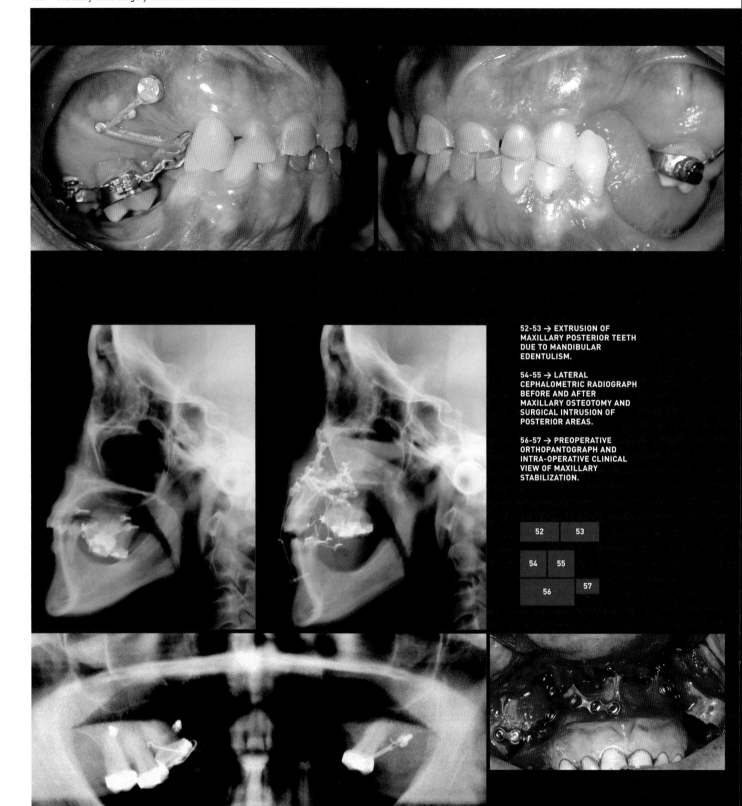

52-53 → EXTRUSION OF MAXILLARY POSTERIOR TEETH DUE TO MANDIBULAR EDENTULISM.

54-55 → LATERAL CEPHALOMETRIC RADIOGRAPH BEFORE AND AFTER MAXILLARY OSTEOTOMY AND SURGICAL INTRUSION OF POSTERIOR AREAS.

56-57 → PREOPERATIVE ORTHOPANTOGRAPH AND INTRA-OPERATIVE CLINICAL VIEW OF MAXILLARY STABILIZATION.

52	53

54	55

56	57

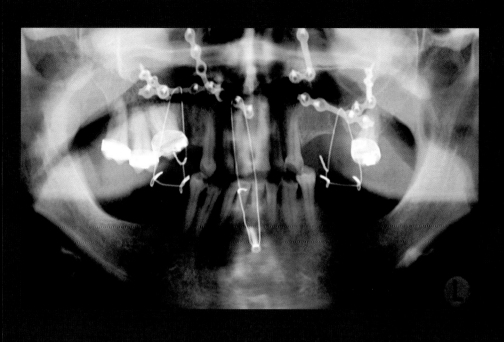

58 → POSTOPERATIVE ORTHOPANTOGRAPH.

59-60 → POST-OPERATIVE CLINICAL CONTROL. NOTE THE RE-ESTABLISHMENT OF A CORRECT INTERARCH DISTANCE.

61 → POSTOPERATIVE ORTHOPANTOGRAPH AFTER MANDIBULAR BONE RECONSTRUCTION WITH CALVARIA BONE GRAFT.

62 → INTRA-OPERATIVE VIEW OF MANDIBULAR BONE RECONSTRUCTION.

58	
59	60
61	62

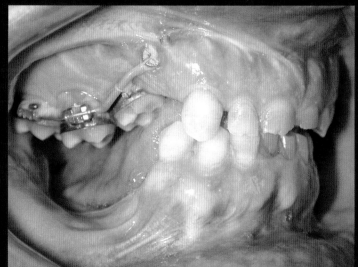

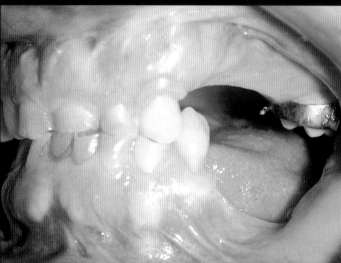

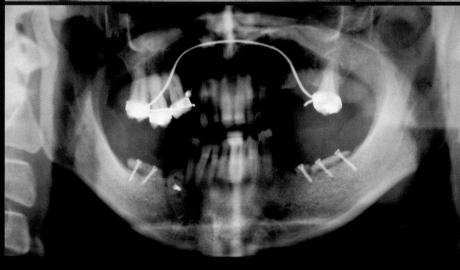

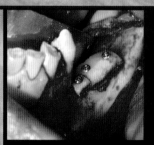

63-64 → HORIZONTAL BONE ATROPHY OF THE ENTIRE MAXILLA AND SURGICAL CORRECTION WITH HORIZONTAL ONLAY GRAFT.

65-66 → VERTICAL BONE ATROPHY OF THE ENTIRE MAXILLA AND SURGICAL CORRECTION WITH VERTICAL ONLAY BONE GRAFT AND BILATERAL SINUS AUGMENTATION SURGERY.

67-68 → VERTICAL AND HORIZONTAL BONE ATROPHY OF THE ENTIRE MAXILLA AND SURGICAL CORRECTION WITH VERTICAL AND HORIZONTAL APPOSITIONAL AND BILATERAL SINUS AUGMENTATION PROCEDURE.

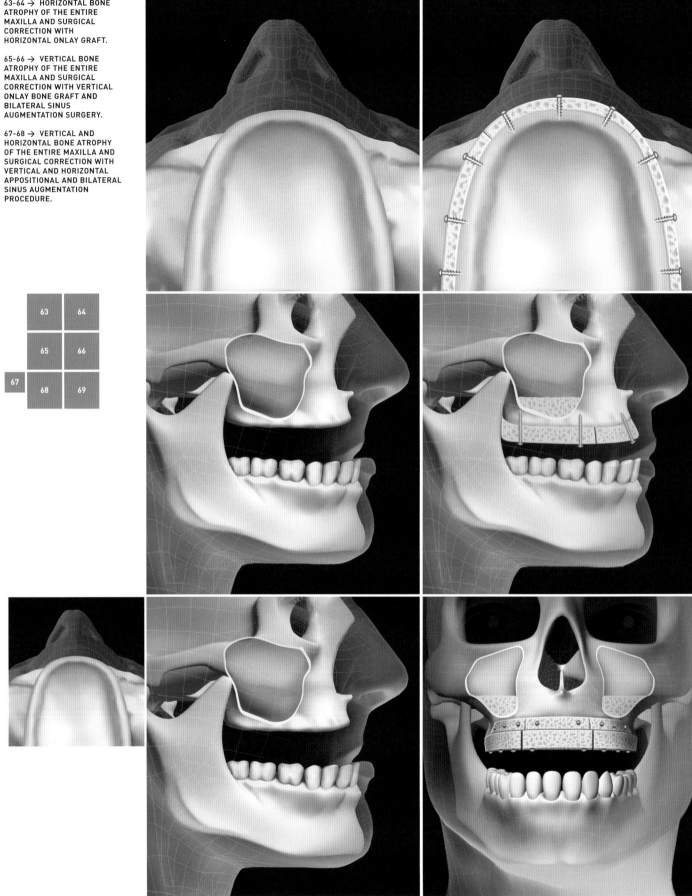

aging aspect, and the basal bone resorption. If a patient with severe vertical (and sagittal) atrophy of the maxilla has a normal profile, with his chin positioned normally on the sagittal plane, the existence of a Class II skeletal relationship might be suspected. In fact, in these patients the Class II relationship is esthetically compensated by counter-clockwise mandibular rotation due to the loss of the anterior vertical dimension. From a practical point of view, only sagittal discrepancies of a maximum of 2 to 3 mm can be compensated by the inclination of the prosthetic elements.

70	71	72
73	74	75
76	77	78
79	80	81

70-75 → MULTI-SECTOR BONE GRAFT WITH THREE-DIMENSIONAL RECONSTRUCTION OF UPPER ALVEOLAR RIDGE TO PRESERVE CORRECT 3D OCCLUSAL RELATIONSHIP.

76-81 → MULTI-SECTOR, THREE-DIMENSIONAL BONE GRAFT WITH FORNIX DEEPENING AT 3 MONTHS.

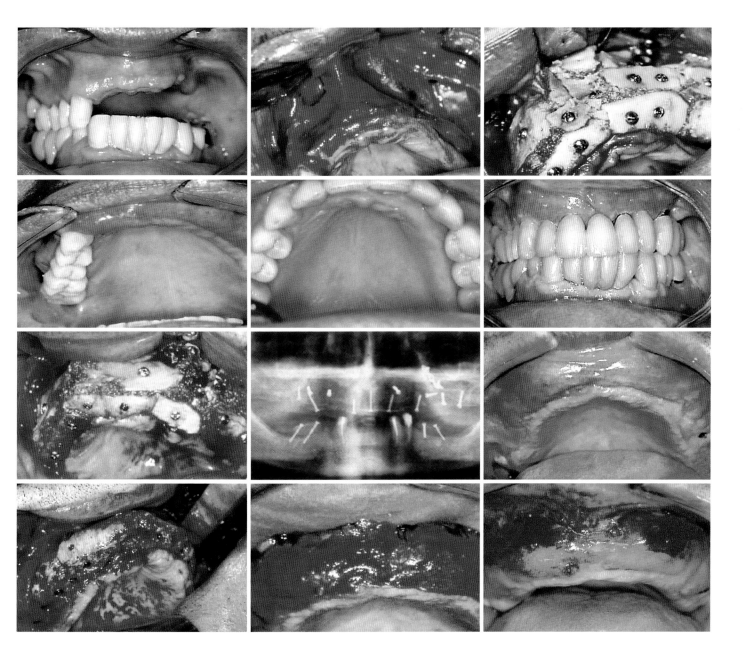

The diagnostic classification of these patients includes all the steps that are routinely performed in orthognathic surgery, i.e.:

- clinical examination of the profile, the facial symmetry, the relationship between the maxilla and the mandible, and the perioral and labial soft tissue;
- a lateral and anterior-posterior cephalometric radiograph to assess three-dimensional skeletal relationship of the opposing jaws;
- presurgical visual treatment objective (VTO) to simulate skeletal movements on the radiograph and to check the need for maxillary, mandibular or chin osteotomies;
- articulated study casts to simulate maxillo-mandibular surgical movement and to fabricate occlusal splints to be used during surgery.

Le Fort I osteotomy technique, moving the maxillary bone forward, downwards and expanding it transversally, associated with autogenous bone grafting in the maxillary sinuses and the nasal fossae, is the elective surgical intervention to treat severe 3D atrophies with an altered relationship between the maxilla and mandible **FIG. 85-99**. In order to reduce the risk of infection and to avoid the formation of postoperative sinus cysts, careful removal of the maxillary sinus mucosa should be performed. The graft is placed to the desired maxillary height, and the amount of bone needed for the future implant rehabilitation is obtained. In some cases, a maxillary osteotomy has also been carried out with a preventive bilateral sinus mucosa lift before the maxillary down-fracture, in order to place the bone graft on the sinus floor, leaving healthy, non-perforated sinus membrane. Although this type of surgical approach is time-consuming and more difficult, it allows the graft to heal more rapidly, with a lower postoperative resorption.

82 → OUTLINE OF MAXILLARY RETRUSION EMPHASIZED BY BONE ATROPHY.

83 → REDUCTION OF VERTICAL SIZE OF MAXILLA ENTAILS ANTICLOCKWISE MANDIBULAR ROTATION AND CONSEQUENT MANDIBULAR PSEUDOPROGNATHISM.

84 → SURGICAL CORRECTION OF SPATIAL POSITION AND MAXILLARY BONE ATROPHY WITH LE FORT I OSTEOTOMY AND INTERPOSITION BONE GRAFT.

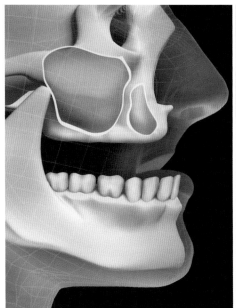
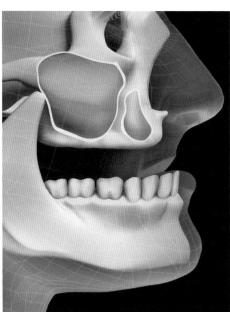
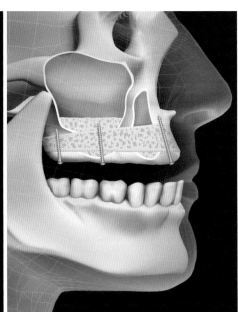

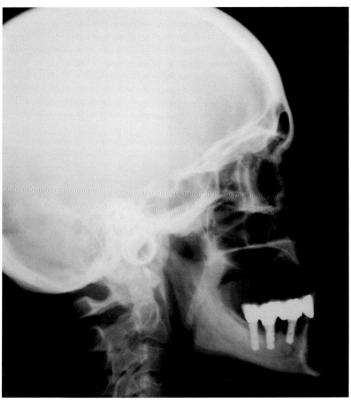
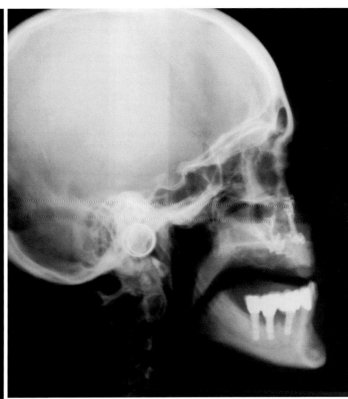

85 A-B → PRE- AND POSTOPERATIVE CEPHALOMETRIC RADIOGRAPH OF PATIENT WITH MAXILLARY RETRUSION, TREATED WITH LE FORT I MAXILLARY OSTEOTOMY TO BRING FORWARD AND LOWER THE MAXILLA USING AUTOGENOUS ILIAC BONE GRAFT PLACED BETWEEN MAXILLARY SINUSES.

86 A-B → PRE- AND POSTOPERATIVE SAGITTAL VIEW. NOTE THE SATISFACTORY LIP SUPPORT AFTER BONE RECONSTRUCTION.

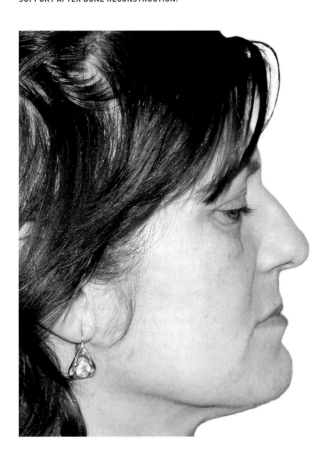
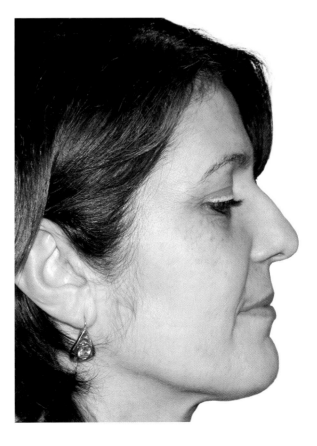

5) EXTREME ATROPHIES

With extremely severe atrophy affecting the basal bone, complex bone reconstructions using microvascular bone flaps, mainly fibula flap, may be advisable **FIG. 100-101**. During these complex bony reconstructions, it is important to use articulated study casts, in order to plan precisely the surgical phase. As already stated, the biology of a revascularized flap is very different from a bone graft, as the bone in a microvascular flap is already vital by definition, and therefore the healing mechanism is comparable to that of fractures, without any resorption linked to creeping substitution. After a few weeks, it is theoretically possible to place implants, although it is advisable to wait at least 3 months.

When the implants are placed, it will be necessary to reshape the fibula graft and assess the need to augment the peri-implant soft tissue **FIG. 102-120**.

LIPOSCULPTURE

As previously mentioned, especially in cases with anterior maxillary bone atrophies, it is often not possible to correct in a satisfactory way the aging aspect of perioral and labial soft tissue. Plastic esthetic surgery techniques, such as liposculpture, may therefore be used for these patients.

INTRODUCTION

Liposculpture is a technique that uses autogenous adipose tissue to correct depressions and increase volume of the cervical-facial area with the final goal of improving the harmony and esthetics.

This technique has been used successfully for over a century; fat grafts in scar areas were described for the first time by Neuber (Neuber 1893).

87 → PATIENT WITH SKELETAL CLASS II RELATIONSHIP.

88 → THE COUNTERCLOCKWISE MANDIBULAR ROTATION, DUE TO LOSS OF MAXILLARY VERTICAL DIMENSION, HIDES THE SKELETAL CLASS II RELATIONSHIP.

89 → SURGICAL CORRECTION OF MAXILLARY BONE ATROPHY WITH LE FORT I OSTEOTOMY TO VERTICALLY LOWER MAXILLA, AND INTERPOSITION BONE GRAFT, TOGETHER WITH MANDIBULAR OSTEOTOMY TO RESTORE CORRECT SKELETAL RELATIONSHIP ON SAGITTAL PLANE.

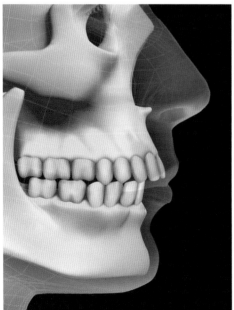
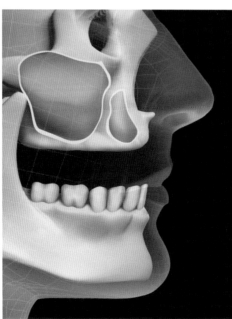
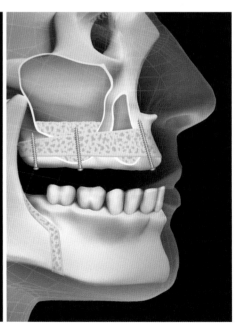

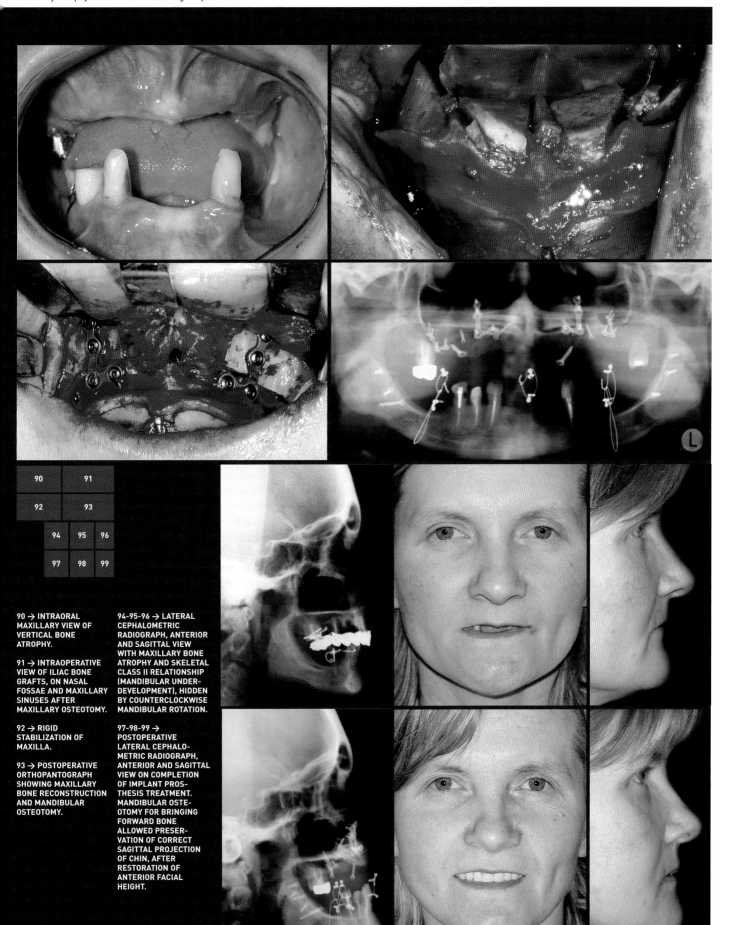

90 → INTRAORAL MAXILLARY VIEW OF VERTICAL BONE ATROPHY.

91 → INTRAOPERATIVE VIEW OF ILIAC BONE GRAFTS, ON NASAL FOSSAE AND MAXILLARY SINUSES AFTER MAXILLARY OSTEOTOMY.

92 → RIGID STABILIZATION OF MAXILLA.

93 → POSTOPERATIVE ORTHOPANTOGRAPH SHOWING MAXILLARY BONE RECONSTRUCTION AND MANDIBULAR OSTEOTOMY.

94-95-96 → LATERAL CEPHALOMETRIC RADIOGRAPH, ANTERIOR AND SAGITTAL VIEW WITH MAXILLARY BONE ATROPHY AND SKELETAL CLASS II RELATIONSHIP (MANDIBULAR UNDER-DEVELOPMENT), HIDDEN BY COUNTERCLOCKWISE MANDIBULAR ROTATION.

97-98-99 → POSTOPERATIVE LATERAL CEPHALO-METRIC RADIOGRAPH, ANTERIOR AND SAGITTAL VIEW ON COMPLETION OF IMPLANT PROS-THESIS TREATMENT. MANDIBULAR OSTE-OTOMY FOR BRINGING FORWARD BONE ALLOWED PRESER-VATION OF CORRECT SAGITTAL PROJECTION OF CHIN, AFTER RESTORATION OF ANTERIOR FACIAL HEIGHT.

Later, in 1910, Lexer reported the use of the same technique for correcting post-trauma depressions in the zygomatic arch (Lexer 1910). During the 20th century, literature continued to report the use of this technique and the results obtained over time.

Liposculpture in the cervical-facial area can be used for purely esthetic reasons (increase of volume of lips, cheekbones, cheeks, chin or the filling of nasolabial and eyelid-jugular grooves) and also in reconstructive surgery, for example for the correction of post-traumatic or iatrogenic scars, depressions and asymmetries caused by badly consolidated fractures, postrhinoplastic nasal deformities, congenital hypoplasy of facial structures, micrognathy, odontogenic maxillary atrophy, and hemi-facial atrophy (Illouz 1986).

SURGICAL TECHNIQUE

Liposculpture surgical technique, as described by Coleman (Fournier 1990; Coleman 1991, 1997) uses fat as an autoge-nous tissue graft using special drawing and insertion modes.

Before the surgical phase, a careful analysis and design of the patient's facial areas to be corrected are essential. The areas from which fat is most frequently taken are: the abdominal wall, buttocks, trochanteric area, internal thighs and the medial area of the knee.

The fat is taken under local anesthesia, and small-sized syringes and cannulae are used to avoid cell trauma. Once fat has been taken, the material is centrifuged to separate the adipose tissue from the non-vital elements such as anesthetic liquid, serum and oil. The separated material is then re-injected into the areas to be corrected, previously anesthetized by combinations of locoregional nerve blocks and local infiltration. For improved survival of the implanted material, small amounts must be injected, distributed among the various levels (subperiostium, intramuscular, subcutaneous, intradermic). After surgery, local swelling or rashes may appear, disappearing within 24 to 36 hours after treatment. Another, though rare, complica-

100 → EXTREME MAXILLARY BONE ATROPHY (RESORPTION OF BASAL BONE).

101 → SURGICAL CORRECTION USING FIBULA MICROVASCULAR FLAP. RED AND BLUE INDICATE ANASTOMIZED FIBULA ARTERIES AND VEINS.

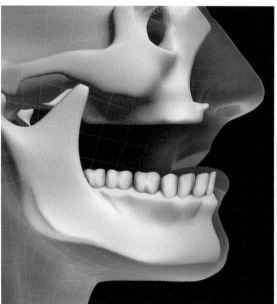

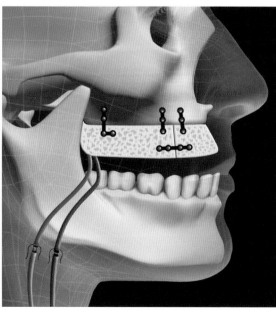

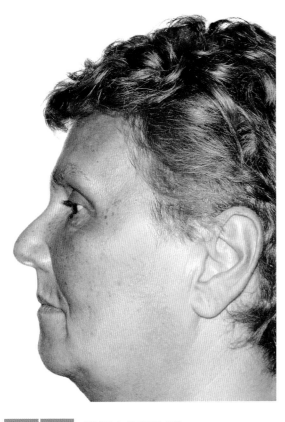
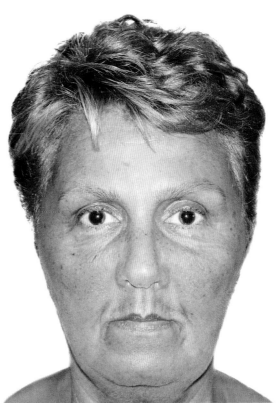

102	103
104	105
	106

102-103 → SAGITTAL AND ANTERIOR VIEW OF CLINICAL CASE WITH EXTREME MAXILLARY BONE ATROPHY.

104 → PREOPERATIVE CEPHALOMETRIC RADIOGRAPH.

105 → INTRAORAL VIEW.

106 → PREOPERATIVE CT SCAN.

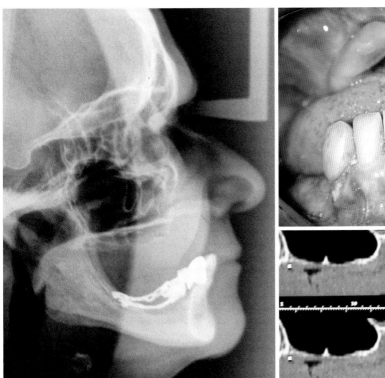
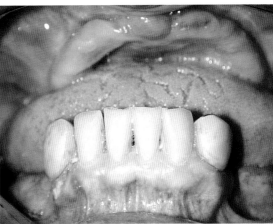
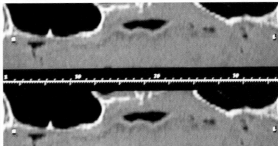

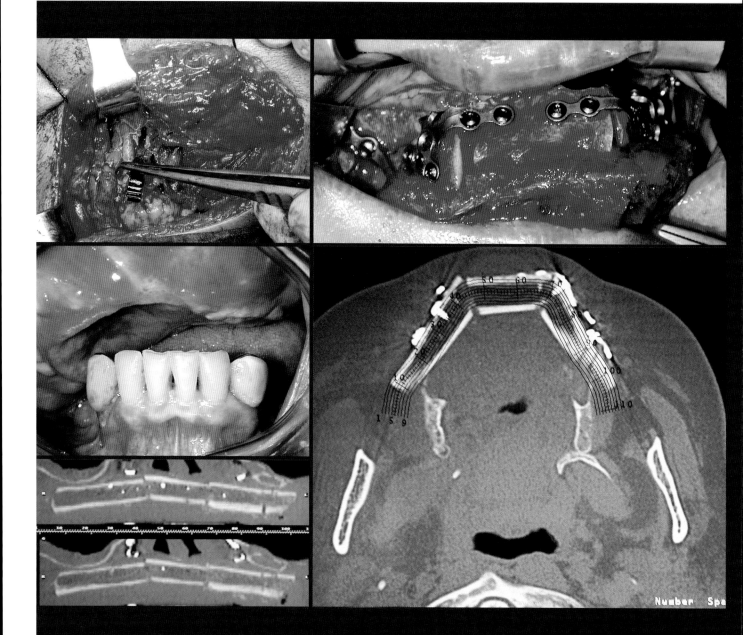

107	108
109	
	111
110	

107 → DETAIL OF VASCULAR MICROANASTOMOSIS.

108 → STABILIZATION OF THE FIBULA GRAFT.

109 → POSTOPERATIVE INTRAORAL CLINICAL VIEW.

110 - 111 → POSTOPERATIVE CT SCAN.

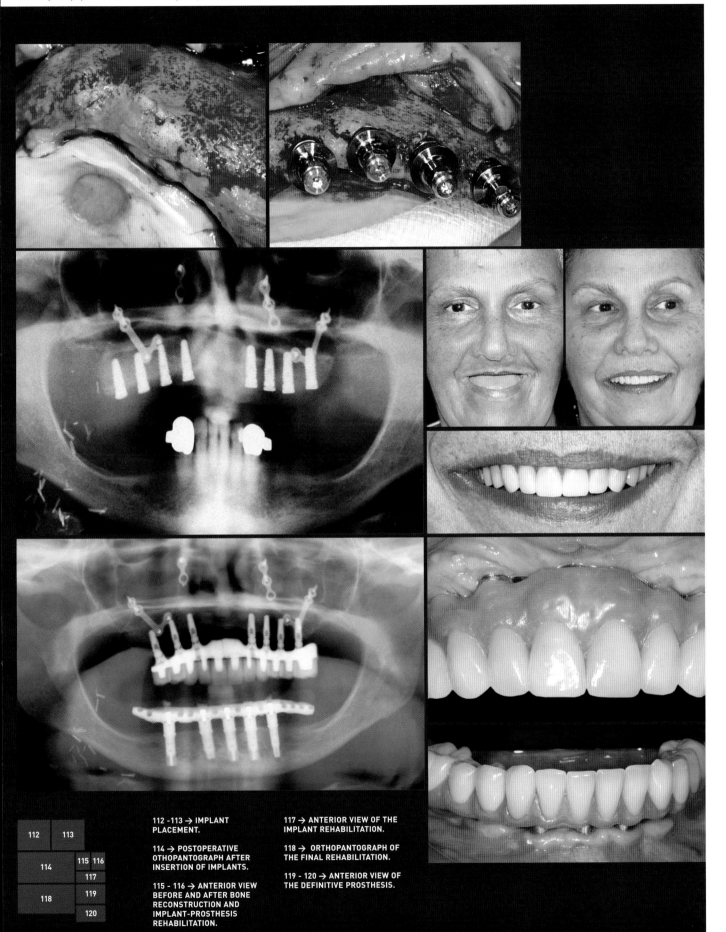

112 -113 → IMPLANT PLACEMENT.

114 → POSTOPERATIVE OTHOPANTOGRAPH AFTER INSERTION OF IMPLANTS.

115 - 116 → ANTERIOR VIEW BEFORE AND AFTER BONE RECONSTRUCTION AND IMPLANT-PROSTHESIS REHABILITATION.

117 → ANTERIOR VIEW OF THE IMPLANT REHABILITATION.

118 → ORTHOPANTOGRAPH OF THE FINAL REHABILITATION.

119 - 120 → ANTERIOR VIEW OF THE DEFINITIVE PROSTHESIS.

SUMMARY TABLE

	Bone atrophy	Reconstructive indication	Type of graft
ATROPHIC POSTERIOR MAXILLA	POSTERIOR REGION BONE ATROPHIES TYPE A	SINUS LIFT	BANK BONE, INTRAORAL WITHDRAWAL OR CORING OF ILIAC CREST DEPENDING ON VOLUME REQUIRED
	POSTERIOR REGION BONE ATROPHIES TYPE B	SINUS LIFT + EXPANSION OF RIDGE OR VESTIBULAR ONLAY GRAFT	HARVESTING OF MONO-CORTEX COMPACT AND SPONGY BONE FROM ILIAC CREST + BONE CHIPS OR HARVESTING OF MANDIBULAR BRANCH FOR BONE DEFICIENCY FOR UP TO 2 TEETH IF SINUS LIFT IS NOT REQUIRED
	POSTERIOR REGION BONE ATROPHIES TYPE C	SINUS LIFT AND ONLAY GRAFTS FOR VERTICAL INCREASE	HARVESTING OF MONO-CORTEX COMPACT AND SPONGY BONE FROM ILIAC CREST + BONE CHIPS
	POSTERIOR REGION BONE ATROPHIES TYPE D	SINUS LIFT AND ONLY GRAFTS FOR VERTICAL AND TRANSVERSE INCREASE	HARVESTING OF MONO-CORTEX COMPACT AND SPONGY BONE FROM ILIAC CREST + BONE CHIPS
ATROPHIC ANTERIOR MAXILLA	ANTERIOR REGION BONE ATROPHIES TYPE A	HORIZONTAL ONLAY GRAFT	HARVESTING OF INTRAORAL COMPACT BONE FROM BRANCH FOR BONE DEFICIENCY FOR UP TO TWO TEETH, OR HARVESTING OF CALVARIA BONE, TOGETHER WITH CORING OF ILIAC CREST, IF NECESSARY, FOR LARGER DEFICIENCIES
	ANTERIOR REGION BONE ATROPHIES TYPE B	VERTICAL ONLAY GRAFT	HARVESTING OF INTRAORAL COMPACT BONE FROM BRANCH OR HARVESTING OF CALVARIA BONE TOGETHER WITH CORING OF ILIAC CREST FOR LARGER DEFICIENCIES
	ANTERIOR REGION BONE ATROPHIES TYPE C	HORIZONTAL AND VERTICAL ONLAY GRAFT	HARVESTING OF CALVARIA BONE ASSOCIATED WITH CORING OF ILIAC CREST FOR LARGER DEFICIENCIES
SEVERE BONE ATROPHY	SEVERE BONE ATROPHY WITH NORMAL MAXILLOMANDIBULAR RELATIONSHIP	ALL RECONSTRUCTIVE STRATEGIES OF REGIONAL DEFECTS	HARVESTING OF COMPACT AND SPONGY BONE FROM ILIAC CREST IS PREFERABLE FOR POSTERIOR DEFICIENCY. HARVESTING OF CALVARIA BONE IS PREFERABLE FOR ANTERIOR DEFICIENCY.
	SEVERE BONE ATROPHY WITH ALTERED MAXILLOMANDIBULAR RELATIONSHIP	LE FORT I OSTEOTOMY WITH INTERPOSITION BONE GRAFTS TOGETHER WITH MANDIBULAR OSTEOTOMY IF REQUIRED	HARVESTING OF BI-CORTEX BONE FROM ILIAC CREST
	EXTREME ATROPHIES (BONE LAMINA PAPYRACEA)	TRANSPOSITION OF FREE FIBULA FLAP	PREPARATION OF FREE FIBULA FLAP

Advantages	Disadvantages	Morbidity
MINIMUM MORBIDITY OF WITHDRAWAL SITE, POSSIBILITY OF OPERATION UNDER LOCAL ANESTHESIA	LIMITED AMOUNT OF BONE FOR INTRA-ORAL WITHDRAWAL	SWELLING IN WITHDRAWAL SITE
LARGE QUANTITY OF BONE, RAPID REVASCULARIZATION, POSSIBILITY OF COMPACT AND SPONGY BONE	LIMITED AMOUNT OF BONE FOR INTRA-ORAL WITHDRAWAL	SLIGHT CLAUDICATION AND PAIN ON WALKING FOR A FEW DAYS
LARGE QUANTITY OF BONE, RAPID REVASCULARIZATION, POSSIBILITY OF COMPACT AND SPONGY BONE	BONE RAPIDLY RESORBED, EXCESS RECONSTRUCTION, NEED FOR EARLY IMPLANT LOAD	SLIGHT CLAUDICATION AND PAIN ON WALKING FOR A FEW DAYS
LARGE QUANTITY OF BONE, RAPID REVASCULARIZATION, POSSIBILITY OF COMPACT AND SPONGY BONE	BONE RAPIDLY RESORBED, EXCESS RECONSTRUCTION, NEED FOR EARLY IMPLANT LOAD	SLIGHT CLAUDICATION AND PAIN ON WALKING FOR A FEW DAYS
MINIMUM RESORPTION	COMPACT BONE THAT IS DIFFICULT TO ADAPT TO THE DEFECT, SLOW REVASCULARIZATION, NEED TO FILL DEFECTS WITH CHIPS	POSSIBLE FORMATION OF SMALL SUBGALEAL HEMATOMA SWELLING IN INTRAORAL WITHDRAWAL SITE
MINIMUM RESORPTION	COMPACT BONE THAT IS DIFFICULT TO ADAPT TO THE DEFECT, SLOW REVASCULARIZATION, NEED TO FILL DEFECTS WITH CHIPS	POSSIBLE FORMATION OF SMALL SUBGALEAL HEMATOMA SWELLING IN INTRAORAL WITHDRAWAL SITE
MINIMUM RESORPTION	COMPACT BONE THAT IS DIFFICULT TO ADAPT TO THE DEFECT, SLOW REVASCULARIZATION, NEED TO FILL DEFECTS WITH CHIPS	POSSIBLE FORMATION OF SMALL SUBGALEAL HEMATOMA
ADVANTAGES AND DISADVANTAGES OF BOTH WITHDRAWAL SITES ARE ASSOCIATED	ADVANTAGES AND DISADVANTAGES OF BOTH WITHDRAWAL SITES ARE ASSOCIATED	MORBIDITY IN THE TWO SITES WHERE BONE WAS HARVESTED IS ASSOCIATED
LARGE VERTICAL INCREASE, POSSIBILITY OF PLACING EXCESS BONE, POSSIBILITY OF CORRECTING MAXILLARY SPATIAL POSITION	THE GRAFT BLOCKS OF BONE ARE EXPOSED TO THE SINUS AIR ENVIRONMENT WITH SUBSEQUENT INCREASED RESORPTION AND RISK OF INFECTION	EXTENSIVE LIFTING OF ABDOMINAL MUSCLES AND GLUTEUS MAXIMUS, INCIDENCE OF DISTURBANCE ON WALKING AND FORMATION OF HEMATOMAS
POSSIBLITY OF RECONSTRUCTING WHOLE MAXILLARY, RESISTANCE TO INFECTION, BONE NOT SUBJECT TO RESORPTION	LONG OPERATION, TECHNICALLY COMPLEX, REQUIRES CONSIDERABLE PSYCHOPHYSICAL COMMITMENT BY PATIENT	CLAUDICANT WALKING FOR ABOUT 2 MONTHS, EVIDENT SCAR, NEED FOR PHYSIOTHERAPY REHABILITATION

tion is represented by the infection of the graft site, which can be treated with antibiotics.

If necessary, surgery may be repeated after about 6 months.

CONCLUSION

Liposculpture is a simple, natural and safe technique, which guarantees a long-lasting result; the use of autogenous material also avoids the onset of allergies and intolerance.

For successful treatment, it is necessary to pay careful attention when drawing, transfer-

ring and inserting the adipose tissue, due to its delicate structure. The area must be well-vascularized for cell survival, and a small amount of tissue must be placed in the various facial levels (Lexer 1910; Wilkinson 1994).

Liposculpture is an important technique in reconstructive and esthetic surgery, which, when used alone or together with other surgical operations, may be a safe means for remodeling the cervical-facial area, as facial elements can be increased three-dimensionally using this surgical intervention.

DEFECT OF IMPLANT SITE

RECONSTRUCTION OF IMPLANT SITE WITH AUTOGENOUS BONE

INSERTION OF IMPLANTS
AFTER 2 TO 3 MONTHS (ILIAC BONE)
AFTER 3 TO 4 MONTHS (CALVARIA BONE)

AFTER 3 MONTHS OF MASTICATORY LOAD
INSERTION OF HEALING SCREWS AND VESTIBULAR PLASTIC SURGERY:

MUCOSAL GRAFT
(IN SECTORIAL RECONSTRUCTIONS);

TRANSPOSED FLAP
(IN MULTI-AREA RECONSTRUCTIONS)

POSSIBLE LIPOFILLING
(FACIAL CONTOURING)

AFTER 2 TO 3 MONTHS
PERI-IMPLANT MUCOSAL GRAFT

BONE ATROPHY OF THE MAXILLA
Time sequence of implant-prosthesis rehabilitation treatment

REFERENCES

1 Bianchi A.
Implantologia ed Implantoprotesi.
Ed. Utet 1999.

2 Brusati R., Chiapasco M., Ronchi P.
Riabilitazione dei mascellari atrofici mediante trapianti ossei, osteotomie, impianti.
Dental Cadmos 1997; 13: 11-7.

3 Carlino F., Giannì A.B., Chiapasco M., Brusati R.
Chirurgia preimplantare nel mascellare superiore.
Implantologia Orale 1998; 2: 9-21.

4 Cawood J.I., Howell R.A.
A classification of the edentulous jaws.
Int. J. Oral Maxillofac. Surg. 1988; 17; 232-6.

5 Chiapasco M., Rossi A.
Chirurgia preimplantare nelle atrofie dei mascellari
in M. Chiapasco, E. Romeo: La riabilitazione implanto-protesica nei casi complessi. Ed. Utet 2003.

6 Chin M., Toth B.A.
Distraction osteogenesis in maxillofacial surgery using internal devices. Review of five cases.
J. Oral Maxillofacial. Surg. 1996; 54: 45-53.

7 Coleman S.R.
Autologous fat transplantation.
Plast. Reconstr. Surg. 1991; 88: 736.

8 Coleman S.R.
Facial recontouring with lipostructure.
Clin. Plast. Surg. 1997; 24.

9 Fournier P.F.
Facial recontouring with fat grafting.
Dermatol. Clin. 1990; 8: 523.

10 Hardesty R.A., Marsh J.L.
Embryologic aspects of bone graft.
In Habal MB, Reddi AH. Bone graft and bone substitute. Philadelphia: WB Saunders, 1992.

11 Hayter J.P., Cawood J.L.
Oral rehabilitation with endosteal implants and free flaps.
Int. Oral Maxillofac. Surg. 1996; 25: 3-12.

12 Hidalgo D.A.
Fibula free flaps: a new method of mandible reconstruction.
Plast. Reconstruction Surg. 1989; 84: 71-9.

13 Hirsch J.M., Ericsson I.
Maxillary sinus augmentation using mandibular bone grafts and simultaneous installations of implants: a surgical technique.
Clin. Oral Impl. Res. 1991; 2: 91-7.

14 Illouz Y.G.
The fat cell "graft" a new technique to fill depressions.
Plast. Reconstr. Surg. 1986; 78: 122.

15 Isaksson S., Ekfeldt A., Alberius P., Blomqvist J.E.
Early results from reconstruction of severely atrophic (Class VI) maxillas by immediate endosseous implants in conjunction with bone grafting and Le Fort I osteotomy.
Int. J. Oral Maxillofac. Surg. 1993; 22: 144-148.

16 Lexer E.
Freie Fettrannsplantation.
Dtsch. Med. Wochenschr. 1910; 36: 640.

17 Neuber F.
Fettransplantation. Berich uber die Verhandlungen der Dt Ges. f Chir. Zentralbl Chir. 1893; 22: 66.

18 Romeo E., Lavarini G., Castelnuovo G.
Aspetti protesici nell'edentulia totale e parziali in M. Chiapasco, E. Romeo La riabilitazione implantoprotesica nei casi complessi.
Ed. Utet, 2003.

19 Sailer H.F.
A new method of inserting endosseous implants in totally atrophic maxillae.
J. Cranio-Maxillo-Fac. Surg. 1989; 17: 299-305.

20 Tetsch P.
Enossale Implantationen in der Zahnheilkunde.
Munich: Hanser, 1991.

21 Triaca A., Carlino F.
Vestibolo plastica con fissazione ossea del lembo. Tecnica personale.
Dental Cadmos 1996; 18: 46-52.

22 Triplett R.G., Sterling R., Schow R.
Autologous bone grafts and endoosseous implants: complementary techniques.
J. Oral Maxillofac. Surg. 1996; 54: 486-94.

23 Van Steenberghe D.
Periodontal aspects of osseointegrated oral implants modum Brånemark.
Dent. Clin. North Am. 1988; 32: 355-65.

24 Wilkinson T.
Fat grafting. In Practical Procedures in Aesthetic Plastic Surgery. New York: Springer-Verlag, 1994.

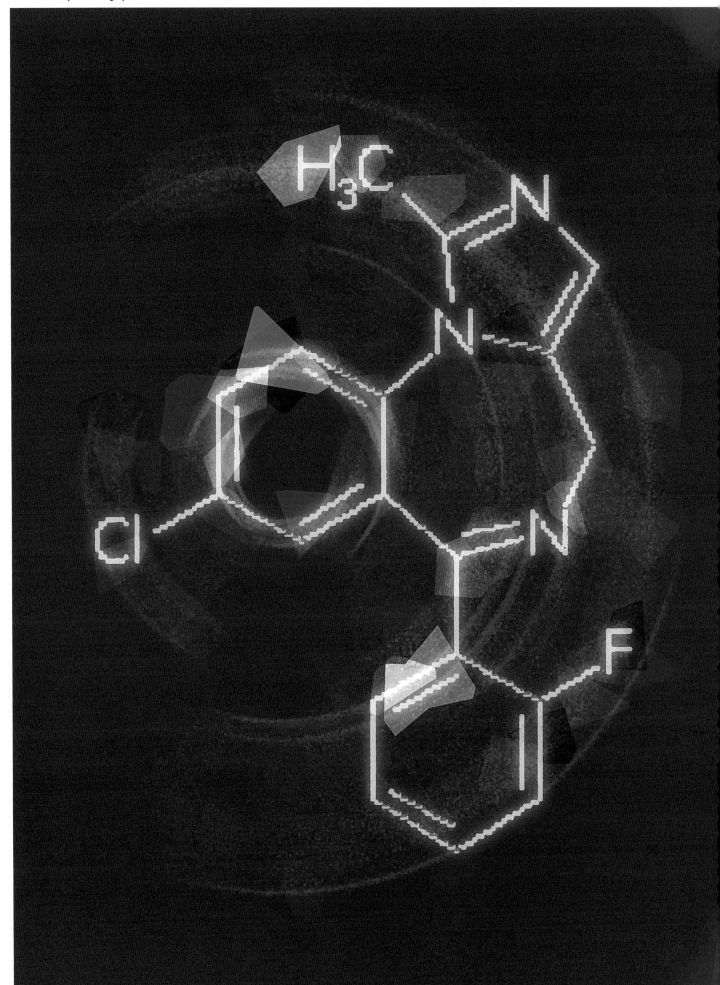

C. TOMMASINO

Anesthesia techniques for sinus augmentation surgery. Conscious sedation using midazolam

08

08

conversation in the operating theatre to a minimum);
- carrying out correct controls of pain stimuli obtained during local anesthesia.

During conscious sedation, the patient autonomously preserves his protective reflexes, cooperates with the surgeon and can be discharged after a short period of time, in this way achieving the concept of office anesthesia. Moreover, patients tend to like conscious sedation and, thus, the frequency of day surgery treatment has significantly increased (Kingon 1990).

Conscious sedation is a technique that produces an intermediate state between wakefulness and hypnosis, and is achieved by the administration of drugs that act on the central nervous system and which possess hypnotic-sedative activity. The essential components for defining conscious sedation (McCarthy et al. 1984) are:
- preservation of consciousness, while the patient can maintain verbal contact and cooperate with the oral surgeon;
- autonomous preservation of the airways' patency and protection reflexes, e.g. swallowing and coughing reflexes;
- neuromuscular relaxation together with a slight analgesic state.

The goals of conscious sedation (Scamann et al. 1985) are:
- to maintain adequate sedation with the minimum risk for the patient, whose vital parameters must be monitored clinically and instrumentally;
- to relieve anxiety and produce amnesia: these aims are achieved by choosing suitable drugs, instructing the patient prior to the operation and preserving low auditory and visual stimulation levels during surgery (including hiding equipment and reducing

CONSCIOUS SEDATION IN ORAL SURGERY

In oral surgery, the possibility that the patient remains sedated and fully conscious, with autonomous control of protective reflexes of his airways and with anterograde amnesia is a considerable advantage for both the oral surgeon and the patient. In 1982, Brophy et al. demonstrated how important amnesia of the surgical procedure was for some dental patients (Brophy et al. 1982).

PATIENTS SUITED TO CONSCIOUS SEDATION

Conscious sedation is a technique that can be used in all cooperative patients (capable of responding positively to simple orders), regardless of age. It is best not to use this technique in patients unable to respond cooperatively and in obese patients.

ANESTHESIOLOGIC EVALUATION AND PREOPERATIONAL EXAMS

The pre-operational anesthesiologic examination aims to assess the patient's state of health in order to choose the most suitable anesthesic technique. Assessing the medical history of the patient and the anesthesiologic exam are aimed at assessing the functional state of the main organs and systems (heart, lungs, kidneys, central nervous system, musculoskeletal system, etc.) and help to predict the risks from anesthesia **TAB. 1**. Preoperative investigations for asymptomatic patients (ASA 1 and 2) undergoing conscious sedation are listed in the table according to age. These guidelines may require variation depending on each individual case **TAB. 2**.

SCALE OF SEDATION

Conscious sedation must ensure that the patient, while sedated and under analgesic treatment, can maintain verbal communication and is able to cooperate with the surgeon. For this reason, it is important to refer to the evaluation scales that ensure the most control possible of the level of sedation.

Below are the most commonly used sedation scales used in oral surgery **TAB. 4-5**, based on the evaluation of parameters that are easy to assess (response to call, speech, expression of face and opening of eyelids).

According to the 'Observer's Assessment of Alertness/Sedation Scale' (OAASS), the optimal level for conscious sedation is indicated by scores 4 and 5 **TAB. 4** (Chernik et al. 1990), while according to the 'Sedation score for the anxious patient', the optimal level is indicated by a score of 3 **TAB. 5** (Oei-Lim et al. 1998).

Careful evaluation of the level of sedation, using scales like those shown, allow the sedative drugs used to be titrated to maintain a constant level of sedation during surgery. Therefore, drugs can be used more safely and efficiently.

BISPECTRAL INDEX

A monitoring system that can objectively assess the level of sedation is the bispectral index (BIS) (Drummond 2000; Sandler et al. 2001). This monitoring system, produced by Aspect Medical Systems (Newton, MA, USA) allows measurement of the level of hypnosis induced by hypnotic-sedative drugs. The system is based on the continuous registration of the electrical cerebral activity (by electroencephalogram, EEG), a signal that varies according to the effects of the hypnotic-sedative agents on the central nervous system (Tommasino & Casati 1999). While a sedative drug, such as midazolam, is being administered, the EEG trace shows a dose-dependent slowing down (the EEG waves increase in height and the frequency decreases). EEG registration is via a sensor (recording electrode) that is placed on the patient's forehead. The signal is sent to an analyser and a processor and is then shown in the form of a number on the BIS monitor. The BIS system analyses the EEG waves using a mathematical model; in technical terms, it carries out a dual spectral analysis (hence the name bispectral). The analysis, which is carried out without any interruption, shows variations in the two parameters in real time: wave height and frequency. This monitoring system, using an extremely complex algorithm, expresses the patient's state of consciousness with a number from 0 to 100; 0 indicates absence of cerebral activity and 100 wakefulness. The numerical value that indicates a good level of conscious sedation is between 70 and 80.

SELECTING THE INTRAVENOUS DRUG FOR CONSCIOUS SEDATION

There are several techniques that have been developed over the years in dental surgery to achieve conscious sedation. These include conscious sedation using nitrous oxide, the use of hypnotic drugs such as barbiturates (methohexital) and propofol, and the use of sedative/anxiolytic drugs such as benzodiazepines.

Conscious sedation produced by benzodiazepine is associated with anterograde amnesia. This effect is evident with midazolam, a benzodiazepine recently introduced onto the market, which represents one of the preferred drugs for obtaining conscious sedation in oral surgery (Jancso & Fodor 1994).

MIDAZOLAM

PHARMACOLOGIC PROFILE

Midazolam belongs to the family of imidozole benzodiazepines with a structure that is different to classical benzodiazepines due to the presence of an imidazole ring. This provides midazolam with the following advantages:

* solubility in aqueous solution with low pH value (< 4);
* stability in solution;
* rapid metabolism.

The chemical structure of midazolam allows the imidazole ring to accept a hydrogen ion at low pH values, producing a positive charge that makes the molecule hydrosoluble, and therefore stable in aqueous solution.

At physiologic pH levels (e.g. after parenteral administration), the molecule loses its charge, becomes lipophilic and rapidly crosses the blood–brain barrier, like other benzodiazepines.

The solubility in aqueous solution explains the absence of symptoms such as pain at the injection site or thrombophlebitic phenomena.

Midazolam, like other benzodiazepines, has anxiolytic, sedative and hypnotic properties, producing an increase in the effect of GABA, which is one of the most important inhibitory neurotransmitters of the central nervous system (Richards et al. 1991).

Benzodiazepines are metabolized by the liver, and the imidazole ring makes the breakdown of midazolam by the enzymatic-hepatic system (cytochrome P450 3A4) much faster. Metabolization has two phases: hydroxylation and glycoconjugation. The hydroxylation process gives rise to three different parmacologically inactive metabolytes (Kronbach et al. 1989). The main metabolyte is a-hydroxymidazolam, which has weak pharmacologic action and does not contribute to midazolam's clinical effects, as it is rapidly glycoconjugated before elimination by the kidneys. The absence of both the metabolyte pharmacologic activity and the enterohepatic recirculation of midazolam explain the lack of secondary pharmacologic effects (Nicholson & Stone 1983).

The plasma concentrations obtained 90 minutes after the intravenous or intramuscular injection of identical doses of midazolam were extremely similar (Crevoisier et al. 1981). Midazolam's distribution ($t_1/2\alpha$) half-life is 4 to 18 minutes, which explains its short duration of action; the elimination half-life ($t_1/2\beta$) varies from 1.7 to 2.4 hours (Dornauer & Roy 1983), and is must shorter than that of diazepam (31.8 hours).

Elimination speed is not connected to the route of administration and is faster in children (Salonen et al. 1987; Payne et al. 1989) and slower in elderly patients (Greenblatt et al. 1984; Servin et al. 1987) or in patients with poor liver function. Studies carried out in patients with cirrhosis and serious liver function deficiency showed a reduction in midazolam plasma clearance and, consequently, an extension of the elimination half-life (MacGilchrist et al. 1986; Trouvin et al. 1988; Pentikaeinen et al. 1989). In patients with chronic kidney failure, the percentage of free midazolam in the plasma, the volume of distribution and the clearance speed of the drug are higher (Vinik et al. 1983).

In these cases, the dose of midazolam must be reduced, as the higher the percentage of free drug, the more the patient is exposed to a higher amount of pharmacologically active product (Vinik et al. 1983).

Anesthesia techniques for sinus augmentation surgery. Conscious sedation using midazolam

137

Class	American Society of Anesthesiologists Definition
Class 1:	Healthy patient
Class 2:	Slight-moderate systemic illness (e.g. high blood pressure controlled pharmacologically, without organ involvement)
Class 3:	Serious systemic illness (e.g. diabetes mellitus with vascular complications, serious heart disease)
Class 4:	Serious systemic illness with life-endangerment (e.g. unstable angina, serious liver and/or kidney failure)
Class 5:	Dying patient, with low survival expectations (e.g. myocardial infarction with cardiogenic shock)

TAB. 1

ASA Classification of anesthesiologic risk
(American Society of Anesthesiologists)

Age	Exams
< 40 years	Hb & Hct, Glycaemia
40 to 60 years:	Hb & Hct, Glycaemia, ECG, Chest x-ray (if smoker)
> 60 years	Hb & Hct, Glycaemia, ECG, Azotemia & Creatinemia, Chest x-ray

Hb: hemoglobin; Hct: hematocrite; ECG: electrocardiogram.

TAB. 2

Basic pre-operative screening in asymptomatic patients

ECG and HR
BP
SpO$_2$
EtCO$_2$

ECG: electrocardiogram
HR: heart rate
BP: blood pressure
SpO$_2$: peripheral oxygen saturation
EtCO$_2$: carbon dioxide from end of expiration

TAB. 3

Instrumental monitoring during conscious sedation

Verbal response	Speech	Facial expression	Eyes	Score
Responds to call, with normal tone	Normal	Normal	Open	5
Slow to respond to call, with normal tone	Slowed down	Slight relaxation	Lowered eyelids	4
Only after several calls	Extremely slowed down	Marked relaxation	Eyelids almost closed	3
Only after physical stimulation	Incomprehensible	Marked relaxation	Eyelids closed	2
Absent	Absent	Marked relaxation	Eyelids closed	1

TAB. 4

Scale of sedation: Observer's Assessment of Alertness/Sedation Score (OAASS)

Consciousness	Collaboration level	Score
Awake and oriented	Anxious, not cooperating	1
Sleepy	Alteration of mood, not fully cooperating	2
Eyes closed, responds to command	Cooperating, allows treatment	3
Eyes closed, can only be woken after slight physical stimulation	Cooperation after several requests	4
Eyes closed, cannot be awoken by slight physical stimulation	No cooperation due to deep sedation	5

TAB. 5

Scale of sedation for anxious patient

EFFECTS ON CENTRAL NERVOUS SYSTEM

Midazolam induces dose-dependent sedation. The level of sedation varies from a sensation of torpor to the induction of deep hypnosis. Midazolam can produce an amnesic effect, that only covers the period of the molecule's pharmacologic activity (anterograde amnesia), without producing retrograde amnesia (Miller et al. 1989).

CARDIO-RESPIRATORY EFFECTS

The effect of midazolam on respiratory and cardiovascular functions are slight for commonly administered doses in surgery and can be compared with those of diazepam. If administered intravenously, midazolam induces a slight, brief reduction in blood pressure, with compensatory increase in heart rate (Conner et al. 1978; Fragen et al. 1978; Forster et al. 1980).

PROLONGING THE SEDATIVE EFFECT

Some drugs, including cimetidine, diltiazem, erythromycin, ketoconazole and verapramil increase midazolam's sedative effect. Patients treated with these drugs must receive a reduced dose of midazolam, to avoid extension of time of actual sedation.

ADMINISTRATION TECHNIQUES FOR MIDAZOLAM

In recent years, different methods have been used to administer midazolam, in order to obtain conscious sedation:
- intravenous bolus;
- intravenous infusion;
- intravenous administration controlled by the patient (patient-controlled sedation, PCS);
- computer-assisted controlled infusion (CACI).

INTRAVENOUS BOLUS

For bolus administration, the suggested dose of midazolam in a healthy adult patient is 0.07 to 0.1 mg/kg. However, the dose required to obtain optimal conscious sedation may vary, especially depending on the patient and on various factors such as age, state of health, and therapeutic drug treatment. The dose of midazolam required to obtain conscious sedation may also vary greatly, a variability that is common to all benzodiazepines, due to the high protein binding in this class of drugs (Dundee & Wilson 1980). In 134 healthy but anxious dental patients (16 to 63 years) treated in day surgery, the dose needed was less than 0.07 mg/kg in 19 cases and higher than 0.1 mg/kg in 59 cases (range used 0.04 to 0.4 mg/kg) and in males, the average dose/kg was much lower than in females (Richards et al. 1993).

Slow administration of midazolam at a dose of 0.14 mg/kg (range 0.05 to 0.27), in patients undergoing conservative dental treatment, induces conscious sedation more rapidly than diazepam, produces anterograde amnesia solely for the dental procedure and allows faster recovery of psychocognitive activities (Barker et al. 1986). In a study by Luyk et al., the administration of an average dose of 5.6 mg of midazolam (range 5.2 to 6 mg) in healthy adults undergoing extraction of the third molar, at a dose of 1 mg/min until conscious sedation was obtained brought about total amnesia of the administration of local anesthesic. No patients lost consciousness and the peripheral oxygen saturation was always higher than 94% (Luyk et al. 1992).

As the sedative and amnesic effect of a single dose of midazolam lasts for about 20 mnutes (Dundee & Wilson 1980), additional doses of the drug must be administered in operations lasting longer, when the patient shows signs that the sedative effect is decreasing. The bolus dose induces an intermittent

Anesthesia techniques for sinus augmentation surgery. Conscious sedation using midazolam

139

effect, with the possibility of alternating hyper-sedation with hyposedation and of inducing sudden variations in the level of sedation.

INTRAVENOUS INFUSION

Continuous intravenous infusion maintains stable plasma concentrations of midazolam and is preferable to repeated administrations, especially when conscious sedation is required for long periods of time.

To rapidly reach the plasma level required, and, therefore the pharmacologic effect required, it is possible to administer an initial bolus, while conscious sedation is maintained by continous midazolam infusion. As shown in studies on healthy volunteers, using this technique means stable plasma concentrations of the drug are reached in a few minutes, and the entire spectrum of desired effects can be achieved, from bland sedation to hypnosis (Allonen et al. 1981).

In a retrospective study on 298 patients undergoing oral surgery (implantology, extractions of third molar, etc.), lasting around 50 minutes, conscious sedation was obtained by an average dose of 10.45 mg (range 1.25 to 40 mg) of midazolam, and the average dose/kg was 0.15 mg (range 0.03 to 0.50 mg). Complete recovery took place in around 94 minutes without complications. Patients cooperated during the operation and were satisfied by the anesthesic technique used (Runes & Strom 1996).

In 102 adult patients undergoing implants, 96% of patients were satisfied with conscious sedation using midazolam and 94% stated that they would choose the same technique for a similar dental treatment. In this study, conscious sedation was carried out using a dose of midazolam between 4.0 and 5.1 (± 2.1 DS) mg/hour. However, it must be considered that in this study, the patients also received an opiate analgesic (fentanyl, 29 to 60 mcg/hour) (Lind et al. 1990).

The continuous intravenous administration was also used successfully in geriatric patients (65 to 92 years of age) and without complications (Campbell & Smith 1997). It is important to remember that, in this age group, infusion speed must be reduced by 25 to 50% compared with the speed used for young patients, as clearance is reduced and elimination half-life is increased (Greenblatt et al. 1984).

When conscious sedation using repeated boluses of midazolam is compared with continuous infusion, anxiolysis is similar in both cases. The amnesic effect tends to disappear more rapidly in the patient who has received repeated boluses compared with the patient who has received continuous drug infusion, and recovery to consciousness is slower after continuous infusion (Luyk et al. 1992).

PATIENT-CONTROLLED SEDATION (PCS)

An alternative technique is patient-controlled sedation (PCS) which can theoretically provide more appropriate levels of sedation.

Several studies in dental patients have examined this mode of administering midazolam, using programmed pumps with suitable 'lock-out' periods. When the two administration techniques for midazolam are compared (continuous infusion vs. PCS), no important differences can be found regarding the hemodynamic parameters (heart frequency and blood pressure) and the patients' oxygen supply. Moreover, both methods determine a good degree of anterograde amnesia and conscious sedation, and the operator cannot distinguish between the two techniques (Zacharias et al. 1994). The dose of midazolam used in PCS, 5.3 ± 2.4 mg (SD), is not statistically different to the one used during continuous infusion controlled by the anesthesiologist (5.0 ± 1.1 mg (SD)) (Rodrigo & Tong 1994). When the patient can choose the midazolam administration interval in PCS, administration at short intervals is preferred (1 vs. 3 minutes) (Rodrigo & Chow 1995).

Patient-controlled sedation, however, seems to be less safe than anesthesiologist-controlled administration. In fact, the Rodrigo and Chow study carried out in 1996 on patients (16 to 30 years of age) undergoing surgery on the third molar, highlighted the fact that patient-controlled administration of midazolam caused the onset of deep sedation in 20% of the patients, with the consequent risk of losing autonomous control of the protective reflexes for the air passages, and making conscious sedation a less safe technique (Rodrigo & Chow 1996).

COMPUTER-ASSISTED CONTROLLED INFUSION

Computer-assisted controlled infusion (CACI) describes the intravenous administration of a drug using a computerized pump with pharmacokinetic software that allows varying levels of drug administration, to maintain a constant plasma concentration, according to a preset goal (Engbergs & Vuyk 1996). This method places attention on the 'blood concentration' and no longer on the amount of drug to be administered according to body weight.

According to the pharmacokinetic model used by the system, the computerized pump can determine the loaded dose needed to reach the required blood concentration and the optimal infusion rate required to maintain the plasma concentration as desired by the operator, who must simply set the target concentrations, both for the induction, then maintenance, after entering the patient's age and weight (Veselis et al. 1997).

This system has the advantage of a more rapid achievement of correct drug concentrations using drugs with a short half-life, allowing rapid modulation of the sedative level (Milne & Kenny 1998). Several drugs can be administered using CACI, and midazolam has

also been administered using this technique. The plasma level of midazolam required to maintain a good level of conscious sedation is 64.5 ± 9.4 ng/ml (Veselis et al. 1997).

In clinical practice, the author's favourite technique is continuous infusion, preceded by the intravenous administration of 1 to 2 mg of midazolam. Continuous infusion allows a constant level of sedation to be maintained over a period of time, without the appearance of lighter sedation (in this case the patient becomes intolerant) or heavier sedation, with the changeover to deep sedation, which frequently induces loss of control of protective reflexes (coughing and swallowing) and a reduction in spontaneous breathing, with the onset of bradypnoea, hypoxia and hypercapnia.

MONITORING

During conscious sedation, the patient is awake, cooperating and preserves his protective reflexes of the airways autonomously. However, if drug administration is not carefully controlled, the patient can go from one sedative level to another (e.g. from conscious sedation to deep sedation, with the consequent loss of protective reflexes). It is therefore necessary to use suitable clinical and instrumental patient monitoring (SIAARTI 1997), and to plan the presence of health workers or doctors who are experts in resuscitation.

Instrumental monitoring ensures an objective control of the patient and, during conscious sedation, should include the continuous recording of an electrocardiogram (ECG) and heart rate (HR), oxygen saturation via pulsoximetry (SpO_2), and carbon dioxide elimination ($EtCO_2$), and the periodical measuring of blood pressure (BP) [TAB. 3]. The incannulation of a vein, which must remain in place until the patient has fully recovered consciousness, is compulsory.

It must be emphasized that peripheral oxygen saturation (SpO_2) is considered to be an essential instrument in dental surgery, even when used for procedures other than conscious sedation. During extraction of the third molar, in fact, the appearance of artery desaturation was noted in both patients under conscious sedation and those under local anesthesia (Rodrigo & Rosenquist 1988; Lowe & Brook 1991). While these desaturations are not clinically important in a healthy patient, they could affect a patient with cardiopulmonary disease.

SpO_2 non-invasively and continuously monitors arterial blood oxygenation, monitors heart rate and provides useful information on both respiratory and cardiovascular functions. Its use is supported by the evidence that clinical monitoring is insufficient in identifying early hypoxia (Torri & Tommasino 1998).

Only careful monitoring of the patient (heart rate, blood pressure, ventilation, oxygenation) will allow early recognition in the vital alterations caused by drugs or physiopathological alterations connected to surgery to be recognised. Clinical and instrumental monitoring must be continued until total recovery of consciousness, while maintaining the desired level of sedation (patient cooperating and sedated) is ensured by the continuous assessment of the patient using sedation scales.

CONCLUSIONS

Due to its particular chemical and pharmacokinetic characteristics, midazolam is especially useful for conscious sedation associated with locoregional anesthesia. The choice of this new benzodiazepine with rapid onset of sedation, short duration of action and hemodynamic stability in oral surgery is mainly due to the following advantages:
- improved titration of dose to be administered and possibility of continuous infusion due to the molecule's hydrosolubility;
- rapid onset of pharmacologic action, after intravenous administration;
- onset of dose-dependent sedative effect, which is easily modulated;
- short elimination half-life and absence of accumulation and/or redistribution phenomena;
- anterograde amnesia;
- rapid discharge of patient.

REFERENCES

1   Allonen H., Ziegler G., Klotz U.
    Midazolam kinetics.
    Clin. Pharmacol. Ther. 1981; 30: 653-61.

2   Barker J., Butchart D.G.M., Gibson J. et al.
    I.v. sedation for conservative dentistry.
    Br. J. Anaesth. 1986; 58: 371-7.

3   Brophy T., Dundee J.W., Heazelwood V. et al.
    Midazolam, a water-soluble benzodiazepine for gastroscopy.
    Anaesth. Intensive Care 1982; 10: 344-7.

4   Campbell R.I., Smith P.B.
    Intravenous sedation in 200 geriatric patients undergoing office oral surgery.
    Anesth. Prog. 1997; 44: 64-7.

5   Chernik D.A., Gillings D., Laine H. et al.
    Validity and reliability of the Observer's Assessment of Alertness/Sedation Scale: study with intravenous midazolam.
    J. Clin. Psychopharmacol. 1990; 10: 244-51.

6   Conner J.T., Katz R.L., Pagano C.W.
    Ro 21-3981 for intravenous surgical premedication and induction of anesthesia.
    Anest. Analg. 1978; 57: 1-5.

7   Crevoisier C., Eckert M., Heizmann P. et al.
    Relation entre l'effet clinique et la pharmacocinetique du midazolam apres l'administration i.v. et i.m. 2eme communication: aspects pharmacocinetiques.
    Arzneim. Forsch. 1981; 16: 2211-15.

8   Dornauer R.J., Roy A.
    Update: midazolam maleate, a new water-soluble benzodiazepine.
    J. Am. Dent. Assoc. 1983; 106: 650-2.

9   Drummond J.C.
    Monitoring depth of anesthesia. Anesthesiology 2000; 93: 876-82.

10 Dundee J.W., Wilson P.B.
    Amnesic action of midazolam.
    Anaesthesia 1980; 35: 459-61.

11 Engbergs F., Vuyk J.
    Target-controlled infusion.
    In: Anaesthesia Rounds, The Medicine Group (Education) Ltd, Abingdon, 1996.

12 Forster A., Gardaz J-P., Suter P., Gemperle M.
    I.v. midazolam as an induction agent for anesthesia. A study in volunteers.
    Br. J. Anaesth. 1980; 52: 907-11.

13 Fragen R.J., Gahl F., Caldwell N.
    A water soluble benzodiazepine, Ro 21-3981, for induction of anesthesia.
    Anesthesiology 1978; 49: 41-3.

14 Greenblat D., Abernethy D., Locniskar A et al.
    Effects of age, gender and obesity on midazolam kinetics.
    Anesthesiology 1984; 61: 27-35.

15 Jancso J., Fodor A.
    Use of Dormicum (midazolam) injection in oral surgery under local anesthesia.
    Fogorv Sz 1994; 87: 329-34.

16 Kingon A.M.
    Intravenous sedation and patient response to minor oral surgery-experience in 408 cases. Dent. Update 1990; 17: 340-3.

17 Kronbach T., Mathys D., Umeno M., Gonzales F.J., Meyer U.A.
    Oxydation of midazolam and triazolam by human liver Cytochrome P450 IIIA4.
    Mol. Pharmacol. 1989; 36: 89-96.

18 Lind L.J., Mushlin P.S., Schnitman P.A.
    Monitored anesthesia care for dental implant surgery: analysis of effectiveness and complications.
    J. Oral Implantol. 1990; 16: 106-13.

19 Lowe T., Brook I.M.
    Oxygen saturation during third molar removal with local anaesthetic alone and in combination with intravenous sedation.
    Br. Dent. J. 1991; 171: 210-11.

20 Luyk NH., Zacharias M., Wanwimolaruk S.
    Bolus dose with continuous infusion of midazolam as sedation for outpatient surgery.
    J. Oral Maxillofac. Surg. 1992; 21: 172-5.

21 MacGilchrist A., Birnie G., Cook A.
    Pharmacokinetics and pharmacodynamics of intravenous midazolam in patients with severe alcoholic cirrhosis.
    Gut 1986; 27: 190-5.

22 McCarthy F.M., Solomon A.L., Jastak J.T et al.
    Conscious sedation: Benefits and risks.
    J. Am. Dental Assoc. 1984; 109: 546-51.

23 Miller R.I., Bullard D.E., Patrissi G.A.
    Duration of amnesia associated with midazolam/fentanyl intravenous sedation.
    J. Oral Maxillofac. Surg. 1989; 47: 155-8.

24 Milne S.E., Kenny G.N.C.
    Future application for TCI systems.
    Anaesthesia 1998; 53: 56-60.

25 Nicholson A.N., Stone B.M.
    Activity of triazolo-benzodiazepine in man.
    Br. J. Clin. Pharm. 1983; 9: 305-306.

26 Oei-Lim V.L.B., Kalkman C.J., Makkes P.C., Ooms W.G.
    Patient-controlled versus anesthesiologist-controlled conscious sedation with propofol for dental treatment in anxious patients.
    Anesth. Analg. 1998; 86: 967-72.

27 Payne K., Mattheyse F.J., Liebenberg D., Dawes T.
    The pharmacokinetics of midazolam in paediatric patients.
    Eur. J. Clin. Pharmacol. 1989; 37: 267-72.

28 Pentikaeinen P.J., Vaelisalmi L., Himberg J.J., Crevoisier C.
    Pharmacokinetics of midazolam following intravenous and oral administration in patients with chronic liver disease and in healthy subjects.
    J. Clin. Pharmacol. 1989; 29: 272-7.

29 Richards A., Griffiths M., Scully C.
    Wide variation in patient response to midazolam sedation for outpatient oral surgery.
    Oral Surg. Oral Med. Oral Pathol. 1993; 76: 408-11.

30 Richards G., Schoch P., Haefely W.
    Benzodiazepine receptors: new vistas.
    The Neurosciences 1991; 3: 191-203.

31 Rodrigo C., Chow K.C.
    A comparison of 1- and 3- minute lockout periods during patient-controlled sedation with midazolam.
    J. Oral Maxillofac. Surg. 1995; 53: 406-10.

32 Rodrigo C., Chow K.C.
    Patient-controlled sedation: a comparison of sedation prior to and until the end of minor oral surgery.
    Aust. Dent. J. 1996; 41: 159-63.

33 **Rodrigo M.R., Rosenquist J.B.**
Effect of conscious sedation with midazolam on oxygen saturation.
J. Oral Maxillofac. Surg. 1988; 46: 746-50.

34 **Rodrigo M.R., Tong C.K.**
A comparison of patient and anaesthetist controlled midazolam sedation for dental surgery.
Anaesthesia 1994; 49: 241-4.

35 **Runes J., Strom C.**
Midazolam intravenous conscious sedation in oral surgery. A retrospective study of 372 cases.
Swed. Dent. J. 1996; 20: 29-33.

36 **Salonen M., Kanto J., Lisalo E., Himberg J-J.**
Midazolam as an induction agent in children: a pharmacokinetic and clinical study.
Anesth. Analg. 1987; 66: 625-8.

37 **Sandler N.A., Hodges J., Sabino M.**
Assessment of recovery in patients undergoing intravenous conscious sedation using bispectral index.
J. Oral Maxillofac. Surg. 2001; 59: 603-11.

38 **Scamann F.L., Klein S.L., Choi W.W.**
Conscious sedation for procedures under local or topical anesthesia.
Ann. Oto. Rhinol. Laryngol. 1985; 94: 21-4.

39 **Servin F., Enriquez I., Fournett M. et al.**
Pharmacokinetics of midazolam used as an intravenous induction agent for patients over 80 years of age.
Eur. J. Anaesthesiol. 1987; 4: 1-7.

40 **SIAARTI.**
Raccomandazioni per il monitoraggio di minima del paziente durante anestesia.
Minerva Anestesiol. 1997; 63: 267-70.

41 **Tommasino C., Casati A.**
Monitoring the brain.
Ballier's Clinical Anesthesiology, 1999; 13: 511-30.

42 **Torri G., Tommasino C.**
Distribuzione degli incidenti critici in anestesia.
Minerva Anestesiol 1998; 64 (suppl 1): 147-55.

43 **Trouvin J.H., Farinotti R., Haberer J.P et al.**
Pharmacokinetics of midazolam in anaesthetized cirrhotic patients.
Br. J. Anaesth. 1988; 60: 762-7.

44 **Veselis R.A., Reinsel R.A., Feshchenko V.A., Wronski M.**
The comparative amnesic effects of midazolam, propofol, thiopental and fentanyl at equisedative concentrations.
Anesthesiology 1997; 87: 749-64.

45 **Vinik H., Reves J., Greenblatt D. et al.**
The pharmacokinetics of midazolam in chronic renal failure patients.
Anesthesiology 1983; 59: 390-4.

46 **Zacharias M., Hunter K.M., Luyk N.H.**
Patient-controlled sedation using midazolam.
Br. J. Oral Maxillofac. Surg. 1994; 32: 168-73.

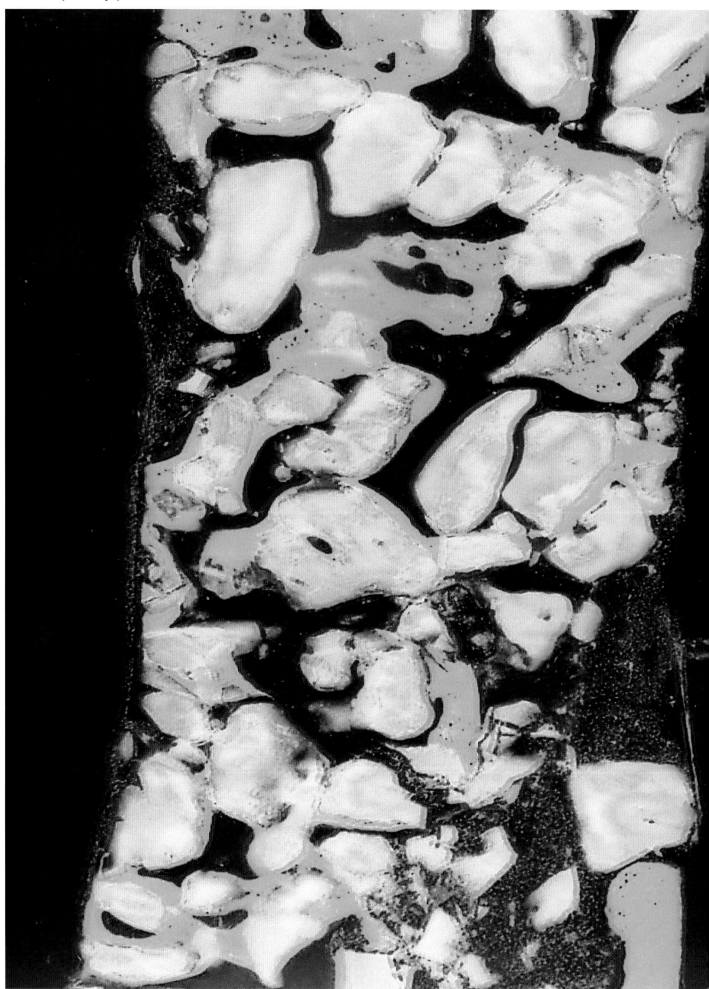

S.S. WALLACE

Clinical indications for different types of graft material

09

09

Insufficient residual alveolar bone height is a common deterrent in the placement of dental implants in the posterior maxilla. Minimal residual crestal bone height may result from alveolar bone resorption following tooth loss, bone loss due to periodontal disease, pneumatization of the maxillary sinus or a combination of the above. Grafting of the floor of the maxillary sinus was first presented in 1977 (Tatum 1977) and first published in 1980 (Boyne & James 1980). We now have 30 years of clinical experience with sinus grafting, as well as over 1400 published articles to use as a database for developing techniques that will improve the outcome while limiting the morbidity of this surgical procedure.

The sinus grafting technique has been modified by many clinicians and techniques today include at least three distinct lateral window entry procedures as well as numerous crestal entry procedures. In addition to changes in surgical techniques, we have also experienced the introduction of various new grafting materials, the utilization of barrier membranes over the lateral window, and the utilization of implants with varying macro- and micro-morphologies, all of which appear to improve the outcome of the sinus elevation procedure. We are currently experiencing the evolution of new technologies such as the use of platelet-rich plasma (PRP), plasma rich in growth factors

(PRGF), recombinant platelet-derived growth factor (PDGF; GEM 21S), bone morphogenetic proteins (BMP; INFUSE BONE GRAFT), and stem cell harvesting technologies to produce tissue-engineered bone, all of which promise to enhance bone formation. One hopes that this evolution will result in ever-higher implant survival rates and/or shorter maturation times for grafts placed in the maxillary sinus.

This chapter will discuss the properties of various grafting materials and membranes and then use an evidence-based approach to present the techniques that have resulted in the highest level of success as has been reported by the outcome parameter of implant survival. The chapter will conclude with a clinical introduction to the most recently introduced regenerative technologies.

EVALUATING SUCCESS

The goals of the sinus elevation are threefold: the predictable formation of vital bone in the pneumatized sinus, the integration of implants into that newly formed bone, and the long-term survival of those implants when placed under functional load. It becomes obvious that the latter two goals are dependent upon successful accomplishment of the first goal, the formation of vital bone. It also becomes obvious that the qualities of the materials utilized to graft the sinus are of importance in achieving a successful result.

Success is best evaluated in terms of successful patient outcomes. Although patient outcomes are occasionally reported, outcomes are often reported in histologic studies as per cent vital bone formation per given time, and in clinical trials, outcome is reported as implant success/survival.

Data pertaining to vital bone production and implant survival in grafted sinuses has been presented in many clinical studies. These studies generally are found to be of limited size and have been performed with different degrees of investigative rigor (levels of evidence). The type of study that would yield the clearest data would be a randomized controlled trial with only one variable. For sinus graft studies the best model would be a randomized controlled bilateral trial comparing two grafts of equal size with all covariables, such as implant type, membrane over window, and time remaining the same. Unfortunately, in over 27 years of sinus graft research, there are only a few studies that meet these parameters. We are, therefore, in a position where we must accept data of a lower level of evidence and statistically adjust for the affects of the existing covariables. Still, even faced with these deficiencies, the evidence regarding bone grafting materials now appears to be quite clear.

A structured, unbiased evaluation of sinus grafting materials may be found in the results published in evidence-based reviews. The reviews select studies according to rigid inclusion criteria and combine the data of the individually selected studies to obtain a larger database and thereby achieve more statistical power. One review (Graziani, 2004) had a very small database, consisting of only randomized controlled trials that unfortunately did not research the variable of graft material. Earlier reviews (Tolman 1995; Tong et al. 1998) had relatively small databases. The Sinus Lift Consensus Conference of 1996 (Jensen et al. 1996) reported on the results obtained by experienced clinicians and, while accurate, is somewhat dated due to the dramatic increase in published reports on various grafting proce-

PARTIAL LIST OF SINUS GRAFTING MATERIALS

TAB. 1

AUTOGRAFTS	INTRAORAL	TUBEROSITY
		CHIN
		RAMUS
	EXTRAORAL	ILIUM
		TIBIA
		CRANIUM
XENOGRAFTS	BOVINE	BIOOSS
		OSTEO/GRAF
	ALGAE	ALGIPORE
ALLOGRAFTS	MINERALIZED	MFDBA
		MCBA
		IRRADIATED CBA
	DEMINERALIZED	DFDBA
ALLOPLASTS	HYDROXYAPATITE	POROUS
		NON-POROUS
	BIOACTIVE GLASS	BIOGRAN
	CALCIUM SULFATE	
	ß-TRI-CALCIUM PHOSPHATES	
	BONE CERAMIC	

dures since 1996. More recently, three exhaustive evidence-based literature reviews were conducted (Wallace & Froum 2003; Del Fabbro et al. 2004; Aghaloo & Moy 2007). This chapter will rely heavily on the results from these evidence-based reviews.

SINUS GRAFT MATERIALS

Autogenous bone was the first grafting material utilized to augment the maxillary sinus. The list of bone replacement grafts (BRG's) utilized to augment or replace autogenous bone as a sinus grafting material is continuously expanding. They fall into the general categories of allografts, xenografts and alloplasts **TAB. 1**. While results with all of these BRGs have been published in the literature, xenografts have by far been the most widely studied.

AUTOGENOUS BONE

The original protocol as described by Boyne (Boyne et al. 1980), and subsequently used by many other clinicians for this procedure (Keller et al. 1994, 1999; Blomqvist et al. 1996; Johansson et al. 1999; Khoury 1999; Wannfors et al. 2000; Kahnberg et al. 2001), utilized 100% autogenous bone harvested from the ilium as a grafting material. This was a logical choice as an autogenous bone graft would contain all the elements necessary to promote vital bone formation, namely minerals, collagen matrix, viable cells, growth factors and BMP. Autogenous grafts, therefore, can be both osteoinductive and osteoconductive. Further, iliac grafts had a history of successful utilization for ridge augmentation procedures and were preferred for their highly cellular composition.

Iliac autografts were utilized both in block form with simultaneous implant placement and in particulate form with simultaneous or

delayed placement, depending upon the ability to achieve primary implant stability in the residual crestal bone.

Other sources for autogenous bone include, extraorally, the tibia and cranium, and intraorally, the ramus, symphysis, and maxillary tuberosity. Of these, the tibial grafts have a high cancellous content, whereas the ramus and symphysis contain mostly cortical bone.

Vital bone formation in sinuses grafted with 100% autogenous bone occurs more rapidly (Tajdoedin et al. 2000, 2002; Valentini et al. 2000) and to a greater extent (Froum et al. 1998) than it does when BRGs are utilized. While the percentage of vital bone that one finds in sinuses grafted with autogenous bone is greater than that seen with BRGs at an early time period, these studies show that bone formation with BRGs is equal to that of bone formation with autogenous bone over time.

The utilization of autogenous bone as a graft material has certain disadvantages. Using a 100% autogenous bone graft requires a second surgical site (intraoral) or possible hospitalization (extraoral), thereby increasing the length of time of the surgical intervention, the surgical risk, and the postsurgical morbidity. Furthermore, clinicians have reported a greater than average degree of graft resorption when using iliac grafts (Moy et al. 1993; Jensen et al. 1998; Garg 2001).

The Sinus Consensus Conference of 1996 (Jensen et al. 1998) reported a difference between implant survival rates in block grafts and in particulate autogenous grafts (84.6% and 92.6% respectively) at 3 years. In one review (Wallace & Froum 2003), the survival rate for implants placed in sinuses grafted with the block grafting technique was found to be 83.3%. This must be compared with the 92.3% survival rate for implants placed in all types of particulate grafts (both autogenous grafts and BRGs) and the overall lateral window implant survival rate of 91.8%. Another review (Del Fabbro et al. 2004) reports an 87.7% survival rate for implants placed in 100% autogenous grafts of all categories.

Explanations for the lower survival rate for implants placed in block grafts may include a demanding surgical procedure that requires stabilization of the block as well as the implants, the tendency of block grafts to resorb, an overall lower percentage of mineralized tissue in the matured graft (see discussion of xenografts) and the covariable effect of the utilization of machine-surfaced implants in many of the block graft studies. The Del Fabbro (Del Fabbro et al 2004) review determined that 69.5% of implants (i.e. more than 50%) placed in block grafts had a machined surface. The greatest cause for failure reported in the Consensus Conference (Jensen et al. 1998) database was idiopathic graft resorption, and this resorption was greatest for grafts of iliac bone and for demineralized bone allografts.

Two consensus statements from the graft material workshop committee at the 1996 Sinus Consensus Conference maintained that autogenous bone was appropriate for sinus grafting and that allografts, alloplasts, and xenografts alone, or in combination, may be effective in selected clinical situations (Jensen et al. 1998). The rationale for this statement was not the poor performance of BRGs, except for demineralized freeze-dried bone allograft (DFDBA), but the limited data that was available at the time. Over the past 11 years, that evidence has been forthcoming.

ALLOGRAFTS

DFDBA has had a long and successful history of use as a grafting material in periodontal defects. The utilization of DFDBA as a sinus grafting material, however, has not demonstrated this level of success. Results from the Sinus Consensus Conference show poor results, as evidenced by lower implant survival rates when used alone (85%) or in combination with

autografts and xenografts (82% and 80%, respectively) (Jensen et al. 1998). A histological report (Jensen & Sennerby 1998) and a clinical report (Langer & Langer 1999) demonstrate both poor-quality bone formation and a relatively low implant survival rate (80%). If the expected result of grafting the sinus is to create a mineralized, stable implant receptor site, a non-mineralized graft material that is susceptible to re-pneumatization (slumping) has been shown to be a less than ideal choice. Turnover of this graft material to vital bone proceeds slowly, as a non-vital remineralization precedes vital bone formation **FIG. 1**.

Studies with mineralized allografts are more limited in nature. One would expect that results with an allograft that retained its mineral content and human bone microstructure would be far superior to that of a demineralized allograft. A randomized controlled trial (Froum et al. 2006) compared the mineralized cancellous bone allograft (MCBA), Puros™, to a known xenograft standard, Bio-Oss®, in 13 bilateral cases. Results showed a higher average percentage of vital bone with the allograft (28.25% vs. 12.44%) accompanied by a lower percentage of residual graft material (7.65% vs. 33%). Figures 2 and 3 **FIG. 2–3** show representative histology taken from the 6-month MCBA core biopsies.

XENOGRAFTS

Of all the investigated bone replacement grafts, the results for xenografts are the most complete and best documented. In the Wallace review (Wallace & Froum 2003), which included 34 lateral window studies, 11 made use of xenografts. The xenografts in this review consisted of deproteinated (anorganic) bovine bone. They were utilized alone, as part of a composite graft with autogenous bone, hydrated with venous blood, or mixed with PRP. The total number of implants placed in this review and followed for a minimum of 1 year post loading was 5267. The survival rate for implants utilizing xenografts was statistically the same as for implants placed in particulate autogenous bone grafts.

The Del Fabbro (Del Fabbro et al. 2004) review was more specific in its study of bone replacement grafts. The most recent review (Aghaloo & Moy 2007) reported implant survival rates in 100% autograft, composite grafts with autogenous bone, 100% alloplast, 100% allograft, and 100% xenograft to be 88%, 92%, 81%, 93.3% and 95.6% respectively.

Comparative studies (Valentini et al. 2000; Hising et al. 2001; Hallman et al. 2002) show higher implant survival rates for 100% xenografts than for 100% autogenous bone or composite grafts of xenograft and autogenous bone.

Additional studies not included in the reviews present histologic and histomorphometric data demonstrating the extent of vital bone production with xenografts, alone or in combination, at varying time intervals. The data is quite positive when compared with results achieved with the 'gold standard' of autogenous bone.

In light of the evidence, the efficacy of xenografts as a BRG for sinus augmentation surgery can not be ignored. As this bone substitute now enjoys widespread use, an understanding of its efficacy and safety is essential.

Native bone in the posterior maxilla is generally of a poor quality/density. As clinicians, we would recognize it as type 3 or 4 bone. An anatomical study (Ulm et al. 1999) reported bone density in the posterior maxilla to be 23 to 26% (as low as 6.73%). Other histomorphometric studies (Moy et al. 1993; Hanisch et al. 1999) report posterior maxillary bone density averages of 45% and 32.6% respectively.

When autografts or demineralized allografts are utilized there is a tendency for both a volumetric resorption in the order of 25% and a transformation of the graft density towards that which would normally be found in the posterior maxilla. The result would then be an implant receptor site with a typical type 3 or 4 bone density.

The efficacy of xenografts as a sinus bone replacement graft may be due to a combination of factors. Foremost would be the osteoconductive capacity of xenografts. In addition, they supply minerals that are necessary for bone formation, their density provides stability to the graft and the implants placed in them, and this density persists long term due to the fact that these grafts do not completely resorb. In fact, histomorphometric and histologic studies show continued remodeling around retained Bio-Oss® particles at 6 and 12 months (Froum et al. 1998; Valentini et al. 2000), 20 months and 7 years (Orsini et al. 2007) and 9 years (Traini et al. 2007).

The osteoconductive properties of xenografts in human sinus grafting have been well documented (Froum et al. 1998; Valentini et al. 2000; Orsini et al. 2007; Traini et al. 2007) and are well demonstrated histologically in Figure 4. They are due to both their chemical composition and their macro- and micromorphology. Histologic sections FIG. 4-6 of sinus graft cores from the Froum (Froum et al. 1998) and Wallace (Wallace et al. 2005) studies reveal bone apposition directly on the surface of xenograft particles. Vital bone 'bridging' of the gaps between xenograft particles is also seen.

Transmission electron microscopy from the Orsini (Orsini et al. 2007) and Traini (Traini et al. 2007) (University of Chieti-Pescara, Department Prof. A. Piattelli) studies demonstrated that the electron-dense layer present at the bone–Bio-Oss® interface at an early time interval of 20 months FIG. 7 was replaced with a direct contact, appearing as an in-growth of bone into the Bio-Oss® structure at 7 years FIG. 8. Similar transmission electron microscopy FIG. 9 and histology FIG. 10 at 9 years show this contin-

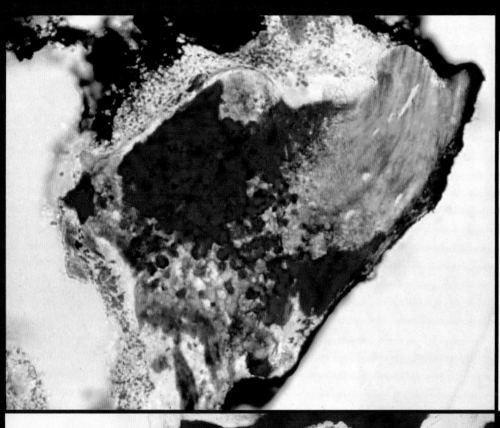

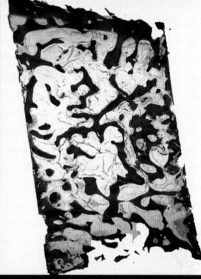

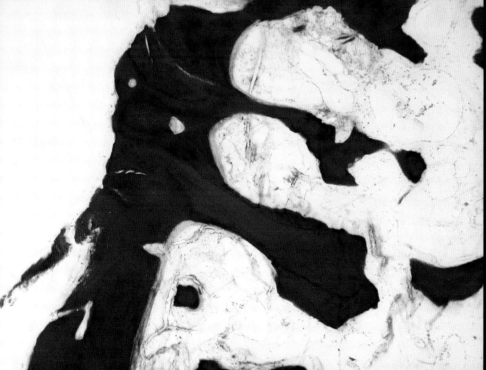

1 → NON-VITAL REMINERALIZATION OF DFDBA. FOCI OF NON-VITAL REMINERALIZATION (RED) WITHIN THE DFDBA COLLAGEN MATRIX (GREEN). STEVENEL'S BLUE AND PICRIC ACID FUCHSIN. ORIGINAL MAGNIFICATION X 40

2 →VITAL BONE FORMATION (RED) IN A MCBA AT 9 MONTHS (25.2%). STEVENEL'S BLUE AND PICRIC ACID FUCHSIN. ORIGINAL MAGNIFICATION X 4.

3 → HIGH POWER VIEW OF BONE FORMATION AROUND MCBA PARTICLES AT 9 MONTHS. STEVENEL'S BLUE AND PICRIC ACID FUCHSIN. ORIGINAL MAGNIFICATION X 20.

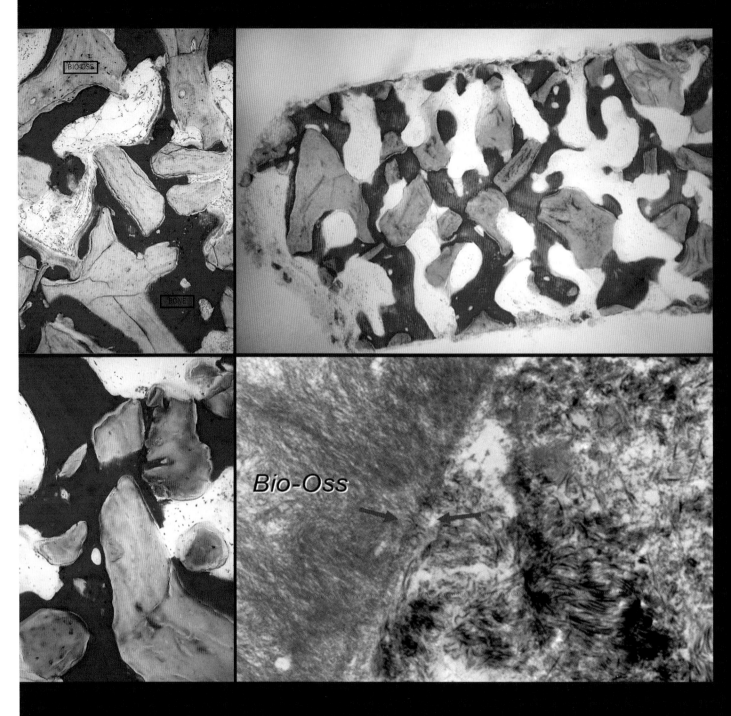

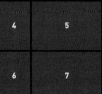

4 → BONE DEPOSITION DIRECTLY ON BIO-OSS PARTICLES. STEVENEL'S BLUE AND PICRIC ACID FUCHSIN. (BIO-OSS – YELLOW, OSTEOID – GREEN, NEW BONE – RED) ORIGINAL MAGNIFICATION X 20.

5 → LOW POWER VIEW DEMONSTRATING 'BRIDGING' OR BONE GROWTH CONNECTING XENOGRAFT PARTICLES AT 6 MONTHS. STEVENEL'S BLUE AND PICRIC ACID FUCHSIN. (XENOGRAFT – BLACK, NEW BONE – RED) ORIGINAL MAGNIFICATION X 4.

6 → VIEW SHOWING DIRECT CONTACT OF NEW VITAL BONE TO XENOGRAFT (BIO-OSS) PARTICLES. (XENOGRAFT – BROWN, NEW BONE – RED) STEVENEL'S BLUE AND PICRIC ACID FUCHSIN. ORIGINAL MAGNIFICATION X 20.

7 → ELECTRON-DENSE LAYER BETWEEN BIO-OSS AND NEWLY FORMED BONE AT 20 MONTHS. TRANSMISSION ELECTRON MICROSCOPY.

ued direct contact and biologic incorporation of the Bio-Oss® with the host vital bone. This indicates that the peri-implant support resulting from these grafts of 100% Bio-Oss® is both biologically acceptable and provides long-term stability.

Minimal re-pneumatization (slumping) was evidenced with xenografts when compared with autografts and allografts in 3-year panoramic radiograph follow-ups of cases submitted to the Academy of Osseointegration Consensus Conference (Jensen et al. 1998). Unpublished data (Wallace et al. Unpublished data) from an NYU sinus study also show no significant change in graft height over a 3-year period.

The fact that xenografts do not completely resorb, coupled with the fact that histology of sinus explants indicates that the xenograft never contacts the implant surface and therefore does not interfere with osseointegration (Valentini et al. 1998; Rosenlicht & Tarnow 1999; Scarano et al. 2004), results in an implant bed that is significantly denser than is found after the use of either autogenous bone or resorbable graft materials. Histomorphometric studies (Froum et al. 1998; Valentini et al. 2000; Yilderman et al. 2000, 2001) all show percentages of vital bone, connective tissue and residual xenograft to be in the order of 25%, 50% and 25% respectively at a time interval of 6 to 12 months after grafting. Due to the presence of this residual 25% xenograft volume, a matured graft that is classified as type 3 or 4 by nature of its vital bone content may function like bone of type 2 density.

Issues of safety when utilizing bone replacement grafts are of concern today because of the worldwide spread of AIDS, the risk of hepatitis transmission, and the outbreak of bovine spongiform encephalopathy in Europe with the subsequent transmission of variant Creutzfeldt–Jakob disease to humans. Although there has never been a case of disease transmission traced to the utilization of particulate

bone replacement grafts, it is important for clinicians to be aware of processing and sterilization procedures for these materials. This knowledge will allow clinicians to be comfortable in selecting these products and in addressing patient's concerns about them.

Regulation and testing of xenograft materials is both thorough and extensive. Raw material is sourced from US cattle and consists of long bones only. The material is processed by high heat or by both heat and chemical means to ensure that it is prion free. Proof of deorganification is obtained through BioRad assay, SDS-PAGE testing and SDS-PAGE and western blotting (Benke et al. 2001; Wenz et al. 2001). Sogal and Tofe (1999) calculated the risk of disease transmission based upon the model of the German Ministry of Health and found the theoretical risk for disease transmission to be 1 infection per 1.3×10^{18} 1-g doses.

SURGICAL TECHNIQUE

While the efficacy of xenografts can not be denied, they must be utilized appropriately. They are osteoconductive, not osteoinductive, therefore the cells and growth factors responsible for bone formation must come from the bony walls of the sinus and the vascular supply found within them. The lateral window should be made as small as is practical for successful membrane elevation and grafting. For maximum efficacy, it is important to elevate the Schneiderian membrane from the medial wall of the sinus to the same level as the proposed graft height so that the graft can be vascularized from this area as well as the remaining lateral wall and the sinus floor **FIG. 11**. Figures 12 and 13 **FIG. 12-13** graphically demonstrate the proper and improper membrane elevation techniques. If the membrane is not elevated from the medial wall a double layer of membrane interferes with the vascularization of the graft. Further, one must expect that bone turnover

Bone

Bio-Oss

8

9

10

8 → AT 7 YEARS THERE IS
DIRECT CONTACT BETWEEN
BIO-OSS PARTICLE AND
VITAL BONE. TRANSMISSION
ELECTRON MICROSCOPY.

9 → 9-YEAR TEM SHOWING
DIRECT CONTACT BETWEEN
HOST BONE AND RESIDUAL
BIO-OSS.

10 → 9-YEAR HISTOLOGY
SHOWING BIOLOGICAL
ACCEPTANCE OF REMAINING
XENOGRAFT PARTICLES.

A. OSTEOBLASTS (ARROWS)
AND OSTEOID NEAR
XENOGRAFT SURFACE. LOW
AND HIGH POWER

B. OSTEOCLASTS (ARROWS)
REMODELING BONE
ADJACENT TO XENOGRAFT
PARTICLE. LOW AND HIGH
POWER.

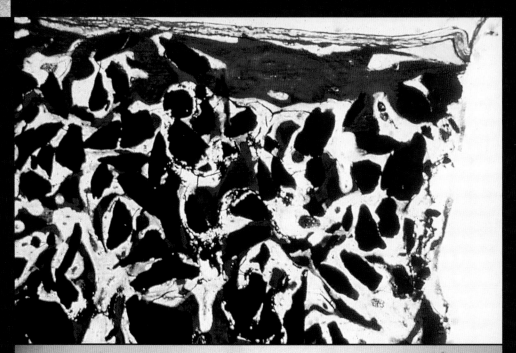

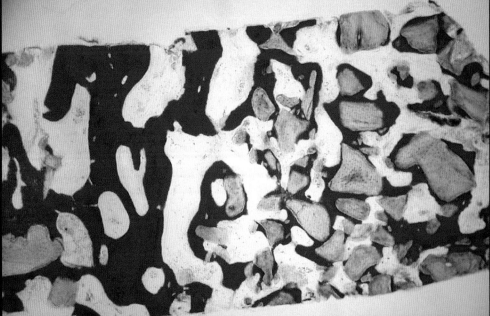

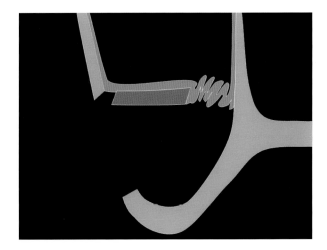

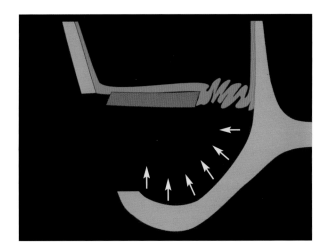

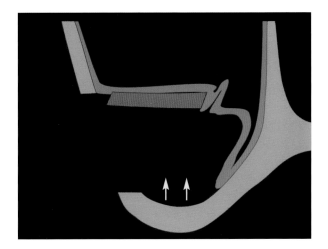

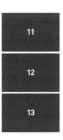

11 → REFLECTION OF THE SCHNEIDERIAN MEMBRANE FROM THE MEDIAL WALL OF THE SINUS. NOTE HEIGHT ON MEDIAL WALL IS EQUAL TO THAT OF LATERAL WINDOW OPENING.

12 → PROPER MEMBRANE ELEVATION EXTENDS UP THE MEDIAL WALL RESULTING IN AN EXCELLENT VASCULAR SUPPLY

13 → IMPROPER MEMBRANE ELEVATION TECHNIQUE CREATES A DOUBLE LAYER OF MEMBRANE OVER THE MEDIAL WALL EFFECTIVELY BLOCKING THE VASCULAR SUPPLY.

will be slower with xenografts than with a similar volume of an osteoinductive autograft. A longer graft maturation period will, therefore, be required to achieve similar amounts of new vital bone (Froum et al. 1998; Valentini et al. 2000).

There is evidence to justify the placement of a barrier membrane over the lateral window once graft placement has been completed. As in a guided bone regeneration procedure, the membrane excludes non-osteogenic connective tissue from the grafted sinus. A randomized controlled trial (Tarnow et al. 2000) utilizing a bilateral sinus model demonstrated that vital bone formation in the membrane-covered sinus will be, on average, twice that of the non-membrane side. This study, as well as controlled trials (Froum et al. 1998; Tawil & Mawla 2001) show higher implant survival rates on the membrane side than on the control side. A review by Wallace (Wallace & Froum 2003) shows implant survival rates for sinuses grafted with particulate grafts to be higher when a barrier membrane is placed over the window (93.6% vs 88.7%). Figure 14 shows direct contact of newly formed bone on the barrier membrane.**FIG. 14** This high level of vital bone formation extends to deeper sections of the core resulting in, on average, twice the vital bone content.

A recent study (Wallace et al. 2005) compared vital bone formation and implant survival with 100% Bio-Oss® sinus grafts when using non-absorbable or bioabsorbable barrier membranes over the lateral window. Average vital bone formation without a membrane, with an absorbable collagen membrane (BioGide), and with an e-PTFE membrane (Gore-Tex) was 12.1%, 17.6% and 16.9% respectively. Further, there was no significant difference in implant survival between the two membrane groups. Histologic appearance and histomorphometric data were similar for the two membrane groups. A representative specimen from the BioGide group **FIG. 15** demonstrates direct

contact between the newly formed bone and the Bio-Oss® particles, inter-particular bridging, and the formation of a new lateral wall adjacent to the now-absorbed collagen barrier membrane (top). **FIG. 15**

NEW TECHNOLOGIES TO ENHANCE BONE FORMATION

Clinicians are always seeking improvements in bone quality and a reduction in graft maturation times. Research has been ongoing for many years to provide answers to these clinical issues. We have seen the development of patient-derived (autogenous) growth factors (PRP, PRGF) that are being utilized today to improve patient outcomes. Over the past decade we have also seen the growth of genetic therapies that have led to the development of recombinant growth factors and BMP. We have also witnessed the development of tissue-engineered bone for use in sinus grafting. This chapter presents an overview of these technologies.

PRP AND PRGF

Both PRP (Marx et al. 1998) and PRGF (Anitua 1999) are derived from autogenous blood at the time of surgery. Small volumes (less than 100 ml) of the patient's blood are drawn at the time of surgery and either a double-spin (PRP) or a single-spin (PRGF) centrifugation is used to fractionate the blood into its constituent red cell, white cell and plasma fractions. The final fractionation with PRP is fully or partially automated (Harvest Technologies, BioMet–Implant Innovations), while that for PRGF (BTI Technologies) is more precisely accomplished with manual pipettes.

As PRP is discussed elsewhere in this text, the following discussion will focus on PRGF.

One of the most important differences between PRP and PRGF is the fact that the

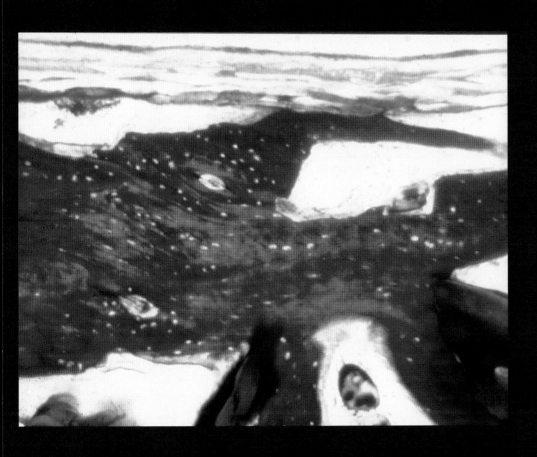

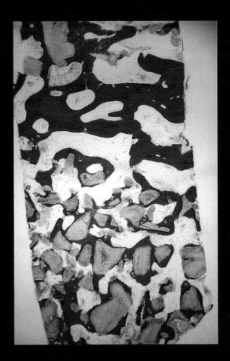

14

15

1 →NEWLY FORMED BONE (RED) IN DIRECT CONTACT WITH AN E-PTFE MEMBRANE (TOP) PLACED AND STABILIZED OVER THE LATERAL WINDOW. STEVENEL'S BLUE AND PICRIC ACID FUCHSIN. ORIGINAL MAGNIFICATION X 20.

2 → VIEW SHOWING VITAL BONE FORMATION (RED) IN GRAFT COVERED WITH A BIOABSORBABLE MEMBRANE. STEVENEL'S BLUE AND PICRIC ACID FUCHSIN. NEW LATERAL WALL (TOP – RED) FORMED BENEATH NOW-RESORBED MEMBRANE. ORIGINAL MAGNIFICATION X 20.

final PRGF product excludes the white blood cell fraction. The white cells contain both inflammatory interleukins and metalloproteases, which both increase the inflammatory response and act to destabilize the fibrin clot network (Samara & Gurbel 2003). Further, PRGF technology allows for the separation of the plasma fraction with the highest concentration of platelets and it does not utilize bovine thrombin for activation.

Both technologies clinically produce platelet concentrations in the order of 4 to 6 times that are found in whole blood. The growth factors found in plasma including PDGF, transforming growth factor-β (TGF-β), fibroblast growth factor (FGF), vascular endothelial growth factor (VEGF), epidermal growth factor (EGF), insulin-like growth factor-1 (IGF-1), and hepatocyte growth factor (HGF) are present, as well as fibronectin, osteonectin and fibrin. Growth factors play an essential role in wound healing and tissue formation. They are stored in the alpha granules of platelets and, when released, trigger multiple biologic events such as chemotaxis, angiogenesis, and cell differentiation.

Extensive evidence exists showing enhanced soft tissue healing in treating diabetic ulcers, burns and other skin lesions (Aldecoda 2001). There are some similar reports in the dental literature along with the clinical observation by this author and others that report more rapid soft tissue healing and a reduction in postoperative morbidity when PRGF is utilized.

It has been reported that the observed increase in growth factors can upregulate bone formation in sinuses grafted with either autogenous bone or bone replacement grafts. While positive results have been seen in soft tissue healing for both PRP and PRGF, statistically significant increases in vital bone formation have infrequently been reported (Marx et al. 1998; Maxor et al. 2004; Kassolis & Reynolds 2005). Other researchers have reported less successful results, and it is the conclusion of

three evidence-based reviews (Sanchez et al. 2003; Wallace & Froum 2003; Boyapati & Wang 2006) that there is insufficient evidence to support the utilization of PRP as an adjunctive therapy for increasing bone formation in maxillary sinus grafting.

RECOMBINANT PLATELET-DERIVED GROWTH FACTOR

After its introduced by Lynch et al (1989), rcombinant platelet-derived growth factor (rhPGDF) has become the most extensively studied protein signaling molecule in dentistry. Human rhPGDF (Regranex Gel > 0.1%) was first approved in 1997 for the treatment of diabetic ulcers. It is now approved in combination with the synthetic matrix β-TCP (β-tricalcium phosphate) as GEM 21S® (Osteohealth, Shirley, NY, USA) for selected use in the oral cavity.

PDGF is naturally present in the alpha granules of platelets, where it is released following injury. After injury, osteoblasts, fibroblasts and macrophages are also sources of PDGF. Once released, PDGF enhances chemotaxis and mitogenesis of osteoprogenitor cells and osteoblasts and also plays an active role in promoting angiogenesis.

In comparison to PRP, which increases the concentration of PDGF 4 to 6 times that found in blood, rhPDGF can achieve a concentration of 1000 times that of the PRP or PRGF concentrate.

Clinical efficacy in treating periodontal defects has been reported (Camelo et al. 2003; Nevins et al. 2003), and GEM 21S® has been FDA approved for this purpose. A recent clinical report (Simion et al. 2007) showed excellent results in ridge augmentation utilizing rhPDGF (Osteohealth) with both bovine bone blocks and Bio-Oss collagen as the carriers.

PDGF appears to be an ideal enhancement factor to use in maxillary sinus grafting due to its ability to stimulate both cell migration and proliferation of osteoblasts and

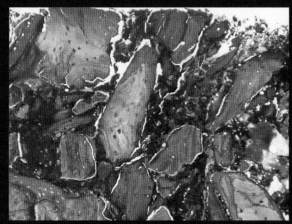
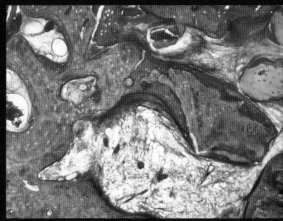

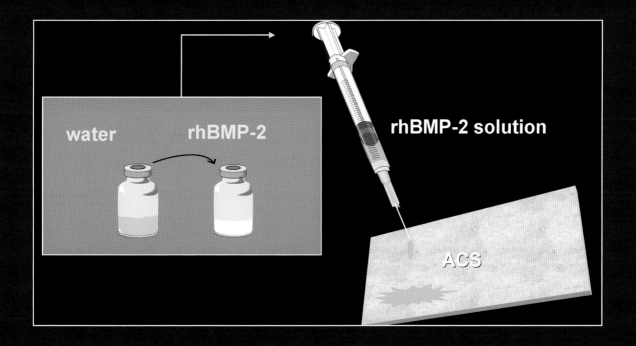

water   rhBMP-2

rhBMP-2 solution

ACS

16 → VITAL BONE FORMATION IN
SINUS CORE AT 6 MONTHS
FOLLOWING GRAFT OF RHPDGF,
WITH BIO-OSS AND MFDBA AS A
CARRIER (COURTESY NEVINS ML).
ORIGINAL MAGNIFICATION X 4.

17 → HIGH POWER OF FIG. 15.
NEWLY FORMED VITAL BONE IN
DIRECT CONTACT WITH THE
CARRIER (COURTESY NEVINS ML).
ORIGINAL MAGNIFICATION X 20.

18 → HYDRATION OF THE
ABSORBABLE COLLAGEN SPONGE
(ACS) WITH RH-BMP-2 SOLUTION
FOR A MINIMUM OF 15 MINUTES.

osteoblast precursor cells. A further positive affect on bone regeneration is achieved through the promotion of angiogenesis.

Currently, the author and other researchers are involved in sinus studies utilizing rhPDGF in combination with Bio-Oss® as the carrier. One study (Artzi et al. 2005) has shown Bio-Oss® to be a more favorable osteoconductor than β-TCP. At present, limited histologic data is available and, at the time of publication, use in sinus grafting is considered an off-label application.

Figures 16 and 17 (courtesy of Myron Nevins) are typical of the histologic results seen in sinus graft application with GEM 21S®. This representative section, taken 6 months after a sinus graft with GEM 21S® rh-PDGF, with a matrix of MFDBA and Bio-Oss®, shows significant vital bone formation on and between the residual grafted matrix particles. **FIG. 16-17**

Gem 21S® is packaged as a dose of 0.3 mg/ml of rh-PDGF-BB in sterile water with 5 cc of the carrier β-TCP. Clinical usage is simple, merely hydrating the carrier with the liquid growth factor.

BMP-2

BMPs comprise a family of osteoinductive proteins some of which are capable of stimulating the existing host mesenchymal cells to form bone. Urist (1965) first described bone morphogenetic activity after producing ectopic bone growth in the rabbit. Further studies led to the purification and cloning of these proteins from bone sources (Wang et al. 1988, 1990; Wozney et all. 1988).

Recombinant forms of BMP have been successfully investigated in the sinus graft model in animals (Nevins et al. 1996; Margolin et al. 1998). Sinus studies in humans include a feasibility study (Boyne et al. 1997), a pilot study (van den Bergh et al. 2000), and a human randomized controlled trial (Boyne et al. 2005).

The human studies have been positive with regard to both safety and efficacy. The multicenter randomized controlled trial by Boyne et al. (2005) compared the bone morphogenetic protein BMP-2 in two concentrations (0.75 and 1.5 mg/ml) with a bone graft control. The BMP-2 in sterile water solution was placed on absorbable collagen sponges (ACS) and allowed a minimum of 15 minutes for the BMP-2 to bind to the collagen receptor sites. After elevation of the Schneiderian membrane, the BMP-2-impregnated ACS were placed in the sinus as the sole grafting material. All test sites were non-perforated and a membrane was not placed over the window. Implant success rates after 36 months of loading for the control group, 0.75 mg/ml group, and the 1.5 mg/ml group were 81%, 88% and 79% respectively. Of further interest was the fact that 15% of the test cases did not produce sufficient bone volume for the placement of dental implants and, when the lower dose was utilized, the maturation time prior to implant placement had to be increased.

One of the major shortcomings experienced with the use of 100% autogenous bone in sinus grafts is the observed tendency of this graft to resorb. This may result in partial re-pneumatization of the sinus with resultant loss in graft volume accompanied by a decrease in density. Many clinicians have resolved this problem by utilizing composite grafts of autogenous bone and a slowly or non-resorbable bone replacement graft (Moy et al. 1993).

Using the above rationale, one might speculate that the results with BMP-2/ACS might be improved by the addition of a slowly resorbable or non-resorbable bone replacement graft. It is imperative at this time to retain the ACS, as the BMP-2 is bound to receptor sites in the collagen that control the release kinetics of the BMP-2. Studies have shown that 95% of the BMP-2 will be retained by the ACS and that this percentage will remain high even after extreme handling (expression of fluid from the sponge) (Hsu et al. 2006). Therefore, any addi-

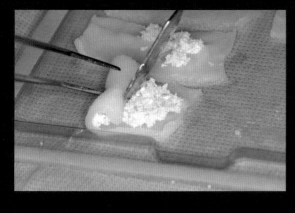

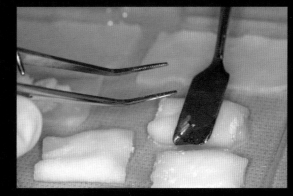

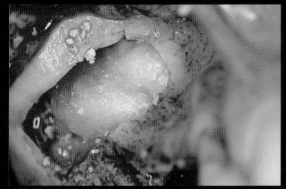

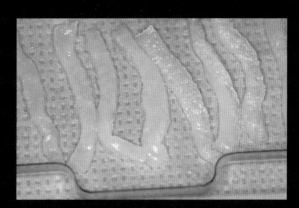

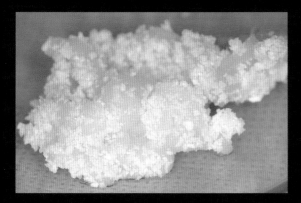

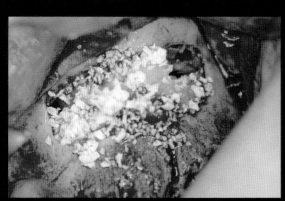

19 → BMP-2 SATURATED ACS COATED WITH BIO-OSS PARTICLES.

20 →BMP-2/ACS/BIO-OSS ROLLED PRIOR TO PLACEMENT IN SINUS.

21 → BMP-2/ACS/BIO-OSS PLACED IN SINUS AFTER ELEVATION OF MEMBRANE.

22 → HYDRATED BMP-2/ ACS CUT IN STRIPS.

23 → HYDRATED BMP-2/ ACS CUT INTO STRIPS AND IS MIXED WITH BIO-OSS PARTICLES.

24 → BMP-2/ACS/BIO-OSS PLACED IN SINUS AFTER ELEVATION OF THE MEMBRANE.

tion of bone replacement graft should occur after the minimum 15 minute hydration time of the BMP-2/ACS **FIG. 18**.

While INFUSE® (Medtronic, MN, USA) has shown efficacy in both sinus grafting (Boyne et al. 2005) and extraction socket therapy (Fiorellini et al. 2005), studies need to be conducted both to determine the minimal effective dose for various applications and to look for ways to increase graft density and promote the maintenance of graft volume. The addition of osteoconductive fillers, such as proven BRGs (xenografts, mineralized allografts) or new mineralized carriers with biologically active surface coatings may play a role as both osteoconductors and as mineralized scaffolds.

The author is presently investigating two clinical applications of the addition of Bio-Oss® to the BMP-2/ACS system to address the aforementioned concerns regarding low density and loss of volume. The first application utilizes the Bio-Oss® particles as a coating (think bread and butter) on the hydrated collagen sponge. The sponges are then rolled and placed into the sinus **FIG. 19–21**. The second application cuts the hydrated ACS into small strips before adding the Bio-Oss® to form a composite prior to insertion into the sinus **FIG. 22–24**. Immediate postoperative DentaScan views show the distribution of the graft **FIG. 25–26**.

A randomized controlled histomorphometric and volumetric human trial testing two concentrations of BMP-2 with an added mineralized bone replacement graft in bilateral sinus grafts will soon be conducted at the New York University Department of Periodontics and Implant Dentistry. It is hoped that this and other studies will help determine the future role of BMP-2 in oral regenerative therapy.

TISSUE-ENGINEERED BONE

The most recent concept being investigated in sinus augmentation is the utilization of tissue-engineered bone as a sinus grafting material. Tissue-engineered bone has the advantage of being an autogenous-derived grafting material that requires a minimal tissue harvest. From a clinical standpoint, the disadvantages are the time required to produce the bone graft and the present cost of this technology-driven therapy.

The technique involves harvesting a small periosteal tissue sample, usually from the cambial layer in the posterior mandible. This tissue is tested for cell viability and is then seeded with cell amplification achieved using standard culture conditions. A three-dimensional matrix may then be used for the formation of calcified bone blocks that are ultimately transplanted to the sinus. Descriptions of this technology may be found in sinus studies by Schmelzeisen et al. (2003), Turhani et al. (2005), and Zizelmann et al. (2007).

Bone formation was shown by Turhani *in vitro* and cancellous bone formation was shown by Schmelzeisen *in vivo*. A major negative aspect was a 90% resorption of the new bone (as compared with 29% in the hip marrow control) shown by Zizelmann at 3 months after the postgrafting procedure.

This technology is in its infancy at the present time and there are still many obstacles to overcome. Again, as in the case with BMP-2, one might consider the utilization of a mineralized bone replacement graft to act as an osteoconductive space maintainer.

A remarkable literature base on sinus augmentation therapy has appeared since the Sinus Consensus Conference of 1996. Questions that went unanswered at that time can now be answered with evidence from a database of over 7000 implants.

However, one must understand that evidence-based dentistry is not meant to preclude

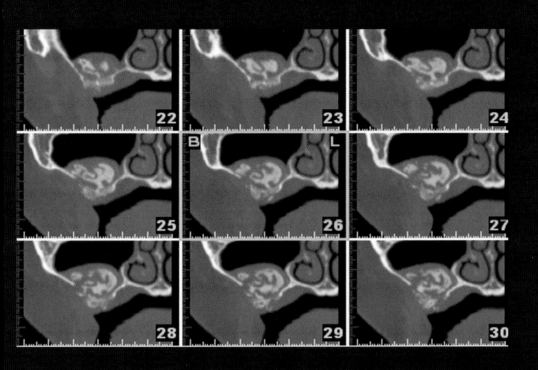

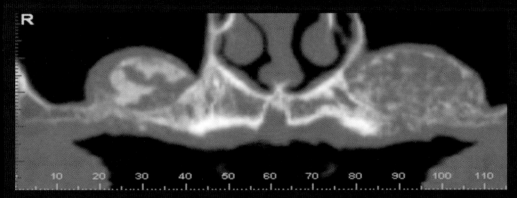

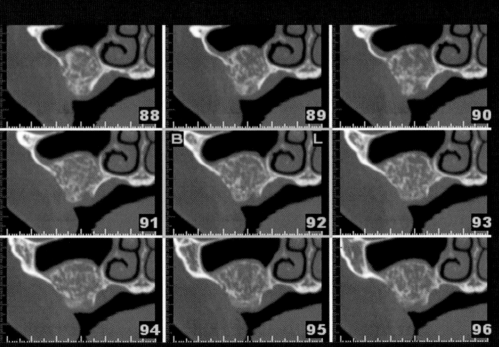

25 → IMMEDIATE POSTOPERATIVE PANORAMIC DENTASCAN VIEW OF BILATERAL SINUS GRAFT.

26 → IMMEDIATE POSTOPERATIVE CROSS-SECTIONAL VIEWS OF BILATERAL SINUS GRAFT WITH RH-BMP-2/ACS/BIO-OSS.

A. 'ROLL' TECHNIQUE.

B. 'PARTICULATE' TECHNIQUE.

the clinical judgment of experienced clinicians. It should be seen as a method to either support, or cause you to re-think your chosen method of therapy on the basis of existing evidence.

Further, the information on graft materials cannot stand alone. Graft materials are but one of the covariables that affect the outcome of the sinus augmentation procedure. To achieve a true understanding of this surgical procedure, the influence of all other covariables, such as the utilization of a barrier membrane and the affect of implant surface micro-morphology must be considered.

REFERENCES

1 Aghaloo T.L., Moy P.K.
Which hard tissue augmentation techniques are the most successful in furnishing bony support for implant placement?
Int. J. Oral Maxillofac. Implants 2007; 22(Suppl): 49-70.

2 Benke D., Olah A., Möhler H.
Protein-chemical analysis of Bio-Oss bone substitute and evidence on its carbonate content.
Biomaterials 2001; 22: 1005-12.

3 Blomqvist J.E., Alberius P., Isaksson S.
Retrospective analysis of one-stage maxillary sinus augmentation with endosseous implants.
Int. J. Oral Maxillofac. Implants 1996; 11: 512-21.

4 Blomqvist J.E., Alberius P., Isaksson S.
Two-stage maxillary sinus reconstruction with endosseous implants: A prospective study.
Int. J. Oral Maxillofac. Implants 1998; 13: 758-66.

5 Boyne P.J., James R.A.
Grafting of the maxillary sinus floor with autogenous marrow and bone.
J. Oral Surg. 1980; 38: 613-6.

6 Del Fabbro M., Testori T., Francetti L., Weinstein R.
Systematic review of survival rates for implants placed in the grafted maxillary sinus.
Int J. Periodontics Restorative Dent. 2004; 24(6): 565-77.

7 Froum S.J., Tarnow D.P., Wallace S.S., Rohrer M.D., Cho S.-C.
Sinus floor elevation using anorganic bovine bone matrix (OsteoGraf/N) with and without autogenous bone: A clinical, histologic, radiographic, and histomorphometric analysis - Part 2 of an ongoing prospective study.
Int. J. Periodontics Restorative Dent. 1998; 18: 529-43.

8 Froum S.J., Wallace S.S., Elian N., Cho S.C., Tarnow D.P.
Comparison of mineralized cancellous bone allograft (Puros) and anorganic bovine bone matrix (Bio-Oss) for sinus augmentation: histomorphometry at 26–32 weeks after grafting.
Int. J. Periodontics Restorative Dent. 2006; 26(6): 543-51.

9 Garg A.K.
Current concepts in augmentation grafting of the maxillary sinus for the placement of dental implants.
Dent. Implantol. Update 2001; 12: 17-22.

10 Graziani F., Donos N., Needleman I., Gabriele M., Tonetti M.
Comparison of implant survival following sinus floor augmentation procedures with implants placed in pristine posterior maxillary bone: a systematic review.
Clin. Oral Implants Res. 2004; 15: 677-82.

11 Hallman M., Sennerby L., Lundgren S.
A clinical and histologic evaluation of implant integration in the posterior maxilla after sinus floor augmentation with autogenous bone, bovine hydroxyapatite, or a 20:80 mixture.
Int. J. Oral Maxillofac. Implants 2002; 17: 635-43.

12 Hanisch O., Lozada J.L., Holmes R.E., Calhoun C.J., Kan J.Y.K., Spiekermann H.
Maxillary sinus augmentation prior to placement of endosseous implants: A histomorpho-metric analysis.
Int. J. Oral Maxillofac. Implants 1999; 14: 329-36.

13 Hising P., Bolin A., Branting C.
Reconstruction of severely resorbed alveolar crests with dental implants using a bovine mineral for augmentation.
Int. J. Oral Maxillofac. Implants 2001; 16: 90-7.

14 Jensen O.T., Sennerby L.
Histologic analysis of clinically retrieved titanium micro-implants placed in conjunction with maxillary sinus floor augmentation.
Int. J. Oral Maxillofac. Implants 1998; 13: 513-21

15 Jensen O.T., Shulman L.B., Block M.S., Iacono V.J.
Report of the sinus consensus conference of 1996. Int. J. Oral Maxillofac. Implants 1998: 13 (supplement).

16 Johansson B., Wannfors K., Ekenbäck J., Smedberg J.-I., Hirsch J.
Implants and sinus inlay bone grafts in a 1-stage procedure on severely atrophied maxillae: Surgical aspects of a 3-year follow-up study.
Int. J. Oral Maxillofac. Implants 1999; 14: 811-8.

17 Kahnberg K.-E., Ekestubbe A., Gröndahl K., Nilsson P., Hirsch J. M.
Sinus lifting procedure: One-stage surgery with bone transplant and implants.
Clin. Oral Implants Res. 2001; 12: 479-87.

18 Keller E., Eckert S.E., Tolman D.E.
Maxillary antral–nasal autogenous bone graft reconstruction of the compromised maxilla: A 12-year retrospective study.
Int. J. Oral Maxillofac. Implants 1999; 14: 707-21.

19 Keller E.E., Eckert S.E., Tolman D.E.
Maxillary antral and nasal one-stage inlay composite bone graft: Preliminary report on 30 recipient sites.
J. Oral Maxillofac. Surg 1994; 52: 438-47.

20 Khoury F.
Augmentation of the sinus floor with mandibular bone block and simultaneous implantation: A 6-year clinical investigation.
Int. J. Oral Maxillofac. Implants 1999; 14: 557-64.

21 Langer B., Langer L.
Use of allografts for sinus grafting.
In: Jensen OT (ed). The Sinus Bone Graft. Chicago: Quintessence, 1999: 69-78.

22 Moy P.K., Lundgren S., Holmes R.E.
Maxillary sinus augmentation: Histomorphometric analysis of graft materials for sinus floor augmentation.
J. Oral Maxillofac. Surg 1993; 51: 857-62.

23 Orsini G., Scarano A., Degidi M., Caputi S., Iezzi G., Piattelli A.
Histological and ultrastructural evaluation of bone around Bio-Oss® particles in sinus augmentation.
Oral Dis. 2007; 13: 586-93.

24 Rosenlicht J., Tarnow D.P.
Human histologic evidence of functionally loaded hydroxyapatite-coated implants placed simultaneously with sinus augmentation: A case report 2½ years post-placement.
Int. J. Oral Implantol. 1999; 25: 7-10.

25 Scarano A., Pecora G., Piattelli M., Piattelli A.
Osseointegration in a sinus augmented with bovine porous bone mineral: Histological results in an implant retrieved 4 years after insertion. A case report.
J. Periodontol. 2004; 75: 1161-6.

26 Tadjoedin E.S., DeLange G.L., Holzmann P.J., Kuiper L., Burger E.H.
Histologic observations on biopsies harvested following sinus floor elevation using a bioactive glass material of narrow size range.
Clin. Oral Implants Res. 2000; 11: 334-44.

27 Tadjoedin E.S., DeLange G.L., Lyaruu D.M., Kuiper L., Burger E.H.
High concentrations of bioactive glass material (BioGran®) vs. autogenous bone for sinus floor elevation.
Clin. Oral Implants Res. 2002; 13: 428-36.

28 Tatum O.H.
Maxillary sinus grafting for endosseous implants.
Presented at the Annual Meeting of the Alabama Implant Study Group. Birmingham, AL April 1977.

29 Tolman D.E.
Reconstructive procedures with endosseous implants in grafted bone: A review of the literature.
Int. J. Oral Maxillofac. Implants 1995; 10: 275-94.

30 Tong D.C., Rioux K., Drangsholt M., Beirne O.R.
A review of the survival rates for implants placed in grafted maxillary sinuses using meta-analysis.
Int. J. Oral Maxillofac. Implants 1998; 13: 175-82.

31 Traini T., Valentini P., Iezzi G., Piattelli A.
A histologic and histomorphometric evaluation of anorganic bovine bone retrieved 9 years after a sinus augmentation procedure.
J. Periodontol. 2007; 78: 955-61.

32 Ulm C., Kneissel M., Schedle A., Solar P., Matejka M., Schneider B., Donath K.
Characteristic features of trabecular bone in edentulous maxillae.
Clin. Oral Implants Res. 1999; 10: 459-67.

33 Valentini P., Abensur D., Densari D., Graziani J.N., Hammerle C. *Histological evaluation of Bio-Oss in a sinus floor elevation and implantation procedure: A human case report.*
Clin. Oral Implants Res. 1998; 9: 59-64.

34 Valentini P., Abensur D., Wenz B., Peetz M., Schenk R.
Sinus grafting with porous bone mineral (Bio-Oss) for implant placement: A 5-year study on 15 patients.
Int. J. Periodontics Restorative Dent. 2000; 20: 245-53.

35 Wallace S.S., Froum S.J.
Effect of maxillary sinus augmentation on the survival of endosseous dental implants. A systematic review.
Ann. Periodontol. 2003; 8: 328-43.

36 Wannfors K., Johansson B., Hallman M., Strandkvist T.
A prospective randomized study of 1- and 2- stage sinus inlay bone grafts: 1 year follow-up.
Int. J. Oral Maxillofac. Implants 2000; 15: 625-32.

37 Wenz B., Oesch B., Horst M.
Analysis of the risk of transmitting bovine spongiform encephalopathy through bone grafts derived from bovine bone.
Biomaterials 2001; 22: 1599-1606.

38 Yilderman M., Spiekermann H., Biesterfeld S., Edelhof D.
Maxillary sinus augmentation using xenogenic bone substitute material (Bio-Oss) in combination with venous blood: A histologic and histomorphometric study in humans.
Clin. Oral Implants Res. 2000; 11: 217-29.

39 Yilderman M., Spiekermann H., Handt S., Edelhoff D.
Maxillary sinus augmentation with the xenograft Bio-Oss and autogenous intraoral bone for qualitative improvement of the implant site: A histologic and histomorphometric clinical study in humans.
Int. J. Oral Maxillofac. Implants 2001; 16: 23-33.

40 Zizelman C., Schoen R., Metzger M.C., Schmelzeisen R. Schramm A., Dott B., et al.
Bone formation after sinus augmentation with engineered bone.
Clin. Oral Implants Res. 2007; 18: 69-73.

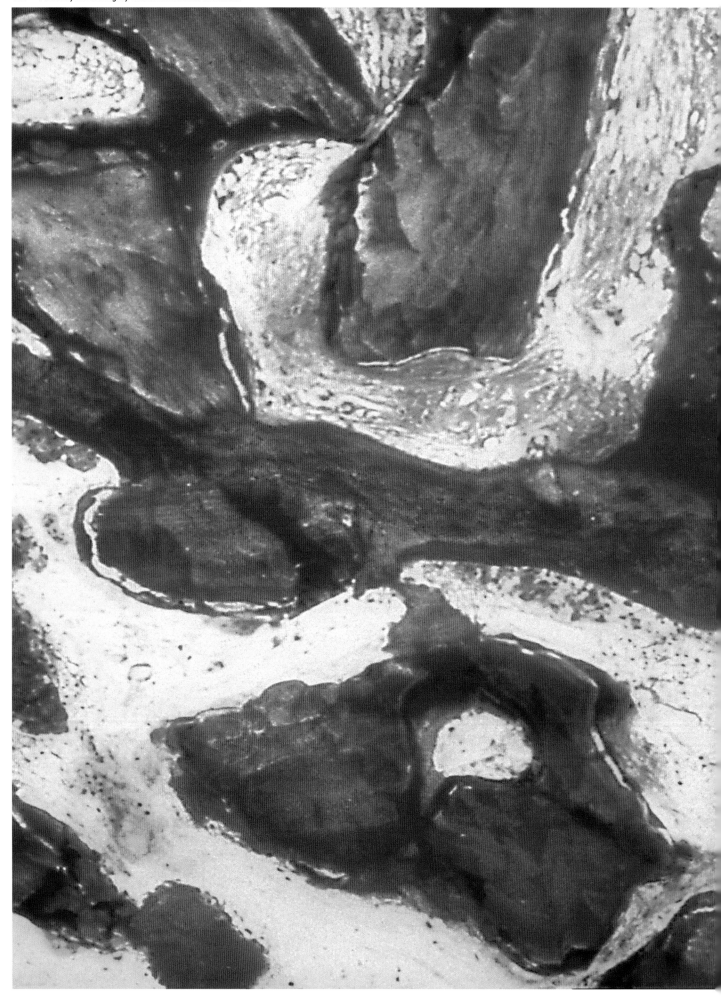

P. VALENTINI

Histologic and clinical results of sinus floor augmentation with bone substitutes

10

10

Sinus floor elevations with bone substitutes, such as freeze dried demineralized bone, freeze dried mineralized bone, hydroxyapatite and xenografts, have frequently been described (Jensen & Greer 1990; Hürzeler et al. 1997a and 1997b; Smiler et al. 1992; Small et al. 1993; Wagner 1991; Ackerman et al. 1994). One bone substitute that has been extensively tested in animal and clinical studies (Hammerle & Karring 2000) is the deproteinized bovine bone graft Bio-Oss® (Bio-Oss®, Geistlich Pharma, Wolhusen, Switzerland). Bio-Oss is derived from bovine bone and processed in such a way that the original characteristics of natural bone are maintained. The architecture of the material, including crystal size, microporosity and surface structure, has been demonstrated to be very similar to human bone (Tidwell et al. 2000).

BIOLOGIC CHARACTERISTICS OF NATURAL BONE MINERAL

The biologic behaviour of natural bone mineral has been extensively described, as outlined below.

OSTEOCONDUCTIVITY

Natural bone mineral has been found to be highly osteoconductive (Zitzmann et al.

2001a; 2001b; Araujo et al. 2001; Maiorana et al. 2000; Piattelli et al. 1999; Hürzeler et al. 1997, 1998; Valentini et al. 1994, 1998, 2000; Schmitt et al. 1997; Wetzel et al. 1995). The reason is assumed to be its high similarity to human bone (Hurzeler et al. 1998). The microstructure, including porosity, surface and crystal size, has been shown to match the characteristics of human bone (Jensen & Greer 1992; Klinge et al. 1992).

SLOW RESORPTION AND LONG-TERM STABILITY

Various studies have demonstrated that natural bone mineral is slowly resorbed by osteoclasts in the normal remodeling process of bone (Zitzmann et al. 2001b; Valentini et al. 2000; Piattelli et al. 1999; Hürzeler et al. 1997a, 1997b, 1998; Pripatnanont et al. 1996; Klinge et al. 1992). Thereby it seems to serve as a long-lasting matrix for new bone and helps to maintain the graft volume (Valentini & Abensur 1997; Triani et al. 2007).

INCREASED MINERAL AMOUNT IN AUGMENTED SITES

Histomorphometric evaluation of sites augmented with natural bone mineral compared with non-grafted bone showed an increased amount of mineral structures in the regenerated area TAB. 1 (Valentini et al. 1998, 2000; Maiorana et al. 2000; Hürzeler et al. 1998; Artzi et al. 2000; McAllister et al. 1998) compared with non-grafted areas. The mineral part of the grafted sites is composed of the bone substitute plus newly formed bone, and the percentage of bone marrow seems to be decreased due to the presence of the bone substitute.

In the following the histological and clinical results of this bone substitute in sinus lift procedures will be discussed.

HISTOLOGIC RESULTS

RESULTS FROM ANIMAL STUDIES

Hürzeler et al (1997a) evaluated natural bone mineral used alone in sinus floor augmentation procedures histologically and histomorphometrically in monkeys. They analysed bone formation and bone implant contact after simultaneous and delayed implant insertion respectively, both under loaded or unloaded conditions. Natural bone mineral particles were embedded in lamellar bone and osteoclasts on the graft particle surfaces suggested ongoing resorption of the particles in the normal remodeling process of bone.

The mineralized bone-to-implant contact in the augmented area measured between 37 and 57%. It was concluded that this material is suitable for sinus augmentation procedures.

Another study evaluated bone mineral density, vertical height stability and extent of natural bone mineral replacement in monkeys (McAllister et al. 1998). Radiographic vertical height of the augmented sinus floor was maintained up to the 18-month time point. Histomorphometric analysis revealed an apparent decrease in the amount of natural bone mineral from 7.5 months to 18 months (19 ± 14% vs. 6 ± 3%). Areas of resorption of the bone substitute particles and replacement with new bone were visible histologically.

RESULTS FROM HUMAN STUDIES

Yildirim et al. (2001) performed sinus floor elevations in 12 patients using a mixture of natural bone mineral and autogenous bone. After 6 to 9 months postoperatively, a total of 36 implants were placed and bone biopsies were taken. Bony integration of the bone substitute particles was visible histologically and the bone was mainly woven. It was concluded from the results that the bony integration of Bio-Oss® was mainly influenced by the individual healing response rather than the maturation of the graft material.

In another clinical study in 10 patients, Maiorana et al. (2001) used a mixture of particulate cancellous bone and marrow and natural bone mineral for sinus floor elevations. Several (5 or 7) months later, implants were placed and histologies were analyzed. Although in the 5-month specimens, areas filled with connective fibrous tissue surrounding the bone substitute particles, in the 7-month biopsies natural bone mineral was integrated and interconnected by newly formed bone. These results indicated that longer periods of healing than 5 months may be favorable.

In a long-term study, Piatelli et al. (1999) histologically evaluated biopsies 6, 9 and 18 months and 4 years after sinus floor elevation with natural bone mineral in a total of 20 patients. By 6 months postoperatively mature new bone surrounding the bone substitute particles had been found. In the 18-months and 4-year specimens, osteoclasts in the process of resorbing new bone and the substitute particles were visible, demonstrating the slow resorption process of the material.

Traini et al. (2007) analysed a 9-year sample retrieved from a grafted sinus. The mean amount of newly formed bone was 46 ± 4.67%, the amount of natural bone mineral remnants was 16 ± 5.89%, and the percentage of marrow spaces was 38 ± 8.93%. A greater number of osteocytes were found in the bone close to natural bone mineral FIG. 9. A greater strength of bone with more osteocytes was reported by Mullender et al. (2005).

Hallmann et al. (2002) compared the use of particulated autogenous bone alone with natural bone mineral alone vs. a mixture of 80% natural bone mineral and 20% autogenous bone in 21 patients in a two-stage procedure. Several (6 to 9) months after grafting, experimental micro-implants for histological evaluation and standard implants for prosthetic treatment were inserted. Six months later the micro-implants were explanted and histologically and histomorphometrically evaluated. There were no statistically significant differences between the bone graft groups regarding bone-implant contact and bone area. Evaluation of implant survival after 1 year of loading showed no difference between the groups. It was concluded that autogenous bone, natural bone mineral alone, as well as a mixture of both, are suitable grafting materials for sinus floor augmentation.

The predictability of implants placed in a sinus augmented with natural bone mineral mixed with demineralized freeze dried bone (DFDB) has been assessed (Valentini & Abensur 1997). Sinus floor elevations (28) were performed in 20 patients in one- or two-stage surgeries. The survival rate of the implants after at least 2 years of loading was evaluated clini-

Overview over histomorphometric study results on the area density in grafted areas
(NBM – natural bone mineral, AB – autogenous bone)

TAB. 1

	% NBM particles	% new bone	% bone marrow / connective tissue	Augmentation material (time of biopsy post-op)
MONKEY (Hürzeler et al. 1997a and b)				
loaded	9–17	30–33	51–61	NBM
unloaded	18–23	27–28	50–54	(8–15 months)
MONKEY (McAllister et al. 1998)				
loaded	62 + 3	19 + 14	29	NBM (7.5 months)
unloaded	70 + 7	6 + 3	24	
HUMAN (Yildirim et al. 2001)				
	29.6	18.9	51.5	NBM+ AB
				(6–9.5 months)
HUMAN (Piatelli et al. 1999)				
loaded	Ca. 30%	Ca. 30%	Ca. 40%	NBM+ AB
unloaded				(6 months – 4 years)
SHEEP (Hallman et al. 2002)				
loaded	41.7 + 26.6	11.8 + 3.6	46.5	NBM
unloaded	39.9 + 8	12.3 + 8.5	47.8	NBM+AB (80:20)
HUMAN (Valentini et al. 2000)				
loaded	21.1 + 7.25	39.2 + 4.4	39.8 + 7.1	NBM (6 months)
unloaded	27.6 + 4.88	27.0 + 11.6	45.4 + 9.12	NBM (12 months)
HUMAN (Valentini et al. 1998)				
loaded	28	28	44	NBM (12 months)

cally. Biopsies were taken in three patients. The implant survival rate was satisfactory following the surgical technique, and the histological evaluation revealed bony integration of the natural bone mineral particles **FIG. 1–2**. However, DFDB failed to show any bony contact **FIG. 3**. From these results the authors recommended using natural bone mineral alone instead of a combination with DFDB.

In a second study, Valentini et al. (2000) evaluated the efficacy of natural bone mineral alone in 15 patients. Twenty sinus augmentation procedures were performed, and 57 implants were inserted 6 months later. In three patients, biopsies were taken 6 and 12 months after grafting. The grafted area was histomorphometrically analyzed and compared with the non-grafted area.

The grafted areas showed a denser mineral scaffold than the non-grafted areas **FIG. 4**. It seemed that the bone substitute particles occupied space at the expense of bone marrow and

Grafted area vs. non-grafted areas after 12 months

TAB. 2

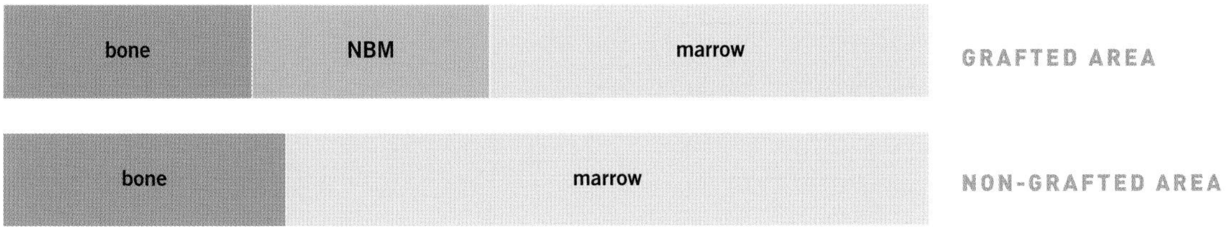

| bone | NBM | marrow | GRAFTED AREA |

| bone | marrow | NON-GRAFTED AREA |

Histomorphometry of grafted areas: 6 months vs 12 months

TAB. 3

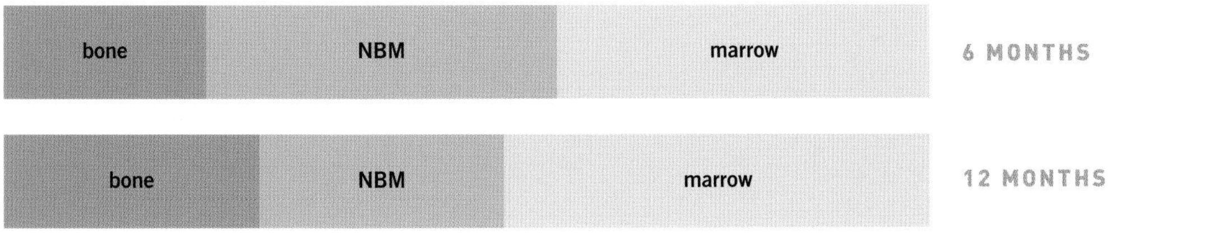

| bone | NBM | marrow | 6 MONTHS |

| bone | NBM | marrow | 12 MONTHS |

Group characteristics

TAB. 4

	Group 1	Group 2	Group 3	Group 4
SURGICAL TECHNIQUE	1 stage	2 stage	1 stage	2 stage
GRAFT MATERIAL	DFDB+NBM	DFDB+NBM	NBM	NBM

connective tissue compartment as the area of new bone corresponded well to the bone area in non-grafted regions **TAB. 2**. There was also a tendency for a decrease in the amount of bone substitute from 6 to 12 months possibly indicating resorption **TAB. 3, FIG. 5**. However, the small patient number did not allow for statistically significant conclusions.

The histomorphometric results and osteoconductivity of this bone substitute material was confirmed by another human case in which an implant was explanted due to unfavorable prosthetic positioning (Valentini et al. 1998). The explantation **FIG. 6** was performed 12 months after sinus grafting and 6 months after implant placement. The density of bone was 28% in the grafted area compared with 27% in the non-grafted area. Bone marrow accounted for 44% in the grafted and 73% in the non-grafted area, with a natural bone mineral area of 28%. Bone-to-implant contact was 73% in the augmented and 63% in the non-grafted region. The most important result was that no natural bone-mineral-to-implant contact was found **FIG. 7**.

CLINICAL RESULTS

In a retrospective study, Valentini & Abensur (2003) evaluated the survival rate of 187 titanium plasma spray-coated cylindrical and machine screw-type implants placed in sinuses grafted with a mixture of 1:1 of natural bone mineral and demineralized freeze dried bone or with natural bone mineral alone. The 58 patients included in this study were divided into four different groups **TAB. 4** and treated with a one- or two-stage technique, according to the volume of residual bone. This determined the possibility of primary stabilization and the duration of treatment, which was 9 or 12 months respectively. The overall implant survival rate was 94.5% after a mean functioning period of 6.5 years (range 2.3 to 9.4 years). The implant survival rate **TAB. 5** was better in sinuses grafted with natural bone mineral alone than with a mixture of natural bone mineral and demineralized freeze dried bone (96.8% vs. 90%). Titanium plasma spray-coated cylindrical implants **FIG. 8** had a better survival rate than screw-type implants in sinuses grafted with a mixture of natural bone mineral and demineralized freeze dried bone, but one-third

TAB. 5

Implant survival rate among groups

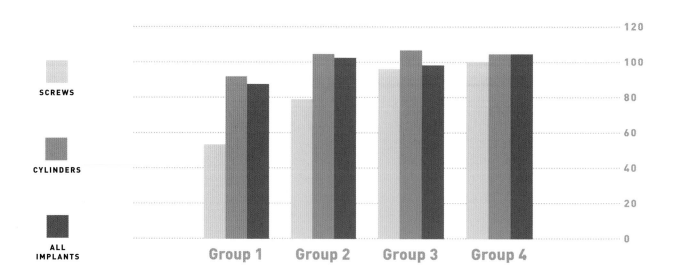

SCREWS

CYLINDERS

ALL IMPLANTS

Group 1   Group 2   Group 3   Group 4

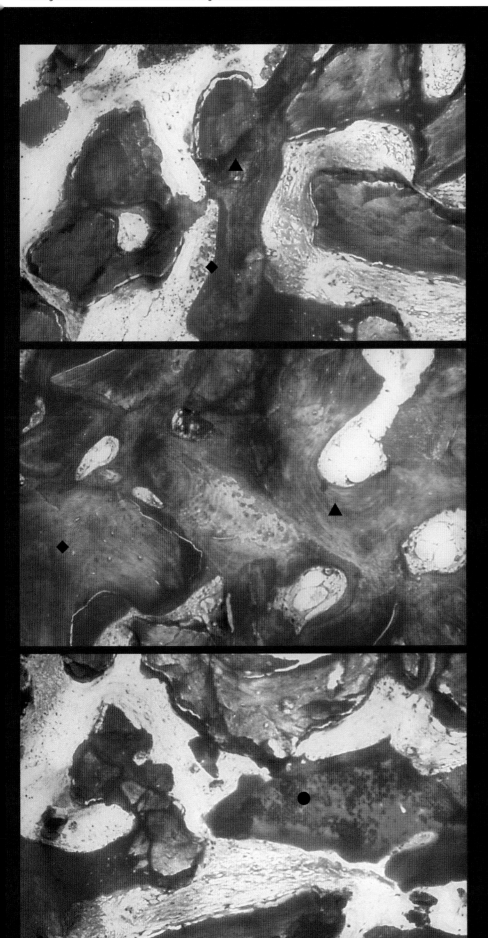

1 → AT 6 MONTHS, NEWLY FORMED WOVEN ( ) BONE SURROUNDS THE GRANULES OF NATURAL BONE MINERAL ( ) AND HAS FORMED BRIDGES BETWEEN THE GRAFTING MATERIAL (ORIGINAL MAGNIFICATION X 25)

2 → AT 12 MONTHS NATURAL BONE MINERAL ( ) IS COMPLETLY EMBEDDED IN A NEW LAMELLAR BONE ( ) (ORIGINAL MAGNIFICATION X 25)

3 → AT 6 MONTHS IT APPEARS THAT DFBD PARTICLES ( ) UNDERGO A PARTIAL RECALCIFICATION BUT THAT NO NEW BONE IS FORMED ON THE SURFACE (ORIGINAL MAGNIFICATION X 25)

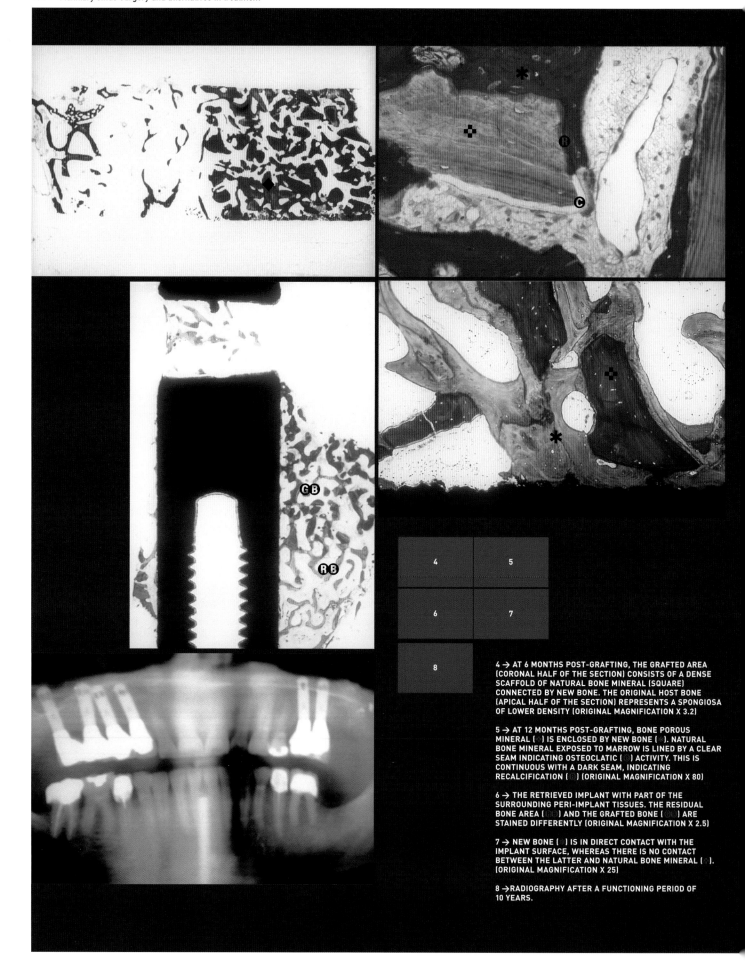

4 → AT 6 MONTHS POST-GRAFTING, THE GRAFTED AREA (CORONAL HALF OF THE SECTION) CONSISTS OF A DENSE SCAFFOLD OF NATURAL BONE MINERAL (SQUARE) CONNECTED BY NEW BONE. THE ORIGINAL HOST BONE (APICAL HALF OF THE SECTION) REPRESENTS A SPONGIOSA OF LOWER DENSITY (ORIGINAL MAGNIFICATION X 3.2)

5 → AT 12 MONTHS POST-GRAFTING, BONE POROUS MINERAL ( ) IS ENCLOSED BY NEW BONE ( ). NATURAL BONE MINERAL EXPOSED TO MARROW IS LINED BY A CLEAR SEAM INDICATING OSTEOCLATIC ( ) ACTIVITY. THIS IS CONTINUOUS WITH A DARK SEAM, INDICATING RECALCIFICATION ( ) (ORIGINAL MAGNIFICATION X 80)

6 → THE RETRIEVED IMPLANT WITH PART OF THE SURROUNDING PERI-IMPLANT TISSUES. THE RESIDUAL BONE AREA ( ) AND THE GRAFTED BONE ( ) ARE STAINED DIFFERENTLY (ORIGINAL MAGNIFICATION X 2.5)

7 → NEW BONE ( ) IS IN DIRECT CONTACT WITH THE IMPLANT SURFACE, WHEREAS THERE IS NO CONTACT BETWEEN THE LATTER AND NATURAL BONE MINERAL ( ). (ORIGINAL MAGNIFICATION X 25)

8 → RADIOGRAPHY AFTER A FUNCTIONING PERIOD OF 10 YEARS.

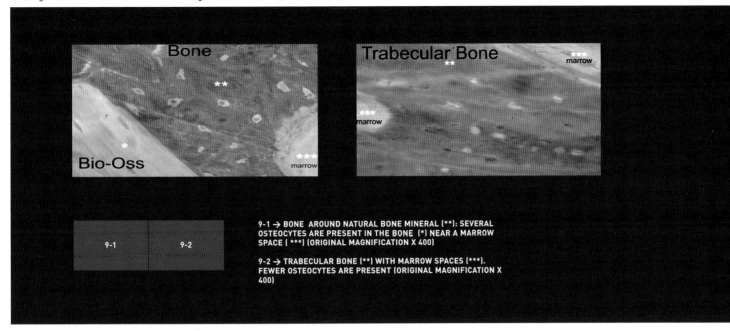

9-1 → BONE AROUND NATURAL BONE MINERAL (**): SEVERAL OSTEOCYTES ARE PRESENT IN THE BONE (*) NEAR A MARROW SPACE (***) (ORIGINAL MAGNIFICATION X 400)

9-2 → TRABECULAR BONE (**) WITH MARROW SPACES (***). FEWER OSTEOCYTES ARE PRESENT (ORIGINAL MAGNIFICATION X 400)

were affected by peri-implantitis. Machine screw-type implants showed a similar survival rate compared with cylinders in sinuses grafted with natural bone mineral alone, without being affected by peri-implantitis.

APPLICATIONS FOR MEMBRANES IN SINUS FLOOR ELEVATIONS

Although the use of membranes for covering the access window to the sinus cavity is a common application, resorbable collagen membranes can be used to cover small- to medium-sized perforations in the Schneiderian membrane (McAllister et al. 1998). Such perforations are a common practical problem. Hallmann et al. (2002) reported on perforated Schneiderian membranes in nine out of 30 sinus augmentation procedures in a clinical study. They used a membrane (Bio-Gide, Geistlich Pharma, Wolhusen, Switzerland) to cover these perforations. Collagen seems to be a suitable material because in moist conditions the collagenous structure sticks to the sinus membrane and seals the tears. Thereby loss of graft particles into the sinus cavity is avoided.

It can be assumed that this may also protect against postoperative infection via the respiratory tract.

CONCLUSIONS

Important evidence for the suitability and efficacy of a bone substitute are the histological results in patients. Various publications are available in which the use of natural bone mineral alone or in combination with autogenous bone has been investigated in sinus floor elevations. Its high osteoconductivity has been confirmed repeatedly. Different histological and histomorphometric analyses allow the conclusion that the bone substitute increases the mineral level of the augmented areas while decreasing the bone marrow space. The mean area density of natural bone mineral varied in the different studies from approximately 10 to 30%. In studies comparing grafted and non-grafted areas, the bone density in both regions was very similar.

It can be speculated that an increased mineral density results in stronger implant anchorage. The results from a study on sheep support this (Haas et al. 1998). In implant pull-out tests 12 to 26 weeks after sinus augmentation, higher initial pull-out strength with natural bone mineral compared with autogenous grafts or the non-grafted control was found. Pull-out forces, both for the bone substitute and for autogenous bone graft, increased to similar values over the 26 weeks. However, the authors did not analyze the area density of the different components (bone substitute, bone marrow, new bone), so conclusions cannot be drawn regarding a causal relationship.

The evidence available demonstrates that sinus floor augmentation procedures can be performed predictably with a suitable bone substitute without the addition of autogenous bone. This can be a major advantage for patients because harvesting of autogenous bone from the chin or hip can be avoided.

REFERENCES

1 Ackermann K.L, Kirsch A., Schober C.
Phykogenes, bovines und korallines Hydroxylapatit als Augmentationsmaterial des recessus alveolaris maxillae: Eine vergleichende Studie.
Z. Stomatol. 1994; 91: 219-24,

2 Araújo MG, Carmagnola D., Berglundh T., Thilander B., Lindhe J.
Orthodontic movement in bone defects augmented with Bio-Oss®.
J. Clin. Periodontol. 2001; 28: 73-80,

3 Artzi Z., Tal H., Dayan D.
Porous bovine bone mineral in healing of human extraction sockets. Part 1: Histomorphometric evaluations at 9 months.
J. Periodontol. 2000; 71: 1015-23.

4 Benezra Rosen V., Hobbs LW, Spector M.
The ultrastructure of anorganic bovine bone and selected synthetic hydroxyapatites used as bone graft substitute materials.
Biomaterials 2002; 23: 921-8.

5 Haas R, Mailath G, Dörtbudak O, Watzek G.
Bovine hydroxyapatite for maxillary sinus augmentation: analysis of interfacial bond strength of dental implants using pull-out tests.
Clin. Oral Implant Res. 1998; 9: 117-22.

6 Hallmann M., Sennerby L., Lundgren S.
A clinical and histologic evaluation of implant integration in the posterior maxilla after sinus floor augmentation with autogenous bone, bovine hydroxyapatite, or a 20:80 mixture.
Int. J. Oral Maxillofac. Implants 2002; 17: 635-43.

7 Hämmerle C, Karring T.
Guided bone regeneration at oral implant sites.
Periodontol. 2000 1998; 17: 151-75.

8 Hürzeler M.B., Kohal R.J., Naghshbandi J., Mota L.F., Conradt J., Hutmacher D., Caffesse R.G.
Evaluation of a new bioresorbable barrier to facilitate guided bone regeneration around exposed implant threads.
Int. J. Oral Maxillofac. Surg. 1998; 27: 315-20.

9 Hürzeler M.B., Quinones C.R., Kirsch A., Gloker C., Schüpbach P., Strub J.R., Caffesse R.G.
Maxillary sinus augmentation using different grafting materials and dental implants in monkeys. Part I. Evaluation of anorganic bovine-derived bone matrix.
Clin. Oral Implant Res. 1997a; 8: 476-86.

10 Hürzeler M.B., Quinones C.R., Kirsch A., Schüpbach P., Krausse A. et al.
Maxillary sinus augmentation using different grafting materials and dental implants in monkeys. Part III. Evaluation of autogenous bone combined with porous hydroxapatite.
Clin. Oral Implant Res. 1997b; 8: 401-11.

11 Jensen O.T., Greer R.O.
Immediate placement of osseointegrating implants into the maxillary sinus augmented with mineralised cancellous allograft and Gore-Tex: second-stage surgical and histological findings.
In: Laney W.R., Tolman D.E. (eds). Tissue Integration in Oral, Orthopedic and Maxillofacial Reconstruction. Chicago: Quintessence, 1992: 321-33.

12 Klinge B., Alberius P., Isaksson S., Jönsson J.
Osseous response to implanted natural bone mineral and synthetic hydroxylapatite ceramic in the repair of experimental skull bone defects.
J. Oral Maxillofac. Surg. 1992; 50: 241-9.

13 McAllister B.S., Margolin M.D., Cogan A.G., Taylor M., Wollins J. *Residual lateral wall defects following sinus grafting with recombinant human osteogenic protein-1 or Bio-Oss in the chimpanzee.*
Int. J. Periodontics Restorative Dent. 1998; 18: 227-39.

14 Maiorana C., Redemagni M., Rabagliati M., Salina S.
Treatment of maxillary ridge reabsorption by sinus augmentation with iliac cancellous bone, anorganic bovine bone, and endosseous implants: a clinical and histologic report.
Int. J. Oral Maxillofac. Implants 2000; 15: 873-8.

15 Maiorana C., Santoro F., Rabagliati M., Salina S.
Evaluation of the use of iliac cancellous bone and anorganic bovine bone in the reconstruction of the atrophic maxilla with titanium mesh: a clinical and histologic investigation.
Int. J. Oral Maxillofac. Implants 2001; 16: 427-432.

16 Mullender M.G., Tan S.D., Vico L., Alexandre C., Klein Nulend J.
Differences in osteocyte density and bone histomorphometry between men and women and between healthy and osteoporotic subjects.
Calcif. Tissue Int. 2005; 77: 291-6.

17 Müller K., Hürzeler M.B., Gläser R.
Kombination von verzögertem Sofortimplantat, Knochenregeneration und subepithelialem Bindegewebs-transplantat zur Verbesserung der Ästhetik.
Implantologie 1996; 4: 337-46.

18 Peetz M.
Characterization of xenogeneic bone material.
In: Boyne P. (ed) Osseous reconstruction of the maxilla and the mandible. Chicago: Quintessence Publishing, 1997: 87-100.

19 Piatelli M., Favero G.A., Scarano A., Orsini G., Piatelli A.
Bone reactions to anorganic bovine bone (Bio-Oss®) used in sinus augmentation procedures: a histologic long-term report of 20 cases in humans.
Int. J. Oral Maxillofac. Implants 1999; 14: 835-40.

20 Pripatnanont P., Nuntanaranont T., Chungpanich S.
Two uncommon uses of Bio-Oss for GTR and ridge augmentation following extractions: two case reports.
Int. J. Periodontics Restorative Dent. 2002; 22: 279-85.

21 Santoro F., Maiorana C.
Osseointegrazione Avanzata.
RC Libri 2001.

22 Schmitt J.M., Buck D.C., Joh S.P., Lynch E., Hollinger J.O.
Comparison of porous bone mineral and biologically active glass in critical-sized defects.
J. Periodontol. 1997; 68: 1043-53.

23 Schlegel K.A., Fichtner G., Schultze.Mosgau S., Wiltfang J.
Histologic findings in sinus augmentation with autogenous bone chips versus a bovine bone substitute.
Int. J. Oral Maxillofac Implants 2003; 18: 53-8.

24 Small S.A., Zinner I.D., Panno F.V., Shapiro H.J, Stein J.I.
Augmenting the maxillary sinus for implants: report of 27 patients.
Int. J. Oral Maxillofac. Implants 1993; 8: 523-8.

25 Smiler D.G., Hohnson P.W., Lozada J.I, Misch C., Rosenlicht J.L., Tatum J.R.H., Wagner J.R.
Sinus lift grafts and endosseous implants: Treatment of the atrophic posterior maxilla.
Dent Clin N Am 1992; 36: 151-86.

26 Tidwell J.K., Blijorp P.A., Stoelinga P.J.W., Brouns J.B., Hinderks F.
Composite grafting of the maxillary sinus for placement of endosteal implants: A preliminary report of 48 patients.
J. Oral Maxillofac. Surg. 1992; 22: 204-9.

27 Traini T., Valentini P., Iezzi G., Piatelli A.
A histologic and histomorphometric evaluation of anorganic bovine bone retrieved 9 years after a sinus augmentation procedure.
J. Periodontol. 2007; 78: 955-61.

28 Valentini P., Abensur D.
Maxillary sinus floor elevation for implant placement with demineralized freeze-dried bone and bovine bone (Bio-Oss®): A clinical study of 20 patients.
Int. J. Periodontics Restorative Dent. 1997; 17: 233-41.

29 Valentini P., Abensur D., Densari D., Graziani J.N., Hämmerle C.
Histological evaluation of Bio-Oss® in a 2-stage sinus floor elevation and implantation procedure.
Clin. Oral Implant Res. 1998; 9: 59-64.

30 Valentini P., Abensur D., Wenz B., Peetz M., Schenk R.
Sinus grafting with porous bone mineral (Bio-Oss®): A study on 15 patients.
Int. J. Periodontics Restorative Dent. 2000; 20: 245-52.

31 Valentini P., Abensur D.J.
Maxillary sinus grafting with anorganic bovine bone: A clinical report of long-term results.
Int. J. Oral Maxillofac. Implants 2003; 17: 556-60.

32 Wagner J.R.
A 3½ year clinical evaluation of resorbable hydroxylapatite OsteoGen (HA Resorb) used for sinus lift augmentation in conjunction with the insertion of endosseous implants.
J. Oral Implantol. 1991; 17: 152-64.

33 Wetzel A.C., Stich H., Caffesse R.G.
Bone apposition onto oral implants in the sinus area filled with different grafting materials.
Clin. Oral Implant Res. 1995; 6: 155-63.

34 Yildirim M., Spiekermann H., Handt S., Edelhoff D.
Maxillary Sinus Augmentation with the Xenograft Bio-Oss and autogenous intraoral bone for qualitative improvement of the implant site: a histologic and histomorphometric clinical study in humans.
Int. J. Oral Maxillofac Implants 2001; 16: 23-33.

35 Zitzmann N., Schärer P., Marinello C.
Long-term results of implants treated with guided bone regeneration: a 5-year prospective study.
Int. J. Oral Maxillofac. Implants 2001; 16: 355-66.

36 Zitzmann N., Schärer P., Marinello C., Schüpbach P., Berglundh T. *Alveolar ridge augmentation with Bio-Oss: a histologic study in humans.*
Int. J. Periodontics Restorative Dent. 2001; 21: 289-95.

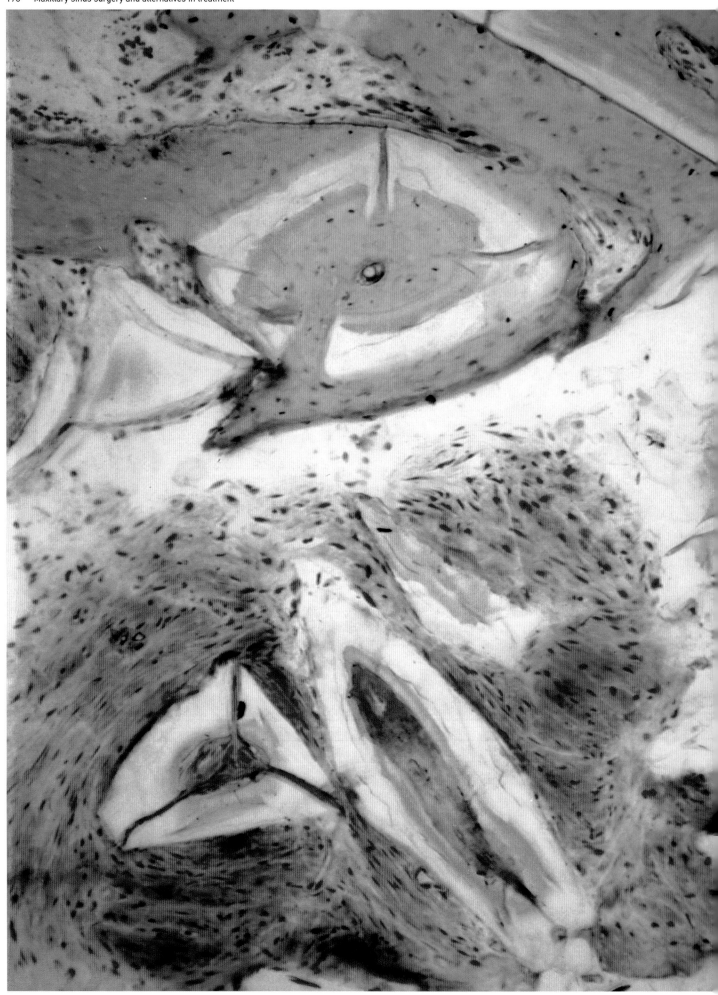

G. CORDIOLI
Z. MAJZOUB

Bioglass
in oral surgery

11

11

INTRODUCTION

Bioceramic materials generally include all inorganic, non-metallic materials intended for use on the human body as graft materials or as elements of prostheses. Depending on the characteristics of the bioceramic material, two types of biologic activity can be expressed:

- Osteoconductive activity: the property of a material acting as a scaffold in which the bone cells and vessels can migrate and proliferate. In histologic terms, bone growth begins from the bone tissue surface and gradually extends towards the material and the center of the defect (centripetal ossification, contact osteogenesis).
- Osteconductive activity: a material's capacity to stimulate the induction of local indifferentiated connective tissue cells or bone precursor cells into bone-forming osteoblasts. In histological terms, bone growth from the defect wall can be seen, but there is also growth in the filled defect and on the material's surface (centrifugal ossification, distance osteogenesis) **FIG.1A-B**.

Certain osteoinductive activity, i.e. a material's property to induce stem cells or osteoprogenitor cells to differentiate in osteoblasts and to induce high levels of osteoblast cell activity, has not been proven for bioceramic materials. The ability to induce bone growth in sites where bone tissue is absent is also present and this is shown by grafting the material in the muscular tissue. Ripamonti (1996) showed an induction of bone tissue in the rectus abdomini of several animals, using porous hydroxyapatite. Yuan et al. (2001) reported induction of bone tissue in dog muscle, using porous glass-ceramic combined with 45S5 BioGlass® as graft material.

Materials with osteoinductive properties are mainly organic, such as bone morphogenetic proteins and cytokines.

The following categories can be identified in the bioceramics family (Alexander et al. 1996):

- Inert bioceramic materials, such as aluminum dioxide, that does not wear and does not trigger immunologic reaction in tissues.
- Resorbable bioceramics, such as β-tricalcium phosphates, which are reabsorbed in the long term and which must then be replaced by natural tissue.
- Resorbable and non-resorbable bioactive bioceramics, such as hydroxyapatite and bioglass that can adhere to hard and soft tissue.

A simple classificaton of ceramic materials for medical use has been drawn up, with their chemical-physical characteristics and their biologic properties **TAB. 1**.

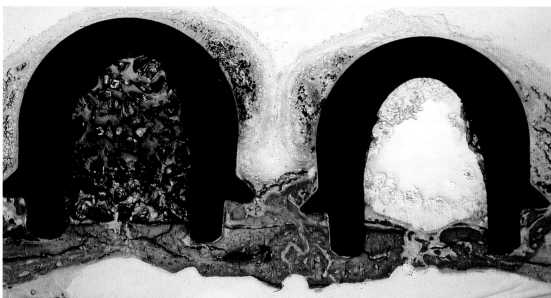

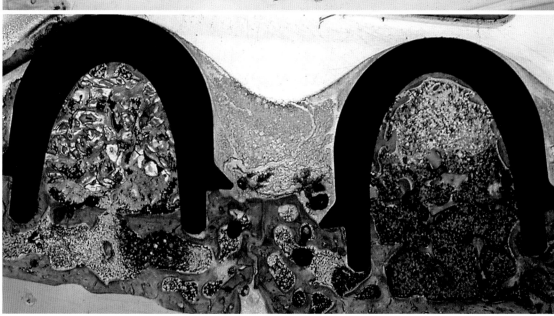

| 1A |
| 1B |

TAB. 1

TYPE OF BIOCERAMIC	TYPE OF ATTACHMENT	EXAMPLE
1	Dense, non-porous, inert or almost ceramic, that adheres via bone growth on the surface (defined as morphological fixation)	Alumina Al_2O_3 (mono and polycrystalline) Zirconium ($ZrSiO_4$)
2	Inert porous ceramic in which bone grows in the porosity, with a mechanical anchorage between material and bone (defined as biologic fixation)	Al_2O_3 (polycrystalline) Hydroxyapatite
3	Dense or porous, resorbable and non ceramics, with active surfaces, which attach directly to the bone tissue by chemical adhesion (named bioactive fixation)	Bioglass Bioactive glass-ceramic Hydroxyapatites Compound bioglass
4	Dense or porous resorbable ceramics that are slowly replaced by bone tissue	Calcium sulfate (plaster of Paris) Tricalcium phosfate calcium phosphate salts

BIOACTIVE MATERIALS

A bioactive material is one that triggers a specific biologic response on the interface of the material, resulting in the induction of adhesion between material and hard and soft tissue (Hench et al. 1972; Hench & Paschall 1974; Hench & Wilson 1984). This concept includes a large range of bioactive materials that have several characteristics and therefore various types of biologic behavior. The category can include bioactive glass such as BioGlass® (US Biomaterials, Baltimore, MD, USA) and PerioGlass® (US Materials), glass-ceramics such as Ceravital®, A/W glass-ceramics, dense hydroxyapatite such as Durapatite® or Calcitite®, and bioactive compounds such as Hapex®. The adhesion strength, the time and chemical-physical mechanisms used to develop these properties with hard and soft tissue are characteristics that vary among the various types of material.

One of the first active bioglasses was 45S5 BioGlass® synthesized by Hench at the end of the 1960s, made up of 45% SiO_2, 24.5% Na_2O, 24.5% CaO and 6% P_2O_5. Other active bioglasses studied are PerioGlass® and BioGran® (3i Implant Innovation, Palm Beach, FL, USA).

The high reactivity of these materials is linked to a sequence of chemical reactions that take place on the interface with vital or liquid tissue material, simulating the body fluid (SBF) plasma composition (Kokubo et al. 1992). The first phase is the loss of alkaline ions, such as Na^+, Ca^{+2} and K^+, from the bioglass surface and their exchange with hydrogen ions (H^+ or H_3O^+) coming from surrounding biologic fluids or from SBF. This exchange of ions takes place rapidly as soon as the bioglass comes into contact with the biologic tissue or with SBF. The loss of the Na^+, Ca^{2+} and K^+ ions causes a local breakage of the silicon and the consequent formation of soluble

$Si(OH)_4$, which in turn join together, creating a surface layer of silicon gel (SiOH) (Kokubo et al. 2003). After these chemical reactions, under a microscope the bioglass surface can be seen to be extremely porous with a pore size of 30 to 40 nm, with an area that develops to more than 100 m^2/g. It has been hypothesized that the loss of soluble silicon from the bioglass surface may be responsible for cell stimulation in the grafted tissue (Anderson et al. 1990). Further to the formation of the silicon gel layer, an amorphous layer of Ca and P ions are deposited on the surface ($CaOP_2O_5$). These have migrated from tissue fluids or from SBF, and incorporate biologic macro-molecules such as serum proteins, growth factors and collagen proteins. This amorphous layer of calcium phosphate ($CaOP_2O_5$) crystalizes, turning into a layer of hydroxy-carbonate apatite (HCA) by incorporation of OH^- and CO_3^{2-} from the surrounding environment. This layer of HCA develops within a few hours of the bioglass implantation. The layer of HCA is therefore responsible for the active bioglass capacity for adhesion to bone and soft tissue. This surface reaction continues until there is exhaustion of the ions in the internal part of the bioglass that serve in ion exchange on its surface. In the end, the layer of residual HCA will be incorporated into the newly formed bone.

The mechanism that causes this nucleation of HCA crystals on the surface of active bioglasses 45S5 BioGlass®, PerioGlass® and BioGran® is still the subject of intense research (Kontonasaki et al. 2002; Hench & Polak 2002) and is the basis of the peculiar characteristics of adhesion to hard and soft tissues of these materials.

This fast reactivity of the material's surface seems to be responsible for the histologic highlighting of the formation of bone tissue around the single particle, which occurs more rapidly than in other ceramic materials. The formation of bone around the single displaced particles far from the bone walls, limiting the defect has also been shown (Wilson & Low 1992). These histologic findings may be the evidence that the undifferentiated cells with osteogenic potential colonise the surface of the active bioglass particles, determining the beginning of the bone formation process simultaneously in various sites of the bone defect.

The sequence of biochemical reactions that occur on the active bioglass in contact with vital tissue or SBF solution has been outlined in table 2 **TAB. 2**.

Several *in vitro* research studies have recently been carried out on the cell-stimulation capacities of the various ions coming from the disintegration of active bioglass. Through microanalysis studies on cDNA, Xynos et al. (2001), demonstrated that ion products of the disintegration of 45S5 BioGlass® acts on the gene expression of human osteoblasts. In further *in vitro* research, Xynos found that the ions produced by the disintegration of BioGlass® 45S5 cause the proliferation of human osteoblasts, increase cellular protein synthesis and induce the mRNA expression of *insulin-like growth factor-II* (*IGF-II*) (Xynos et al. 2000). Loty et al. (2001), using fetal rat osteoblasts cultivated on active bioglass, showed the importance of the bioglass surface composition in promoting the differentiation of osteogenetic cells and the consequent formation of the bone matrix, which results in strong adhesion of the material to the bone tissue. Maroothynaden & Hench (2001) carried out *in vitro* and *in vivo* studies, showing that 45S5 BioGlass® induces a better proliferation and differentiation of bone cells. This phenomenon may be a factor that prevents the demineralization of bone tissue caused by age or under conditions of non-gravity. Oonoshi et al. (2000) demonstrated in an experimental study on animals that when applied in bone defects, BioGlass® 45S5 stimulates greater bone regeneration than synthetic hyroxyapatite and glass-ceramic. Gorustovich et al. (2002) found an increase in peri-implant bone formation in the marrow when particles of 45S5 BioGlass® were inserted at the same time as the implants.

1	INITIAL BIOGLASS SURFACE
2	EXCHANGE OF ALKALINE IONS NA⁺, CA²⁺, K⁺
3-4	DISINTEGRATION AND REPOLYMERIZATION OF THE SILICON SURFACE
5	PRECIPITATION OF AMORPHOUS LAYER OF CALCIUM PHOSFATE
6	ENUCLEATION AND CRYSTALLIZATION OF CALCIUM PHOSFATE INTO HCA
7	ABSORPTION OF PROTEINS, GROWTH FACTORS, ETC.
8	MACROPHAGE ACTION
9	ADHESION OF UNDIFFERENTIATED CELLS
10	CELL DIFFERENTIATION
11	ADHESION OF DIFFERENTIATED CELLS
12	CRYSTALLIZATION OF MATRIX

TAB. 2

Table of biochemical reaction sequences that develop on the active bioglass surface.

The variation in the stoichiometric composition of Bioglass® components brings about changes in their capacity for adhesion to tissues and is therefore different from other bioactive ceramic materials (Oonishi et al. 1995).

CLINICAL APPLICATIONS OF ACTIVE BIOGLASS

After BioGlass® was introduced at the end of the 1960s, and defined as the first synthetic material capable of adhering to hard and soft tissues (Hench et al. 1972; Wilson & Noletti 1990) the clinical applications of this material and other similar ones were then mainly directed to the reconstruction and the treatment of bone defects in various medical sectors.

One of the first clinical applications of BioGlass® or compound materials with bioglass was the reconstruction of middle ear ossicles (Merwin 1986).

In orthopedic and maxillofacial surgery, active bioglass has been used alone or together with various types of material (composite bioglass) for the reconstruction of bone segments or for filling bone defects (Schubert et al. 1988; Giannini et al. 1992; Wilson et al. 1993; Pavek et al. 1994; Kinnunen et al. 2000; Schulte et al. 2000; Aitasolo et al. 2001).

Bioactive glass has recently been the subject of intense experimental and clinical research in bone reconstruction applications in oral surgery, in periodontology and implantology [TAB. 3].

BIOGRAN®

A small-particle active bioglass with structural characteristics that are different from other active bioglass has recently been introduced into experimental and clinical practice. BioGran® is a resorbable amorphous bioglass in the form of granules 300 to 355 µm in size. Its chemical composition is 45% SiO_2, 24.5% CaO, 24.5% NaO_2 and 6% P_2O_5 (the same as BioGlass® and PerioGlass®). Its specific nature, however, is due to its capacity to increase bone repair, not only via the osteoconductive properties of its particle surface but also due to its osteostimulative capacities leading to bone formation inside the granules, even far from the bone wall limiting the defect (Ducheyne & Qiu 1990; Schepers et al. 1991, 1993, 1998a, 1998b; Schepers & Ducheyne 1993, 1997; Wheeler et al. 1998; Cancian et al. 1999). In this way, osteogenesis takes place on the surface and inside the granules [FIG. 2]. Based on these premises, which are perhaps improved in comparison with other types of bioglass, BioGran® is being used in multiple applications in the periodontal and implantology fields. After examining the literature on human clinical applications of BioGran® [TAB. 4] we can deduce that the use of this graft material has overall shown it to have a high osteoregenerative capacity in the treatment of periodontal bone defects and in the treatment of bone defects or bone atrophies in the maxilla and mandible [FIG. 3A-C]. Recently, however, in an experimental study on animals carried out to examine the long-term influence of Bio-Oss® and BioGran® on bone formation using the guided tissue regeneration (GTR) technique, Stavropoulos et al. (2003) histologically showed that in sites grafted with the materials, there was a lower amount of bone compared with non-grafted control sites and that the material's chips were mainly surrounded by connective tissue.

Author	Publication	Method	Parameters	X-ray	Conclusions
Knapp et al.	Int. J. Periodontics Restorative Dent. 2003	12 horizontal and vertical ridge increases with reinforced e-PTFE membranes and bioglass graft	Measurement of ridges before and after re-entry, biopsies at re-entry. 50% of membrane exposure	Yes	Bioglass graft with e-PTFE membrane does not bring about a notable increase in the bone volume of ridge deficiencies
Novaes et al.	Implant Dent. 2002	Case report: immediate post-extraction implant with use of membrane and bioglass graft	Clinical evaluation	Yes	After 6 months, the peri-implant defect was completely filled by mineralized tissue
Norton & Wilson	Int. J. Maxillofac. Implants 2002	Clinical cases with bioglass grafts in post-extraction sites and for the filling of ridge defects and the insertion of implants in grafted sites	Success of implants, histology of grafted sites	Yes	96.8% of success of implants at 3 years, the graft material has a reduced stimulative effect on the bone
Froum et al.	J. Periodontol. 2002	Comparison of bioglass and DFDBA bioglass in post-extraction sites in a human model	Histology at 8 months	No	Vital bone: 59.5% bioglass 34.7% DFDBA 32.4% control
Yukna et al.	J. Periodontol. 2001	Comparison between bioglass graft and use of e-PTFE membrane in the treatment of 27 grade II furcation lesions.	Periodontal indices and re-entry at 6 months	Yes	All the grade II furcations were transformed into grade I. No difference between the two types of treatment
Park et al.	J. Periodontol. 2001	38 periodontal bone defects, 21 grafts with Bioglass®, 17 check-ups	Periodontal indices	Yes	The use of Bioglass® grafts improves the CAL and BPD
Camargo et al.	Oral Surg. Oral Med. Oral Pathol. Oral Radiol. Endod. 2000	Postextraction graft with Bioglass® and coverage with calcium sulfate	Histology at 6 months with recovery	No	Test sites for more bone, less vertical resorption and similar horizontal resorption compared with control sites
Nevins et al.	Int. J. Periodontics Rest. Dent. 2000	5 periodontal defects treated with PerioGlass	Periodontal indices. Histology	Yes	Right-hand filling of defects. New bone in apical part of defect. No signs of periodontal regeneration except in one case.
Anderegg et al.	J. Periodontol. 1999	15 patients with mandibular molar furcation defects treated using open flap and active Bioglass® or flap alone	Periodontal indices	Yes	More positive results in defects treated with Bioglass® in grade II furcations
Lovelace et al.	J. Periodontol. 1998	Comparison of Bioglass® and DFDBA in treating periodontal defects after 6 months of healing	Periodontal indices	Yes	Similar results with the two graft materials
Low et al.	Int. J. Periodontics Restorative Dent. 1997	12 patients with periodontal defects grafted with Bioglass®	Periodontal indices at 3, 6 and 24 months	Yes	Average survery reduction of 3.33 mm. CAL gain of 1.92 mm Right-hand filling of defect of 3.47 mm
Zamet et al.	J. Clin. Periodontol. 1997	44 periodontal bone defects, split mouth, test site, bioglass graft site check-up, open flap curettage.	Periodontal indices at 3, 6, 9 and 12 months	Yes CADIA	improved PD, CAL, CADIA in test sites.
Shapoff et al.	Compendium Cont. Educ. Dent. 1997	37 bone defects treated with Bioactive glass and autogenous bone, bioactive glass and DFDBA. 6 month follow-up	Periodontal indices at 6 months	Yes	Significant clinical non-differences. At 6 months it is difficult to distinguish the Bioglass®

TAB. 3

Studies in literature on the use of active bioglass in bone and pariodontal tissue repair processes

CADIA, computer assisted densitometric image analysis; CAL, clinical attachment level; DFDBA, demineralized freeze-dried bone allograft; e-PTFE, expanded polytetrafluoroethylene; PD, probing depth

CONCLUSIONS

The biologic properties of bioglass have been the subject of several *in vitro* and *in vivo* studies in various branches of medicine. They have shown a particular efficiency in promoting the reconstruction of bone tissue, owing to their osteostimulative capacities. This osteogenetic potential is linked to the characteristics of the material's surface and the properties expressed by the bioglass disintegration products, which activate six families of genes in the bone cells. These genes stimulate cellular division and the matrix and growth factor synthesis by the bone

TAB. 4

Human clinical studies on the use of BioGran® in periodontology and in reconstructive bone surgery

CAL, clinical attachment level

Author	Newspaper	Experiment	Parameters	X-ray	Conclusions
Throndson & Sexton	Oral Surg. Oral Med. Oral Pathol. Oral Radiol. Endod. 2002	Extraction of 3rd mandibular molar. Split mouth design Test site with BioGran® graft, control site no filling	Periodontal clinical evaluation	Yes	Improved CAL on distal surface of 2nd molar in test sites. Bone levels equal
Tadjoedin et al.	Clin. Oral Implants Res. 2002	Sinus lift con split mouth. Test site 80–100% BioGran® with 0–20% autogenous bone. Autogenous bone control site	Histological		Bone density: Test site 27% at 4 months, 36% at 6 months, 39% at 15 months. Control site: 39% at 4 months, 41% at 6 months, 42% at 15 months
Cordioli et al.	Clin. Oral Implants Res. 2001	12 sinus lifts with BioGran® graft and autogenous bone in 4:1 proportion	Biopsies at 9/12 months. Implant follow-up 12 months	Yes	Bone density 30.6%. Implant success 100%
Tadjoedin et al.	Clin. Oral Implants Res. 2000	10 bilateral sinus lifts with one sinus filled with 1:1 BioGran® and autogenous bone, the other sinus is filled with bone only. Insertion of deferred implants	Histology and parameters of bone turnover at 4, 5, 6 and 16 months		41% bone density at 4 months, 42% at 5 months, 44% at 6 months, 46% at 16 months. Excavation of granules at 4 months and complete substitution at 16 months
Leonetti et al.	Implant Dent. 2000	Summers technique with BioGran® graft and insertion of implants	Clinical	Yes	Predictable method for inserting implants in the longer posterior-superior sectors
Rosenberg et al.	J. Esthet. Dent. 2000	12 pairs of periodontal bone defects. Split mouth design. Bioglass graft test site, no graft control site	Periodontal indices and re-entry at 6 months	Yes	Improved CAL and improved bone filling in test sites
Furusawa & Mizumuna	Implant Dent. 1997	25 sinus lifts and grafts with BioGran®	Histology and microanalysis after 7 months	Yes	Bone formation with similar biomechanical characteristics to control autogenous bone in all cases
Schepers et al.	Implant Dent. 1993	106 bone defects of varying types		Yes, at 2, 3, 6 months	After 3 months, the material begins to integrate with the bone tissue. At 6 months, material cannot be seen

cells. Several *in vitro* studies and animal experiments have shown the considerable potential of this bioglass in promoting bone regeneration. Further research is still needed concerning human clinical applications, in the form of randomized controlled clinical studies, long-term clinical studies and histologic data.

REFERENCES

1   Alexander H., Brunski J.B., Cooper S.L., Hench L.L., Hergenrother R.W, Hoffman A.S., Kohn J., Langer R., Peppas N.A., Ratner B.D., Shalaby S.W., Visser S.A., Yanmas I.V.
Classes of materials used in medicine. In Biomaterials Science: An introduction to Materials in medicine, Ratner B.D., Hoffman A.S., Schoen F.J., Lemons J.E. (eds.) Academic Press, New York 1996; 37-130.

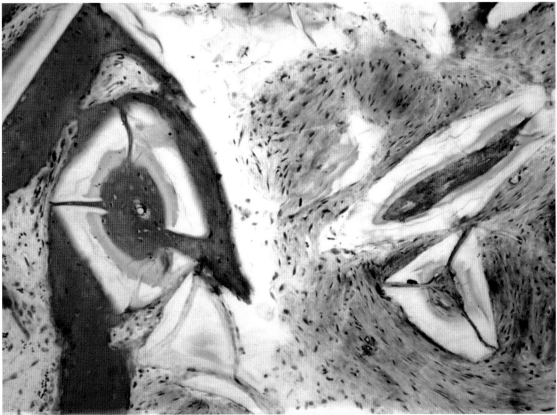

2 → HISTOLOGIC PICTURE OF BIOGRAN® GRANULES GRAFTED INTO A BONE DEFECT. NOTE THE BONE FORMATION IN THE GRANULE EXCAVATION THAT COMMUNICATES THROUGH SMALL FISSURES IN THE SURROUNDING TISSUE. THERE IS CONTINUITY BETWEEN THE EXTERNAL AND INTERNAL BONE TISSUE. OTHER GRANULES ARE STILL INCAPSULATED BY CONNECTIVE TISSUE. ONE OF THESE HAS AN OSTEOID TISSUE FORMATION INTERNALLY (ORIGINAL MAGNIFICATION 100 X).

3 A → LEFT MAXILLARY SINUS AUGMENTATION WITH AUTOGENOUS BONE GRAFT AND BIOGRAN® (RATIO 1/7).

3 B → PRE-OPERATIONAL DENTASCAN.

3 C → DENTASCAN BEFORE IMPLANT CONNECTION.

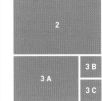

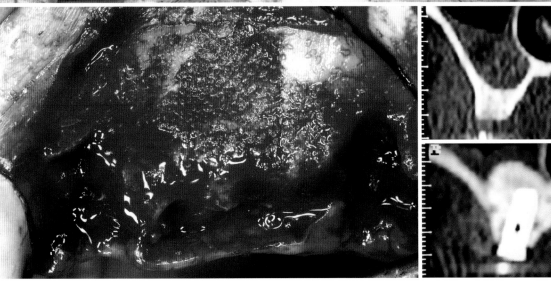

2   Anderegg C.R., Alexander D.C., Freidman M.
    *A bioactive glass particulate in the treatment of molar
    furcation invasions.*
    J. Periodontol. 1999; 70: 384-7.

3   Anderson O.H., Karlsson K., Kangasniemi I.
    *Calcium phosphate formation at the surface of bioactive
    glasses* in vivo.
    J. Non-Crystalline Solids 1990; 119: 290-6.

4   Camargo P.M., Lekovic V., Weinlaender M., Klokkevold P.R.,
    Kenney E.B., Dimitrijevic B., Nedic M., Jancovic S., Orsini M.
    *Influence of bioactive glass on changes in alveolar process
    dimension after exodontia.*
    Oral Surg. Oral Med. Oral Pathol. Oral Radiol. Endod.
    2000; 90: 581-6.

5   Cancian D.C., Hochuli-Vieira E., Marcantonio R.A.,
    Marcantonio R.A. Jr.
    *Use of BioGran and calcitite in bone defects: Histological
    study in monkeys (*Cebus apella*).*
    Int. J. Oral Maxillofac. Implants 1999; 14: 859-64.

6   Cordioli G.P., Mazzocco C., Brugnolo E., Majzoub Z.
    *Maxillary sinus floor augmentation using bioactive glass
    granules and autogenous bone with simultaneous implant
    placement: clinical and histological findings.*
    Clin. Oral Implant Res. 2001; 12: 270-8.

7   Ducheyne P., Qiu Q.
    *Bioactive ceramics: The effect of surface reactivity on bone
    formation and bone cell function.*
    Biomaterials 1990; 20: 2287-303.

8   Froum S., Cho S-C, Rosenberb E., Rohrer M., Tarnow D.
    *Histological comparison of healing extraction socket implanted
    with bioactive glass or demineralized freeze dried bone
    allograft: a pilot study.*
    J. Periodontol. 2002; 73: 94-102.

9   Furusawa T., Mizunuma K.
    *Osteoconductive properties and efficacy of resorbable bioactive
    glass as a bone-grafting material.*
    Implant Dent. 1997; 6: 93-101.

10 Giannini S., Moroni A., Pompili M., Ceccarelli F., Cantagalli S.,
    Pezzuto V., Trinchese L., Zaffe D., Venturini A., Pigato M.
    *Bioceramics in orthopaedic surgery: state of the art and pre-
    liminary results.*
    Ital. J. Orthop. Traumatol. 1992; 18: 431-41.

11 Gorustovich A,. Rosenbusch M., Guglielmotti M.B.
    *Characterization of bone around titanium implants and
    bioactive glass particles: An experimental study in rats.*
    Int. J. Maxillofac. Implants 2002; 17: 644-50.

12 Hench L.L. & Paschall H.A.
    Histochemical responses at a biomaterials interface.
    J. Biomed. Mater. Res. 1974; 5: 49-64.

13 Hench L.L. & Wilson J.
    Surface-active biomaterials.
    Science 1984; 226: 630-6.

14 Hench L.L., Polak J.M.
    Third-generation biomedical materials.
    Science 2002; 295: 1014-7.

15 Hench L.L., Sprinter R.J., Allen W.C., Greenlee Jr. T.K.
    Bonding mechanisms at interface of ceramic prosthetic materials.
    J. Biomed. Mater. Res. 1972; 2: 117-41.

16 Kinnunen I., Aitasalo K., Pollonen M., Varpula M.
    Reconstruction of orbital floor fracture using bioactive glass.
    J. Craniomaxillofac. Surg. 2000; 28: 229-34.

17 Knapp C.I., Feuille F., Cochran D.L., Mellonig T.J.
    *Clinical and histologic evaluation of bone-replacement grafts
    in the treatment of localized alveolar ridge defecys. Part 2:
    Bioactive glass particulate.*
    Int. J. Periodontics Restorative Dent. 2003; 23: 129-37.

18 Kokubo T., Kim H.M., Kawashita M.
    Novel bioactive materials with different mechanical properties.
    Biomaterials 2003; 24: 2161-75.

19 Kokubo T., Kushitaini H., Sakka S., Kitsugi T., Yamamuro Y.
    *Solutions able to reproduce in vivo surface-structure changes
    in bioactive glass ceramic A-W.*
    J. Biomed. Mater. Res. 1992; 26: 1147-61.

20 Kontonasaki E., Zorba T., Papadopoulou L., Pavlidou E.,
    Chatzistavrol X., Paraskevopoulos K., Koidis P.
    *Hydroxy Carbonate Apatite formation on particulate Bioglass®
    in vitro as a function of time.*
    Cryst. Res. Technol. 2002; 37: 1165-71.

21 Leonetti J.A., Rambo H.M., Throndson R.R.
    *Osteotome sinus elevation and implant placement with narrow
    size bioactive glass.*
    Implant. Dent. 2000; 9: 177-82.

22 Loty C., Sautier J.M., Tan M.T., Oboeuf M., Jallot E.,
    Boulekbach J., Greenspan D., Forest R.
    *Bioactive glass stimulate in vitro osteoblasts differentiation
    and creates a favorable template for bone tittue formation.*
    J. Bone Miner. Res. 2001; 16: 231-9.

23 Lovelace T.B., Mellonig J., Meffert R.M., Jones A.A.,
    Nummikoski P.
    *Clinical evaluation of bioactive glass in the treatment of
    periodontal osseous defects in human.*
    J. Periodontol. 1998; 69: 1027-35.

24 Low S.B., King C.J., Krieger J.
    *An evaluation of bioactive ceramic in the treatment of
    periodontal osseous defects.*
    Int. J. Periodontics Restorative Dent. 1997; 17: 359-5.

25 Maroothynaden J., Hench L.L.
    *Bioglass® stimulation of embryonic long-bones in altered
    loading enviroments.*
    J. Gravit. Physiol. 2001; 8: 79-80.

26 Merwin G.E.
    Bioglass middle ear prosthesis: preliminary report.
    Ann. Otol. Rhinol. Laryngol. 1986; 95: 78-82.

27 Nevins M.L., Camelo M., Nevins M., King C.J., Oringer R.J.,
    Schenk R.K., Fiorellini J.P.
    *Human histologic evaluation of bioactive ceramic
    in treatment of periodontal defects.*
    Int. J. Periodontics Restorative Dent. 2000; 20: 458-67.

28 Norton M.R. & Wilson J.
    *Dental implants placed in extraction sites implanted with
    bioactive glass: human histology and clinical outcome.*
    Int. J. Maxillofac. Implants 2002; 17: 249-57.

29 Novaes Jr A.B., Papalexiou V., Luczyszyn S.M., Muglia V.A.,
    Souza S.L., Taba Jr M.
    *Immediate implant in extraction socket with acellular dermal
    matrix graft and bioactive glass: a case report.*
    Implant Dent. 2002; 11: 343-8.

30 Oonishi H., Hench L.L., Wilson J., Sugihara F., Tsuji E.,
    Matsuura H., Kin S., Yamamoto T., Mizokawa S.
    *Quantitative comparison of bone growth behavior in granules
    of Bioglass®, A-W glass-ceramic and hydroxyapatite.*
    J. Biomed. Mater. Res. 2000; 51: 37-46.

31 Oonishi H., Kushitani S., Iwaki H., Saka K., Ono H., Tamura A., Sugihara T., Hench L.L., Wilson J., Tsuji E.
Comparative bone formation in several kinds of bioceramic granules. In: Wilson J., Hench L.L., Greespan D.C. (eds). Bioceramics 8. Amsterdam: Elsevier. 1995: 137-44.

32 Park J.S., Suh J.J., Choi S.H., Moo I.S., Cho K.S., Kim C.K., Chai J.K.
Effects of pretreatment clinical parameters on bioactive glass implantation in intrabony periodontal defects.
J. Periodontol. 2001; 72: 730-40.

33 Pavek V., Novak Z., Strnad Z., Kudrnova D., Navratilova B.
Clinical application of bioactive glass-ceramic BAS-O for filling cyst cavities in stomatology.
Biomaterials 1994; 15: 353-8.

34 Ripamonti U.
Osteoinduction in porous hydroxyapatite implanted in heterotopic sites of different animal models.
Biomaterials 1996; 17: 31-5.

35 Rosenberg E.S., Fox G.K., Cohen C.
Bioactive glass granules for regeneration of human periodontal defects.
J. Esthet. Dent. 2000; 12: 248-57.

36 Schepers E., Barbier L., Ducheyne P.
Implant placement enhanced by bioactive glass particles of narrow size range.
Int. J. Maxillofac. Implants 1998a; 13: 655-65.

37 Schepers E., De Clercq M., Ducheyne P., Kempeneers R.
Bioactive glass particulate material as a filler for bone lesions.
J. Oral Rehabil. 1991;18: 439-52.

38 Schepers E., Huygh A., Barbier L., Ducheyne P.
Microchemical analysis of bioactive glass particles of narrow size range. In: LeGeros R., LeGeros J. (eds). Bioceramics 11. NewYork: World Scientific 1998b; 559-62.

39 Schepers E.J.G., Ducheyne P.
Bioactive glass particles of narrow size range for the treatment of oral bone defects: a 1-24 month experiment with several materials and particles size and size range.
J. Oral Rehabil. 1997; 24: 171-81.

40 Schepers E.J.G., Ducheyne P.
The application of bioactive glass particulate of narrow size range as a filler material for bone lesions: a 24 months animal experiment. In: Bioceramic. Proceedings of the 6th International Symposium on Ceramics in Medicine. Philadelphia: Butterworth-Heinemann Ltd 1993; 6: 401-4.

41 Schepers E.J.G., Ducheyne P., Barbier L., Schepers S.
Bioactive glass particles of narrow size range: a new material for the repair of bone defects.
Implant Dent. 1993; 2: 151-6.

42 Schubert T., Purath W., Liebscher P., Schulze K.J.
Clinical indications for the use of jena bioactive, mechanically modifiable glass ceramics in orthopedics and traumatology.
Beitr. Orthop. Traumatol. 1988; 35: 7-16.

43 Schulte M., Schultheiss M., Hartwig E., Wilke H.J., Wolf S., Sokiranski R., Fleiter T., Kinzi L., Claes L.
Vertebral body replacement with a bioglass-polyurethane composite in spine metastases: clinical, radiological and biomechanical results.
Eur. Spine J. 2000; 9: 437-44.

44 Shapoff C.A., Alexander D.C., Clark A.E.
Clinical use of a bioactive glass particulate in the treatment of human osseous defects.
Compend. Contin. Educ. Dent. 1997; 18: 352-63.

45 Stavropoulos A., Kostopoulos L., Nyengaard JR., Karring T.
Deproteinized bovine bone (BioOss®) and bioactive glass (Biogran) arrest bone formation when used as adjunct to giuded tissue regeneration (GTR).
J. Clin. Periodontol. 2003; 30: 636-43.

46 Tadjoedin E.S., de Lange G.L., Holzmann P.J., Kulper L., Burger E.P.
Histological observations on biopsies harvested following sinus floor elevation using a bioactive glass material of narrow size range.
Clin. Oral Implants Res. 2000; 11: 334-44.

47 Tadjoedin E.S., de Lange G.L., Lyaruu D.M., Kuiper L., Burger E.P.
High concentrations of bioactive glass material (Biogran) vs. Autogenous bone for sinus floor elevation.
Clin. Oral Implants Res. 2002; 13: 428-36.

48 Throndson R.R., Sexton S.B.
Grafting mandibular third molar extraction sites: a comparison of bioactive glass to a nongrafted site.
Oral Surg. Oral Med. Oral Pathol. Oral Radiol. Endod. 2002; 94: 413-9.

49 Wheeler D.L., Stokes K.E., Hoellrich R.G., Chamberland D.L., McLoughlin S.W.
Effect of bioactive glass particle on osseous regeneration of cancellous defects.
J. Biomed. Mater. Res. 1998; 15: 527-33.

50 Wilson J., Low S.B.
Bioactive ceramics for periodontal treatment: comparative studies in the patus monkey.
J. Applied Biomater. 1992; 3: 123-9.

51 Wilson J., Noletti D.
Bonding of soft tissue to Bioglass®.
Handbook of bioactive ceramics 1990.

52 Wilson J., Clark A.E., Hall M., Hench L.L.
Tissue response to Bioglass® endosseous ridge maintenance implants.
J. Oral Implantol. 1993; 19: 295-302.

53 Xynos I.D., Edgar A.J., Buttery L.D., Hanch L.L., Polak J.M.
Gene-expression profiling of human osteoblasts following treatment with the ionic products of Bioglass® 45S5 dissolution.
J. Biomed. Mater. Res. 2001; 55: 151-7.

54 Xynos I.D., Edgar A.J., Buttery L.D., Hanch L.L., Polak J.M.
Ionic products of bioactive glass dissolution increase proliferation of human osteoblasts and induce insulin like growth factor II mRNA expression and protein synthesis.
Biochem. Biophys. Res. Commun. 2000; 24: 461-5.

55 Yuan H., de Bruijn J.D., Zhang X., van Blitterswijk C.A., de Groot J.D.
Bone induction by porous glass ceramic made from Bioglass® (45S5).
J. Biomed. Mater. Res. 2001; 58: 270-6.

56 Yukna R.A., Evans G.H., Aichelmann-Reidy M.B., Mayer E.T.
Clinical comparison of bioactive glass bone replacement graft material and expanded polytetrafluoroethylene barrier membrane in treating human mandibular molar class II furcations.
J. Periodontol. 2001; 72: 125-33.

57 Zamet J.S., Darbar U.R., Griffiths G.S., Bulman J.S., Bragger U., Burgin W., Newman H.N.
Particulate Bioglass® as a grafting material in the treatment of periodontal intrabony defects.
J. Clin. Periodontol. 1997; 24: 410-8.

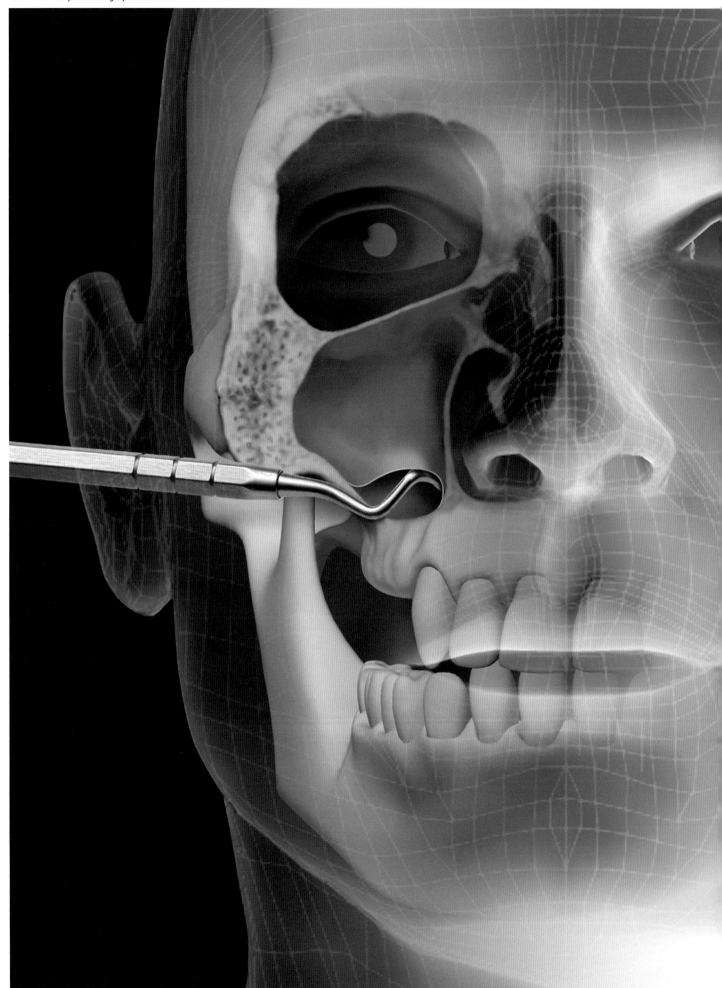

T. TESTORI
S.S. WALLACE

Surgical procedures:
lateral window approach

12

12

anesthesia. An ideal anesthetic drug is articaine hydrochloride 4% (400 µg/l) with epinephrine (adrenaline) 1:100,000. Due to its high protein linkage, this molecule delivers a more rapid onset than other anesthetics and gives effective, long-lasting anesthesia.

FLAP DESIGN

Before making the access flap, the following factors must be taken into consideration:
*   mesio-distal position of the sinus
*   location of the sinus floor
*   ideal position of the antrostomy
*   position and amount of the keratinized gingiva
*   presence/absence of teeth.

The length of the incision must take into consideration any bone regeneration therapies that the surgeon may need to perform during the surgery. However, maxillary sinus elevation does not affect the transverse relationship between the maxilla and the mandible FIG. 1.

The incision must be full thickness and can be midcrestal or palatal in position, the latter variant is recommended if there is a muscular insertion on the ridge, if the keratinized gingiva is insufficient, or if it is less than 2 to 3 mm from the center of the ridge to the mucogingival junction. The presence of keratinized

ANESTHESIA

Proper anesthesia is an essential requirement to guarantee optimal patient comfort during surgery and to better control the surgical site. Subperiostal anesthesia via slow infiltration is recommended, maintaining a speed of 1 ml/min, in order to achieve maximum efficacy and duration.

To aid in surgical access, the authors strongly suggest that an infiltration should also be carried out on the labial commissure, to prevent the patient's defensive reactions, which tend to contract the cheeks, thereby reducing access to the surgical site. The standard technique entails vestibular and palatal plexus

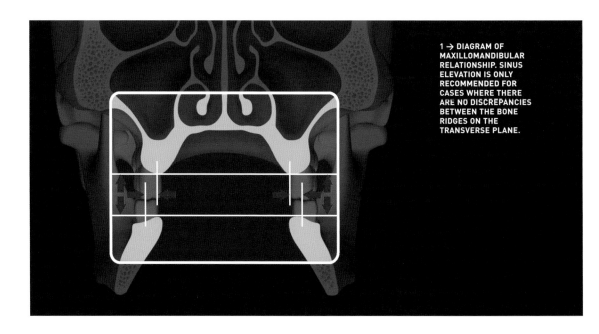

1 → DIAGRAM OF MAXILLOMANDIBULAR RELATIONSHIP. SINUS ELEVATION IS ONLY RECOMMENDED FOR CASES WHERE THERE ARE NO DISCREPANCIES BETWEEN THE BONE RIDGES ON THE TRANSVERSE PLANE.

tissue on both edges of the incision aids suturing, and the palatal positioning of this incision should be limited so that it is possible to maintain vascular support and avoid necrosis in the palatal portion of the flap.

If the sinus extends into the first premolar, a hockey-stick incision should be made that is mesial to the canine and beveled into the attached gingiva starting from the line-angle between the vestibular side and the approximal line angle of the tooth.

If the sinus is located in the first/second premolar area, the incision will begin distally from the canine.

Depending on the clinical situation, the incision may be sulcular or submarginal.

The former is recommended if there are natural teeth with no periodontal disease and if the incision ends with a microsurgical suturing technique **FIG. 2**. If the teeth are prepared, an incision apical to the probing depth is preferable, especially in thin periodontal biotypes.

If bone is to be taken from the tuberosity, the crestal incision can extend over it to allow for the simultaneous exposure of the donor site **FIG. 3**.

The vertical releasing incision must be made parallel to the vascular supply and depends on the antero-posterior extent of the sinus and the position of the planned antrostomy.

FLAP ELEVATION

When performing the full-thickness mucoperiosteal flap elevation, the elevator must be adherent to the bone surface, so that the periosteum remains undamaged.

Correct design and flap elevation allow excellent control of hemostasis, which in turn is dependent on several factors **TAB. 1**.

Once the lateral wall is exposed, the cortical bone over the window (which has few vascular channels) can easily be distinguished from the more vascular (cancellous) bone located anterior and crestal to the sinus. In some cases, the posterior-superior alveolar artery can be seen as it emerges through the lateral wall in an anterior-posterior direction **FIG. 4**.

If the area bleeds excessively, gauze should be used and pressed for 5 minutes on the vestibular fornix area.

In cases where the preoperative computerized tomography (CT) scan shows a lack of vestibular bone or a sinus communication, the surgeon must proceed carefully. During flap elevation, it is necessary to dissect the flap from the sinus membrane **FIG. 5A-C**.

• Evaluation of the patients' clinical history; check for drugs that may interfere with coagulation
• Utilize sedation to obtain a reduction in heart rate and blood pressure
• Operate on inflammation-free tissue
• Utilize correct anesthesia
• Correct flap design and elevation, preserve periosteum
• Complete surgery in less than 1.5 hours

TAB. 1

Obtaining optimal hemostatis

ANTROSTOMY

The position of the antrostomy is determined by the size and location of the maxillary sinus.

The antrostomy can easily be carried out with cooled sterile saline irrigation, using a high-speed (50,000 rpm) straight surgical handpiece and a tungsten carbide bur with a 2.3 mm diameter. When the membrane is visible as a blue shadow, it is advisable to switch to a diamond bur (ISO 2.3), which is less likely to create a perforation in the event of accidental contact with the thin sinus membrane. A high-speed handpiece with a No. 8 diamond bur can also be used. If the cortical wall is thin and the membrane appears as soon as the flap has been elevated (blue shadow), it is appropriate to begin immediately with the less aggressive diamond bur.

It has been shown that the utilization of piezoelectric surgery when making the antrostomy and performing the initial membrane elevation reduces the incidence of accidental membrane perforation from the rotary instrumentation average from 25% to 7% or below (Vercellotti et al. 2001; Wallace et al. 2007; Blus et al. 2008) **FIG. 6A-B**.

If the lateral wall is more than 2 mm thick, the cortical bone can be eroded using a piezoelectric osteoplasty insert or a manual bone scraper (Safescraper® BioMet 3i, West Palm Beach, FL, USA) that allows for the reduction of the thickness of the bone and collection of the bone chips, which may be used as an autogenous graft material.

The antrostomy is normally oval in shape and should not have sharp edges that may cause perforations of the Schneiderian membrane during the elevation. However, the shape may vary depending on the presence of septa, and may even be kidney-shaped to efficiently manage the presence of any maxillary septa (also called Underwood's septa) **FIG. 7A-B**. Another technique is to divide the antrostomy into two

separate osteotomies to gain access to both sides of the septum. In some cases, it is possible to cut off the base of the septum and remove it, or lift it with the membrane. The size of the antrostomy depends on the vertical elevation required and the number of implants that are to be placed. On average, an antrostomy size of 20 mm mesio-distally and 15 mm apico-coronally is sufficient to guarantee easy surgical access. When the surgeon's experience level is such that he/she can safely elevate the membrane with reduced access, a smaller, more conservative access window can be made. This will retain a larger source of blood supply to the lateral wall and perhaps enhance the maturation of the graft.

The technique can be modified in relation to the position and the course of the vascular anastomosis in the bony lateral wall.

Vascularization of the grafting material placed in sinus floor elevation procedures occurs via the following three routes (Solar et al. 1999).

- Extraosseous anastomosis (EA) occurs via the terminal branch of the posterior superior alveolar artery (PSAA) branch of the maxillary artery (MA), with an extraosseous terminal branch of the intraorbital artery (IOA), another branch of the MA. It runs at a mean height of 23 to 26 mm from the alveolar margin. An extraosseous vestibular vascular anastomosis was observed in 44% of cases. The vessels may cause hemorrhage during flap preparation and periosteum-releasing incisions.
- Intraosseous anastomosis (IA) or alveolo-antral artery occurs via the second branch of PSAA (dental branch) with the IOA. It runs at a distance of 18.9 to 19.6 mm from the alveolar margin.
- Branches of these three vessels (PSAA, IOA and IA) in the sinus membrane.

The middle portion of the Schneiderian membrane is supplied by the sphenopalatine artery, the terminal branch of the MA.

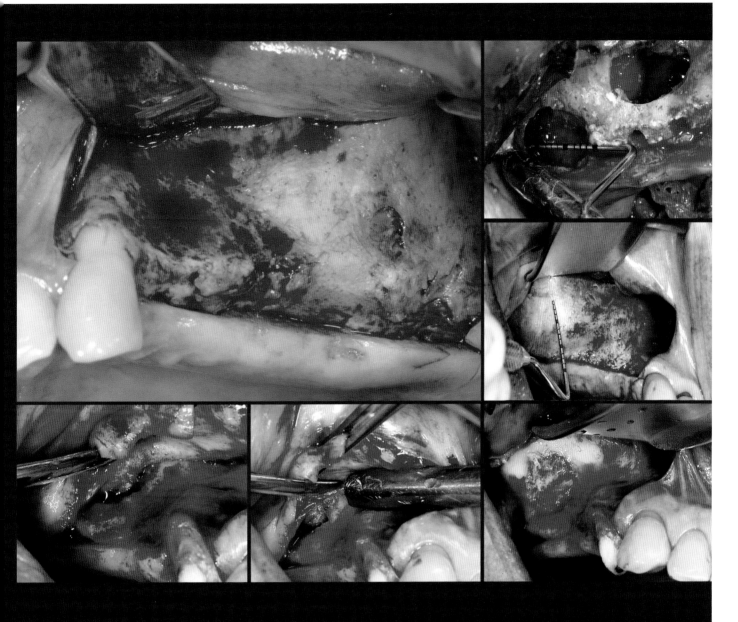

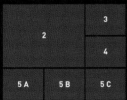

2 → WHEN ADJACENT TEETH ARE PERIODONTALLY HEALTHY THE RECOMMENDED HORIZONTAL INCISION MAY BE INTRASULCULAR AROUND THE NATURAL TEETH, CRESTAL OR SLIGHTLY TO THE PALATE.

3 → IF BONE IS TO BE HARVESTED FROM THE TUBEROSITY, THE HORIZONTAL INCISION MAY EXTEND DISTALLY UNTIL THE DONOR SITE IS EXPOSED.

4 → ELEVATING THE FLAP MAY REVEAL THE INTRAOSSEOUS ANASTOMOSIS.

5 A → INITIAL ELEVATION SHOWS A COALESCENCE BETWEEN THE PERIOSTEUM AND THE PERIOSTEAL PART OF THE SCHNEIDERIAN MEMBRANE. THE TISSUE LAYERS ARE CAREFULLY SEPARATED BY SPLIT-THICKNESS DISSECTION TO AVOID PERFORATING THE SINUS MUCOSA.

5 B → LATER STAGES OF FLAP ELEVATION.

5 C → FLAP COMPLETELY DISSECTED FROM THE SINUS MUCOSA, WITHOUT PERFORATION.

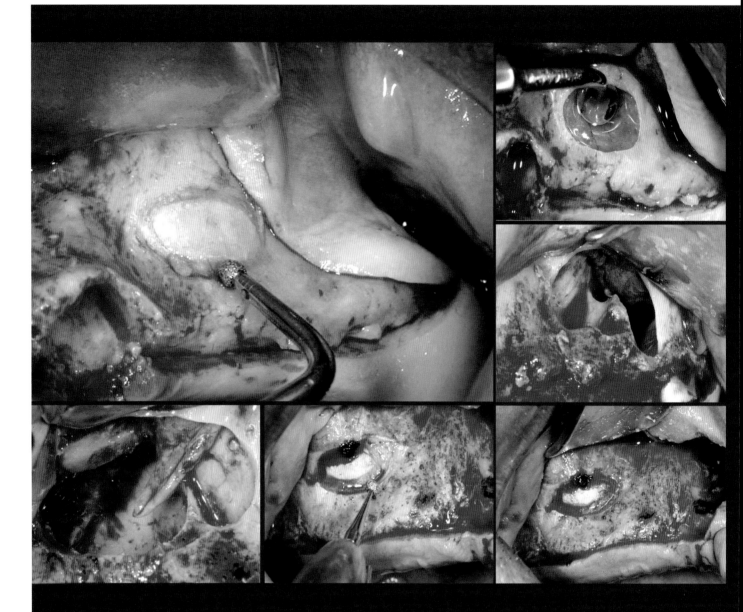

6 A → PREPARATION OF ANTROSTOMY USING PIEZOELECTRIC INSERTS.

6 B → INITIAL PHASE OF SINUS ELEVATION, USING PIEZOELECTRIC INSTRUMENTS.

7 A → IN THE EVENT OF LARGE SINUS SEPTA, THE ANTROSTOMY SHAPE MAY BE ALTERED.

7 B → FULLY ISOLATED BONE SEPTUM.

8 A-B → REPAIR OF ANTROSTOMY USING ROTARY INSTRUMENTATION. IF THE ARTERY IS SEVERED, IT IS POSSIBLE TO CONTROL BLEEDING BY ELECTRO-CAUTERIZATION, TAKING CARE TO AVOID DAMAGING THE SINUS MEMBRANE.

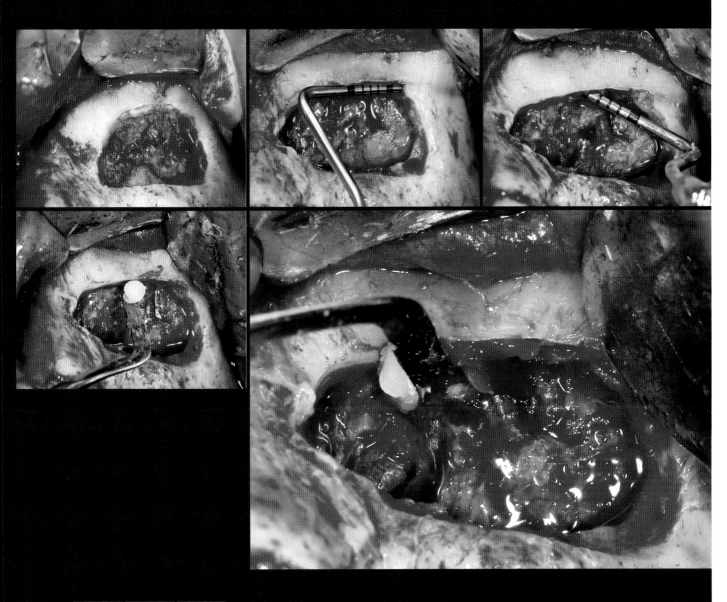

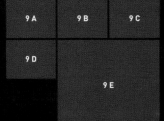

9 A → INTRAOSSEOUS ANASTOMOSIS OF THE ARTERY CAN BE SEEN ALONG THE UPPER EDGE OF THE ANTROSTOMY.

9 B → THE DIAMETER OF THE VESSEL IS MEASURED WITH A PERIODONTAL PROBE FOR TEACHING PURPOSES TO SHOW THE SIZE OF THE VESSEL. IN THIS CASE, THE DIAMETER WAS 0.75 MM.

9 C → PROBING OF THE MESIAL VASCULAR TRUNK.

9 D-E → IF THE INTRAOSSEOUS ANASTOMOSIS IS LACERATED AND NOT TREATED, SIGNIFICANT BLEEDING OR HEMATOMAS MAY OCCUR AT THE END OF THE VASOCONSTRICTIVE EFFECT OF THE ANESTHESIA. IN THE EVENT OF THE VESSEL BEING CUT, USE OF BONE WAX OR CAUTERIZATION IS RECOMMENDED TO CONTROL BLEEDING.

10 → ANGLE BETWEEN THE LATERAL AND MEDIAL WALL OF THE SINUS: NARROW ANGLES RESULT IN HIGHER PERFORATION RATES.

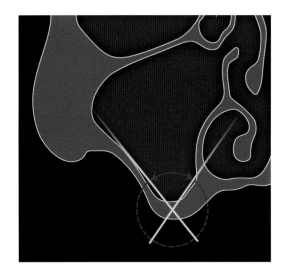

The antrostomy can be moved coronally to avoid damaging the artery, which normally has an anterior-posterior course. If the antrostomy must be made over the vessel, piezoelectric surgery can be used to keep the vessel intact.

The diameter of the intraosseos vessel is normally between 0.5 and 1 mm and can be assessed using a periodontal probe.

If the artery is severed during surgery, to avoid bleeding and possible hematoma formation it may be necessary to electro-cauterize the two trunks of the vessels with specific bipolar devices FIG. 8A-B. An alternative is to use Bone Wax (Johnson & Johnson, Brussells, Belgium) on each end FIG. 9A-E. Once the vasoconstrictive effect of the local anesthesia has ended, a severed, but untreated anastomosis may cause postoperative bleeding.

TAB. 2

Position of antrostomy

Apical: height of graft required, location of PAS artery
Coronal: 3 mm above the sinus floor
Mesial: as close to anterior wall as possible
Distal: determined by number of implants to be placed

At the beginning of the learning curve, the linear dimensions of the antrostomy should extend 20 mm mesiodistally and 15 mm craniocaudally, then reaching a more conservative antrostomy of about 15 mm mesiodistally and 10 mm craniocaudally for the positioning of three implants.

TAB. 3

Incidence of perforations in relation to the maxillary sinus anatomy

ANGLE BETWEEN THE LATERAL AND MEDIAL WALL	PERCENTAGE OF PERFORATIONS
Less than 30°	62.5%
Angle between 30° and 60°	28.6%
Angle greater than 60°	0%

TAB. 4

Types of antrostomy

ELEVATED ANTROSTOMY	
Indications	in clinical cases with good surgical access and the thickness of the cortical wall allows reflection (< 2 mm)

COMPLETE ANTROSTOMY	
Indications	in cases with more difficult surgical access and/or thick vestibular wall (> 2 mm)
	presence of septa
	shallow sinuses in the vestibular-palatal direction at the recess

The distal margin of the antrostomy is positioned in relation to the number of implants to be placed. The coronal part of the antrostomy is best made 3 to 4 mm above the sinus floor. The mesial part of the antrostomy should be as far forward as possible, 3 to 4 mm from the sloping anterior wall, as the anterior recess is usually narrow and is the site of a high incidence of surgical difficulties during membrane elevation **TAB. 3**.

A New York University (NYU) study showed a correlation between the percentage of perforations and the anatomy of the sinus, with the perforation rate in the narrow, anterior sinus being much higher than in the wider, posterior area (Cho et al. 2001). On a perpendicular CT section, it is possible to calculate the angle formed by the alveolar vestibular and palatal walls. If the angle is less than 30 degrees, the perforation percentage is much higher **FIG. 10, TAB. 2**.

Another anatomic factor that can affect the percentage of perforations is the presence of septa, normally encountered in 31 to 48% of cases (Ulm et al. 1995; Velásquez-Plata et al. 2002; Kim et al. 2006; Shibli et al. 2007; Zijderveld et al. 2008).

A CT-scan study has shown that septa tend to be lower on the lateral wall and become higher in proximity to the medial wall (Velazquez-Plata et al. 2002).

There is also correlation between the membrane thickness and the incidence of perforation. An NYU study (Cho et al. 2002) on 65 CT evaluations dividing the membranes into thin (less than 1.5 mm) and thick (more than 1.5 mm), found that the total perforation rate was 31% with thin membranes and 16.6% with thick membranes.

Once the osteotomy has been completed, the mobility of the antrostomy is tested by pressing slightly on the edges. Any residual bone bridges must be removed along the antrostomy perimeter to release the window, and sharp edges should be eliminated as they may cause membrane perforation during elevation.

There are two basic types of antrostomy. An elevated antrostomy leaves the cortical wall intact and adherent to the Schneiderian membrane. It is lifted inside the maxillary sinus and acts as the future sinus floor. To gain better access and vision, it is easier to partly or totally remove the vestibular bony wall, this procedure is called a complete antrostomy. Removal of the window portion of the lateral wall has not been shown to affect the clinical outcome of the procedure (Smiler 1997) **TAB. 4**.

SINUS MEMBRANE ELEVATION

When elevating the membrane it is critical to keep the elevators directly in contact with the bone at all times.

Sinus membranes with a thickness less than 3 or 4 mm can be elevated and do not represent a contraindication for sinus augmentation.

Using either manual or piezoelectric elevators the membrane is first carefully elevated, usually starting on the sinus floor and then extending to the anterior and posterior. The final elevation is up the medial wall to the full height of the expected graft placement **FIG. 11A-F**.

Perforations are statistically more frequent in the mesio-superior corner. To avoid such complications, it is recommended to extend the antrostomy mesially to allow direct access to the anterior sinus wall.

Elevation should proceed only where the membrane detaches easily. If the surgeon should encounter resistance to elevation, it is advisable not to continue pressing with a blunt instrument. Mucosal adherences to the underlying bone must be severed using sharp instruments, keeping them in close contact with the bone.

Depending on the anatomic configuration of the sinus, the surgeon can choose the instrument with the most suitable angle for elevating the membrane.

The sinus membrane's integrity can be tested by asking the patient to breathe in deeply while observing the membrane lifting. However, it is necessary to remember that small perforations cannot be detected using this type of test.

The sinus membrane must be elevated until the medial wall of the sinus can be seen. Elevating the membrane without exposing the medial sinus wall may result in a re-pneumatization of the sinus medially and result in insufficent bone for implant placement. Moreover, an elevation that reaches the medial wall exposes a greater area of bone surface, which enhances vascularity and also produces sufficient bone volume to allow for prosthetically guided implant placement (Peleg et al. 1999).

There are different biologic and prosthetic reasons that justify membrane elevation up to the medial sinus wall:

- vascularization is increased by exposing a greater bone surface area, an area from which the healing mechanisms start
- it improves graft stability, preventing re-pneumatization of the sinus
- it allows correct prosthetically guided implant positioning
- it maintains physiologic drainage with a new sinus floor
- the graft material should not elevate the sinus membrane any further as this uncontrolled elevation may cause accidental graft loss inside the sinus due to membrane perforation.

In cases of extreme pneumatization, the wall with the largest surface and, therefore, the largest vascular supply is the medial sinus wall. In fact, the surface of the medial sinus wall is larger than the bone surface of both the crestal and lateral walls combined. In cases with an extremely thin membrane it is advisable to protect the sinus membrane with a resorbable collagen barrier membrane before placing the graft.

A volumetric study of the maxillary sinus has found that on average, 5.46 cm^3 of material is needed to develop 15 mm of graft vertically (Uchida et al. 1998), a volume of 3.5 cm^3 is usually adequate for placing three 13 mm long implants.

The presence of mucous retention cysts, with the classic radiographic appearance of a 'rising sun', is not a contraindication for sinus augmentation procedures, as they can be treated during surgery. One possible treatment is needle-aspiration carried out using a normal calibre 22 syringe that aspirates the serum content of the cyst, hence collapsing the cyst walls. This procedure can be carried out before or during membrane elevation, depending on the diameter and position of the cysts. Large cysts near to the antrostomy are easier to needle-aspirate before elevating the membrane. It is difficult to elevate a membrane in the presence of a large-sized cyst because of downward pressure due to its weight or the possibility that, once elevated, it may block the osteum.

PREPARATION OF IMPLANT SITE

If there is a minimum of 3 to 4 mm of the residual crestal bone of good quality, it is possible to place the implants simultaneously. In clinical cases with type 3 and 4 crestal bone, undersizing the implant site is recommended. While preparing the implant site it is advisable to protect the sinus membrane with a periosteal elevator, to avoid damaging the membrane with the burs.

If the residual crestal bone is less than 3 or 4 mm, it is advisable to elevate the sinus membrane first and place the implants in a staged approach.

In some cases with good bone quality (type 2 bone), implants can be inserted simultaneously, even if there is only 1 to 3 mm of residual crestal bone (Peleg et al. 2006; Mardinger et al. 2007).

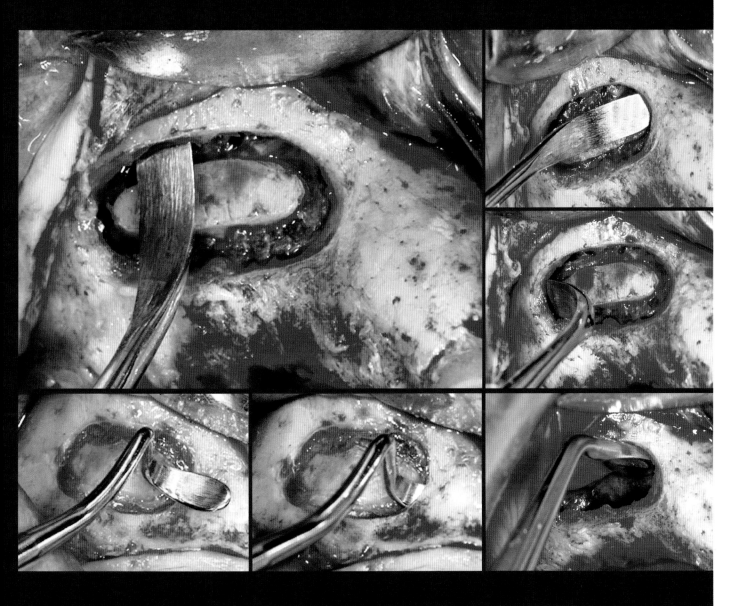

	11 B
11 A	11 C

| 11 D | 11 E | 11 F |

11 A → INITIAL PHASE OF SINUS ELEVATION WITH MANUAL INSTRUMENTS. THE INITIAL APPROACH IS BEST MADE ALONG THE APICAL EDGE OF THE ANTROSTOMY.

11 B-C → INITIAL PHASES OF SINUS ELEVATION MESIALLY AND DISTALLY. SPECIFIC ELEVATORS ARE DESIGNED TO REACH THE ANTERIOR AND POSTERIOR RECESSES.

11 D-E → ELEVATORS MUST BE KEPT IN DIRECT CONTACT WITH THE BONE TO AVOID PERFORATING THE MEMBRANE.

11 F → THE ELEVATION IS CONTINUED, TO EXPOSE THE MEDIAL SINUS WALL.

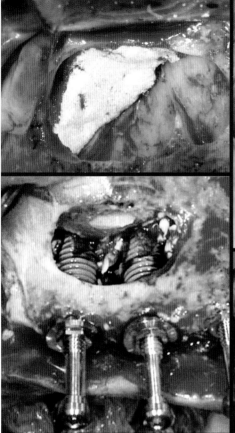
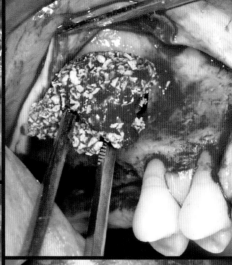
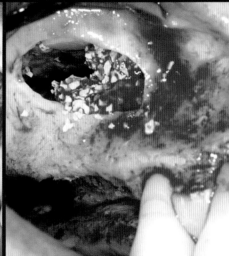
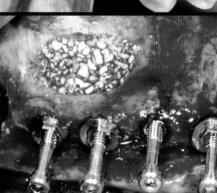
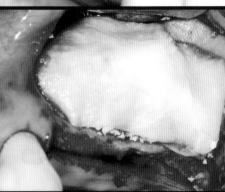

SURGICAL PROCEDURE OF GRAFT AND IMPLANT PLACEMENT

12 A		
	12 B	12 C
12 D	12 E	12 F

12 A → A COLLAGEN MEMBRANE MAY BE PLACED TO PROTECT THE SINUS MEMBRANE FROM MICRO-LACERATIONS DURING GRAFT INSERTION. THE ADVANTAGE OF USING A COLLAGEN MEMBRANE LIES IN ITS TENDENCY TO ADHERE AND STICK TO THE SINUS MUCOSA.

12 B → INITIAL PHASE OF GRAFT PLACEMENT (ABBM).

12 C → THE GRAFT IS FIRST PLACED IN THE ANTERIOR RECESS AND ALONG THE MEDIAL SINUS WALL.

12 D → IMPLANT POSITIONING.

12 E → GRAFTING IS COMPLETED. IT MUST BE REMEMBERED THAT THE MATERIAL MUST BE COMPACTED AGAINST THE BONE WALLS IN ORDER NOT TO LEAVE VOIDS.

12 F → PLACEMENT OF A BIOABSORBABLE BARRIER MEMBRANE ABOVE THE ANTROSTOMY.

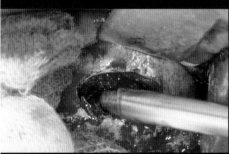
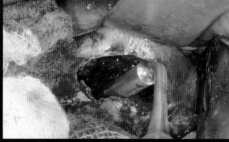
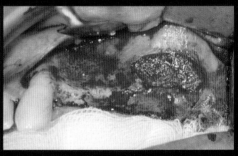

ISOLATION OF THE SURGICAL FIELD AND SURGICAL PLACEMENT OF THE GRAFT USING SPECIFIC INSTRUMENTS

12 G	12 H	12 I

12 G → ISOLATION OF THE SURGICAL FIELD WITH STERILE GAUZES AND PLACEMENT OF GRAFT USING SPECIFIC INSTRUMENTS (CARRIERS): IN THIS WAY, PLACEMENT IS MORE PRECISE AND ANY BACTERIAL CONTAMINATION IS PREVENTED.

12 H → USE OF SPECIFIC COMPACTOR FOR IMPROVED ADAPTATION OF GRAFT MATERIAL.

12 I → FILLING IS COMPLETE WHEN THE LATERAL WALL CONTOUR IS RESTORED.

Recent systematic reviews (Wallace & Froum 2003; Del Fabbro et al. 2004) showed that there is no statistically significant difference between simultaneous and delayed implant placement protocols.

PLACING THE GRAFT AND THE IMPLANTS

The graft material should be positioned starting from the least accessible areas, taking care to place the graft in contact with the bony walls to aid in the healing process. The sinus membrane, if thin, may be protected with a collagen membrane. The anterior and posterior recesses are filled first, followed by the area along the medial sinus wall. The graft should not elevate the membrane any further and must not be compacted too densely, as this may prevent vascularization, especially with biomaterial grafts.

Placement of graft material should be limited distally and apically, to the extent needed to place the planned number of implants, as overfilling may lengthen the graft maturation time.

Subsequently the implants are placed in the prepared implant sites. Rough-surface implants have shown a higher survival rate than those with smooth surfaces (Wallace & Froum 2003; Del Fabbro et al. 2004).

The graft is then finalized, filling the residual space up to the lateral wall of the sinus.

Correct maxillary sinus elevation, observing the above-mentioned procedures, does not change sinus physiology and does not produce any change to the tone of voice (Tepper et al. 2003).

A resorbable membrane is then placed over the antrostomy **FIG. 12A-I**. Several clinical studies (Tarnow et al. 2000; Tawil & Mawla 2001; Wallace et al. 2005) have shown that the placing of a membrane results in a higher percentage of vital bone and a higher implant

survival rate. A recent NYU study also showed that there is no difference between using a collagen membrane rather than an expanded polytetrafluoroethylene (e-PTFE, Gore-tex) membrane (Wallace et al. 2005). The collagen membrane's adherence capacity allows it to be placed without fixation screws and, as it is resorbable, it avoids subsequent removal procedures.

When choosing the ideal graft material, a recent clinical study (Testori et al. 2008), carried out on patients undergoing sinus elevation with either 100% autogenous bone or 100% deproteinized bovine bone grafts, showed that there is no statistically significant difference between the two graft materials in terms of implant survival. When considering follow-up results up to 60 months, the cumulative implant survival rate reached 97.1% in cases treated with deproteinized bovine bone and 96.4% in cases treated with autogenous bone taken from extraoral sites **TAB. 5-6**.

A correct and incorrect augmentation procedure is shown in **FIG. 13A-J, 14A-F**.

SUTURING

The flap must close passively, without tension. If necessary, periosteal releasing incisions can be made to help achieve passive closure. This should only be necessary when performing simultaneous ridge augmentation procedures, as a pure sinus graft does not increase the contour of the ridge.

The first suture should be placed at the mesial corner, between the horizontal and the vertical incision.

Horizontal mattress sutures or continuous sutures can be used on the ridge.

The type of suture to be used depends on the type of tissue: non-resorbable monofilament is recommended for keratinized gingiva, whereas resorbable sutures are recommended for alveolar mucosa.

CORRECT
PROCEDURES
FOR MAXILLARY
SINUS
ELEVATION

13 A → ANTROSTOMY CARRIED OUT USING ROTARY INSTRUMENTS.

13 B → ANTROSTOMY IS COMPLETED, AND SINUS MEMBRANE ELEVATION USING MANUAL INSTRUMENTS.

13 C → ANTERIOR VIEW OF THE ELEVATION, THE ELEVATOR REACHES THE MEDIAL SINUS WALL.

13 D → PREOPERATIVE PHOTO.

13 E → ANTROSTOMY.

13 F → MEMBRANE ELEVATION.

13 G → PLACEMENT OF THE GRAFT.

13 H → PLACEMENT OF THE MEMBRANE.

13 I → MATURATION OF THE GRAFT.

13 J → PLACEMENT OF THE IMPLANT.

13 A	13 B	13 C	
13 D	13 E	13 F	13 G
13 H	13 I	13 J	

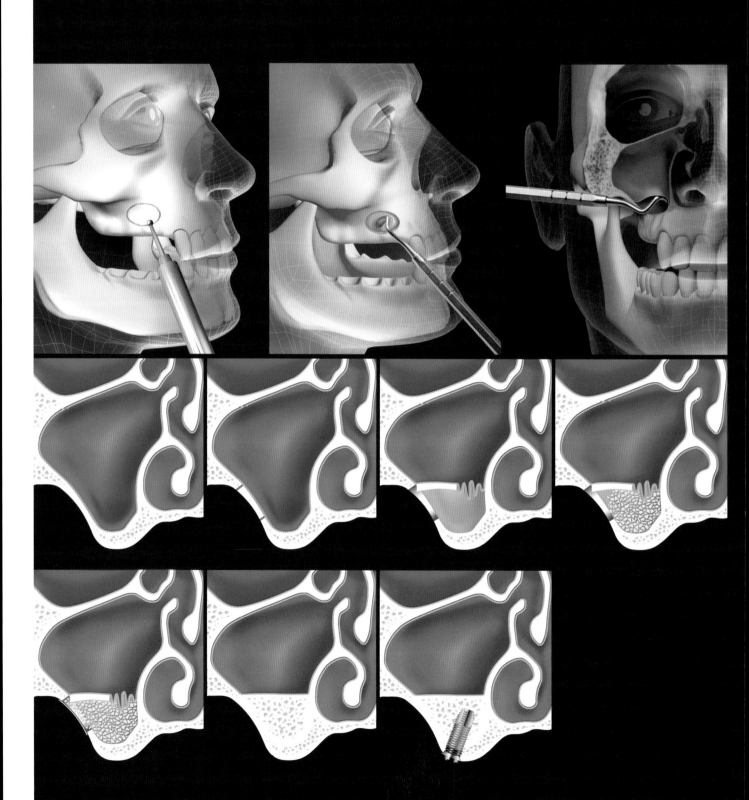

INCORRECT PROCEDURES FOR MAXILLARY SINUS ELEVATION

INCORRECT MANAGEMENT OF THE SINUS MEMBRANE WITH PARTIAL AUGMENTATION. IN ADDITION TO CAUSING SINUS RE-PNEUMATIZATION, IT PREVENTS THE CORRECT POSITIONING OF THE IMPLANT.

14 A → PARTIAL ELEVATION.

14 B → PLACEMENT OF THE GRAFT.

14 C → RE-PNEUMATIZATION AND LATER MATURATION OF GRAFT.

14 D → LOSS OF GRAFT VOLUME.

14 E → INCORRECT POSITIONING OF THE IMPLANT.

14 F → CLINICAL CASE THAT SHOWS PARTIAL FILLING OF SINUS WITH MEDIALIZATION OF THE MEMBRANE AND INCOMPLETE ELEVATION OF THE LATTER.

14 A	14 B	14 C
14 D	14 E	14 F

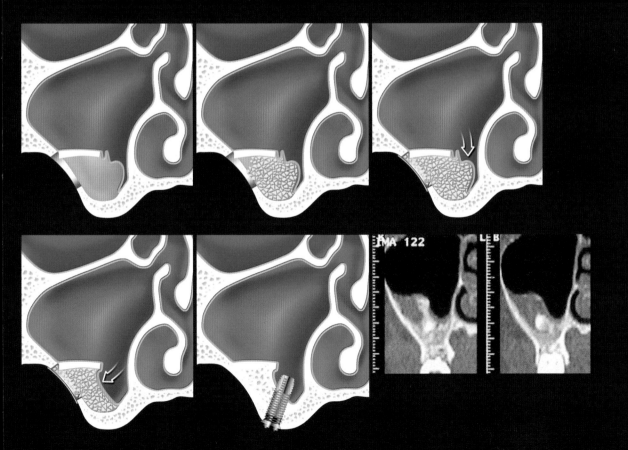

COMPLICATIONS DURING SURGERY

Complications during sinus evevation surgery are infrequent and generally easily managed. The two most common intraoperative complications are perforation of the Schneiderian membrane (11%) and intraoperative bleeding (2%) (Zijderveld et al. 2008).

A relatively infrequent intraoperative complication is hemorrhage from the posterior/superior alveolar artery. This can be controlled by electro-cauterization, being careful not to cause necrosis of the sinus membrane. If the anastomosis is intraosseous, Bone Wax may be used to stop the bleeding.

The most frequent intraoperative complication is the perforation of the Schneiderian membrane. Occurrence of this complication ranges from 7% to 56% of cases when using rotary instrumentation (Jensen et al. 1998; Khoury 1999; Wannfours et al. 2000; Ziccardi & Betts 1999; Kirch et al. 1999; Kasabah et al. 2003), and was reported to be as low as 3.8% using piezoelectric surgery.

In the event of a membrane perforation, the surgeon must continue the elevation, but at a distance from the perforation so as to release the tension along the perforation itself. Working near the perforation usually causes the size of the perforation to increase.

Life table analysis of cases treated with 100% deproteinized bovine bone (Bio-Oss®)

TAB. 5

Follow-up, months of load	Number of patients	Number of implants inserted	Duration	Number of failed implants	Implant survival rate	Cumulative survival rate
healing	15	35	0	1	97.1%	97.1%
0 to 12	15	34	0	0	100%	97.1%
12 to 24	15	34	0	0	100%	97.1%
24 to 36	15	34	8	0	100%	97.1%
36 to 48	12	26	5	0	100%	97.1%
48 to 60	10	21	11	0	100%	97.1%
> 60	3	10	9	0	100%	97.1%

Life table analysis of cases treated with 100% autogenous bone

TAB. 6

Follow-up, months of load	Number of patients	Number of implants inserted	Duration	Number of failed implants	Implant survival rate	Cumulative survival rate
healing	10	56	0	0	100%	100%
0 to 12	10	56	0	0	100%	100%
12 to 24	10	56	9	2	96.4%	96.4%
24 to 36	9	47	3	0	100%	96.4%
36 to 48	7	44	20	0	100%	96.4%
48 to 60	4	24	16	0	100%	96.4%
> 60	2	8	8	0	100%	96.4%

A classification of perforations, which divided them into five categories according to their relationship to the location of the antrostomy, was presented and later amended by the same authors (Vlassis & Fugazzotto 1999; Fugazzotto & Vlassis 2003). These articles also gave advice on how to complete the membrane elevation. All perforations occurring along the most superior part of the antrostomy are included in class I. The second category contains perforations along the lateral and inferior walls of the antrostomy.

When treating class I perforations, the surgeon must release tension along the perforation by not working too close to it. Further release and elevation of the membrane will allow it to collapse on itself and close the laceration. A collagen barrier membrane can be used over the perforation area. Class II perforations are further subdivided depending on the presence or absence of intact sinus membrane (> 4 to 5 mm) around the laceration. In class IIA, with the perforation along the front edge of the antrostomy with an anteriorly expanding maxillary sinus, it is possible to widen the antrostomy and expose the adjacent intact membrane, which can be readily elevated to close the perforation by collapsing the healthy membrane above the laceration.

In class IIB, which includes cases where the perforation is located in an area that does not allow an intact portion of membrane to be exposed around it, a pouch technique has been suggested (Fugazzotto & Vlassis 2003; Proussaefs & Lozada 2003).

A more recent study by the authors presented four different repair strategies in the management of very large perforations with clinical, radiographic, and histologic evidence of success (Testori et al. 2008).

All of these techniques involve stabilization of the repair membrane so that it does not shift in the immediate postoperative period **FIG. 15A-D, 16A-D, 17A-I**.

These include:
- folding the membrane outside the lateral wall
- utilization of tacks and sutures
- utilization of a modified Loma Linda pouch technique.

In the event of large lacerations, it is possible to continue the surgery by utilizing a pouch technique (Proussaefs & Lozada 2003; Testori et al. 2008). In this case a resorbable collagen membrane is inserted into the maxillary sinus and stretched along the maxillary sinus walls. The edges of the membrane are kept outside the antrostomy and are turned over along the vestibular bone margin. The graft is then placed in the 'pouch' and a resorbable membrane is placed over the antrostomy and graft. The flap is then sutured according to standard protocol.

When placing particulate grafts in cases with large perforations, it may is useful to mix the graft with platelet rich plasma (PRP) or venous blood. This will improve the handling of the now coagulated graft. This is recommended only for handling purposes, as the benefits of PRP in graft maturation are controversial (Froum et al. 2002; Boyapati & Wang 2006).

Furthermore, most studies report that there are no differences in implant survival when comparing non-perforated with perforated and repaired sinus grafting procedures (Schwartz-Arad et al. 2004; Shlomi et al. 2004; Ardekian et al. 2006; Karabuda et al. 2006; Testori et al. 2008). There is also no correlation between membrane perforations and the incidence of postoperative complications (Raghoebar et al. 2001).

If excess graft material is placed that is beyond the predetermined volume indicated by the membrane elevation (overpacking), it is possible for the membrane to tear, with subsequent loss of the graft material into the sinus cavity. In the event of massive graft loss into the sinus cavity, removal of all the material is

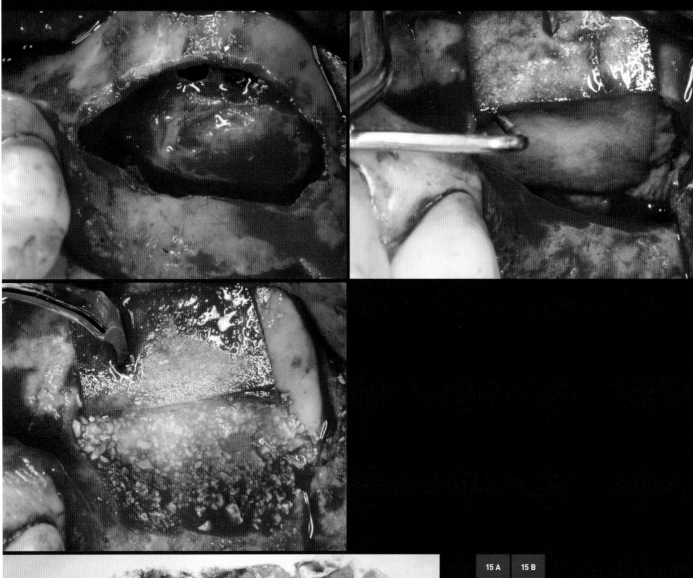

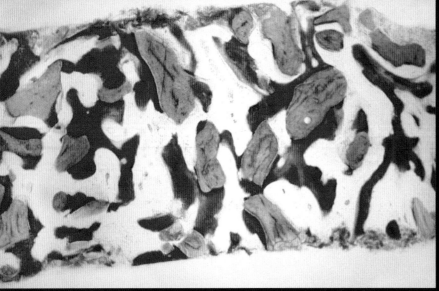

15 A → THE SINUS MEMBRANE PERFORATION IS VISIBLE ON THE SUPERIOR BORDER OF THE ANTROSTOMY.

15 B → REPAIR MEMBRANE (BIOMEND, ZIMMER) IS IN PLACE, WITH A PORTION OUTSIDE THE SINUS WINDOW AND THE REMAINDER FOLDED INTO THE SINUS TO MAKE A NEW ROOF.

15 C → PARTICULATE GRAFT MATERIAL (BIO-OSS) IN PLACE.

15 D → HISTOLOGY AT 9 MONTHS. BIO-OSS PARTICLES (YELLOW) ARE IN DIRECT CONTACT WITH NEWLY FORMED VITAL BONE (RED). OSTEOID (GREEN) LINES MANY SURFACES (STEVENEL'S BLUE AND VAN GEISON PICRIC FUCHSIN; ORIGINAL MAGNIFICATION X 10).

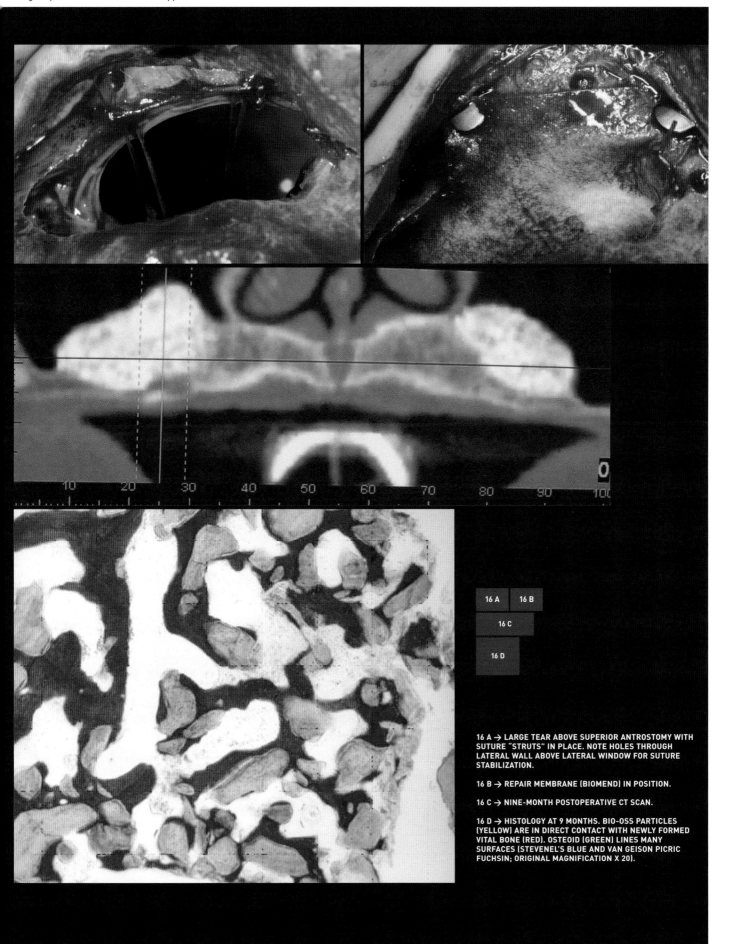

16 A → LARGE TEAR ABOVE SUPERIOR ANTROSTOMY WITH SUTURE "STRUTS" IN PLACE. NOTE HOLES THROUGH LATERAL WALL ABOVE LATERAL WINDOW FOR SUTURE STABILIZATION.

16 B → REPAIR MEMBRANE (BIOMEND) IN POSITION.

16 C → NINE-MONTH POSTOPERATIVE CT SCAN.

16 D → HISTOLOGY AT 9 MONTHS. BIO-OSS PARTICLES (YELLOW) ARE IN DIRECT CONTACT WITH NEWLY FORMED VITAL BONE (RED). OSTEOID (GREEN) LINES MANY SURFACES (STEVENEL'S BLUE AND VAN GEISON PICRIC FUCHSIN; ORIGINAL MAGNIFICATION X 20).

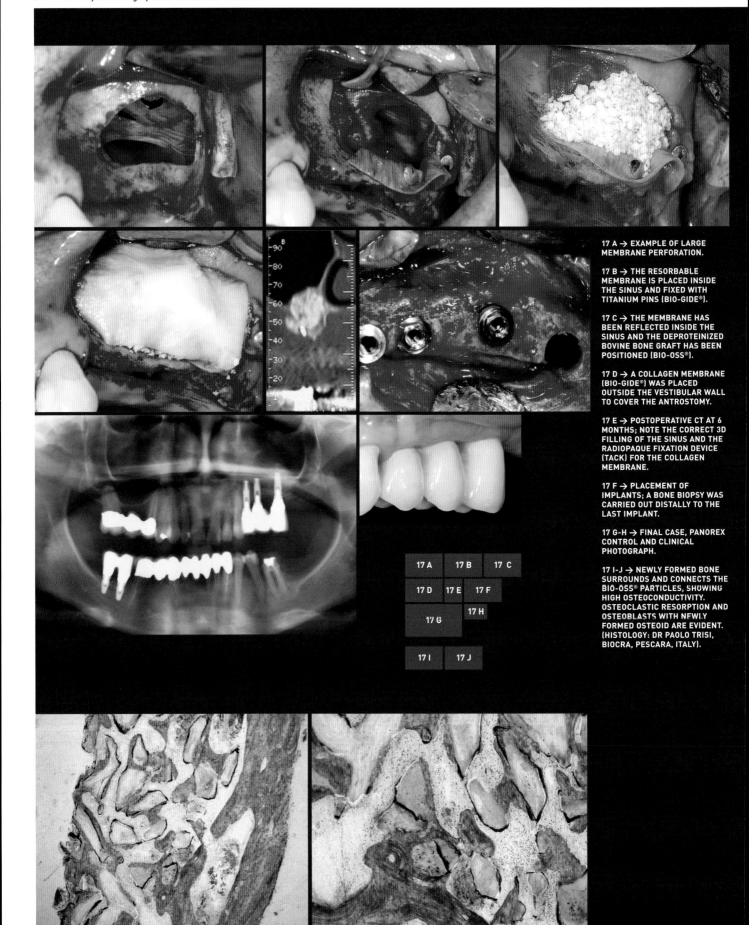

17 A → EXAMPLE OF LARGE MEMBRANE PERFORATION.

17 B → THE RESORBABLE MEMBRANE IS PLACED INSIDE THE SINUS AND FIXED WITH TITANIUM PINS (BIO-GIDE®).

17 C → THE MEMBRANE HAS BEEN REFLECTED INSIDE THE SINUS AND THE DEPROTEINIZED BOVINE BONE GRAFT HAS BEEN POSITIONED (BIO-OSS®).

17 D → A COLLAGEN MEMBRANE (BIO-GIDE®) WAS PLACED OUTSIDE THE VESTIBULAR WALL TO COVER THE ANTROSTOMY.

17 E → POSTOPERATIVE CT AT 6 MONTHS; NOTE THE CORRECT 3D FILLING OF THE SINUS AND THE RADIOPAQUE FIXATION DEVICE (TACK) FOR THE COLLAGEN MEMBRANE.

17 F → PLACEMENT OF IMPLANTS; A BONE BIOPSY WAS CARRIED OUT DISTALLY TO THE LAST IMPLANT.

17 G-H → FINAL CASE, PANOREX CONTROL AND CLINICAL PHOTOGRAPH.

17 I-J → NEWLY FORMED BONE SURROUNDS AND CONNECTS THE BIO-OSS® PARTICLES, SHOWING HIGH OSTEOCONDUCTIVITY. OSTEOCLASTIC RESORPTION AND OSTEOBLASTS WITH NEWLY FORMED OSTEOID ARE EVIDENT. (HISTOLOGY: DR PAOLO TRISI, BIOCRA, PESCARA, ITALY).

ORIGINAL MAGNIFICATION 25X

ORIGINAL MAGNIFICATION 50X

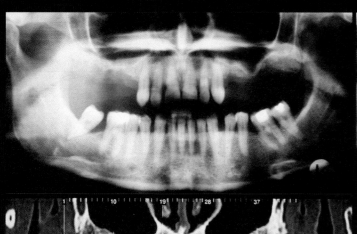
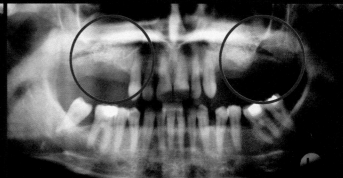

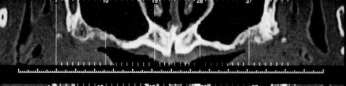
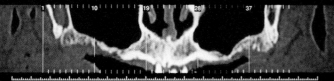
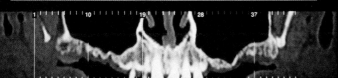

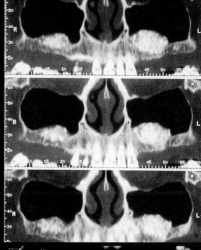

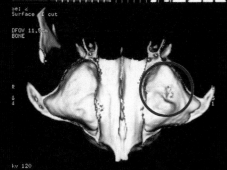

18 A	19 A
18 B	19 B
18 C	19 C
	19 D

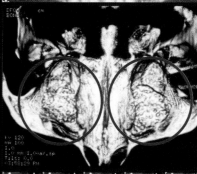

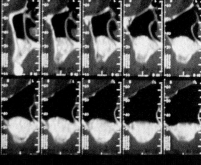

18 A → PREOPERATIVE PANORAMIC OR CROSS SETION OF A CLINICAL CASE.

18 B → PREOPERATIVE CT SECTION.

18 C → THREE-DIMENSIONAL VIEW OF MAXILLA: CIRCLE INDICATES AN AREA OF BONE DEHISCENCE WITH DIRECT CONTACT BETWEEN ORAL MUCOSA AND SINUS MEMBRANE.

19 A → POSTOPERATIVE ORTHOPANTOGRAPH: THE RADIOPAQUE AREAS REPRESENT THE PREVIOUSLY PLACED GRAFT MATERIAL.

19 B → PANORAMIC POSTOPERATIVE CT VIEW.

19 C → POSTOPERATIVE PERPENDICULAR RECONSTRUCTION. NOTE THE CORRECT 3D FILLING OF THE MAXILLARY FLOOR.

19 D → POSTOPERATIVE RECONSTRUCTION OF THE MAXILLARY SINUS. NOTE THE CORRECT 3D FILLING OF THE SINUSES.

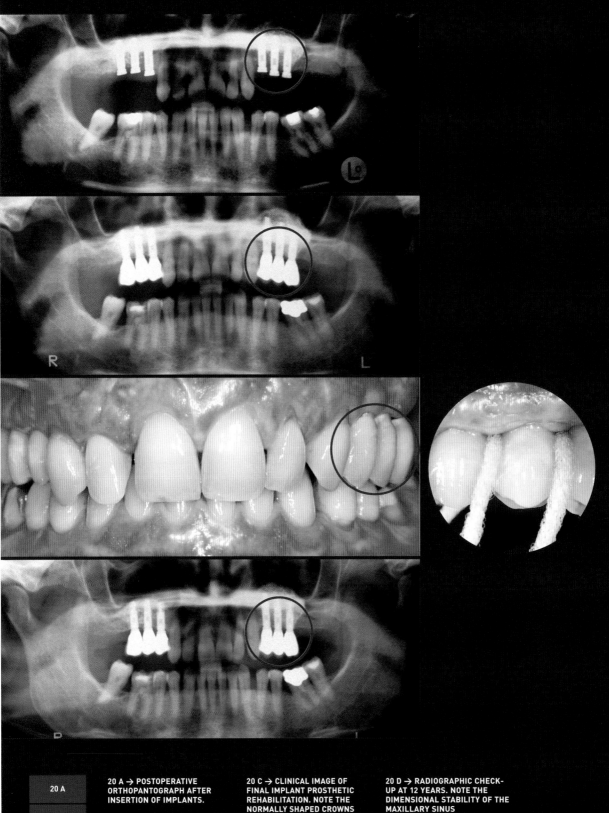

| 20 A |
| 20 B |
| 20 C |
| 20 D |

20 A → POSTOPERATIVE ORTHOPANTOGRAPH AFTER INSERTION OF IMPLANTS.

20 B → ORTHOPANTOGRAPH OF FINAL CLINICAL CASE IN WHICH THE GRAFTED SPACE CAN STILL BE SEEN.

20 C → CLINICAL IMAGE OF FINAL IMPLANT PROSTHETIC REHABILITATION. NOTE THE NORMALLY SHAPED CROWNS WITH CORRECT PROSTHETIC EMERGENCE PROFILES.

20 D → RADIOGRAPHIC CHECK-UP AT 12 YEARS. NOTE THE DIMENSIONAL STABILITY OF THE MAXILLARY SINUS AUGMENTATION USING A HIGHLY MINERALIZED GRAFT.

required. A significant loss of graft containment not seen during the surgery may be the cause of postoperative complications. These may include postoperative sinusitis and/or infection. Further, the remaining graft material may be of such poor density and deficient volume that implant placement may not be possible.

A complete clinical case with the correct clinical indications and surgical procedures is shown **FIG. 18A-C, 19A-D, 20A-D**.

REFERENCES

1 Ardekian L., Oved-Peleg E., Mactei E., Peled M.
   The clinical significance of sinus membrane perforation during augmentation of the maxillary sinus.
   J. Oral Maxillofac. Surg. 2006; 64: 277-82.

2 Blus C., Szmukler-Moncler S., Salama M., Salama H., Garber D.
   Sinus bone grafting procedures using ultrasonic bone surgery: 5-year experience.
   Int. J. Periodontics Restorative Dent. 2008; 28: 221-9.

3 Boyapati L., Wang H.L.
   The role of platelet-rich plasma in sinus augmentation: a critical review.
   Implant Dent. 2006; 15: 160-70.

4 Cho S.-C., Wallace S.S., Froum S.J., Tarnow D.P.
   Influence of anatomy on Schneiderian membrane perforations during sinus elevation surgery: three-dimensional analysis.
   Pract. Proced. Aesthet. Dent. 2001; 13: 160-3.

5 Cho S.-C., Yoo S.K., Wallace S.S., Froum S.J., Tarnow D.P.
   Correlation between membrane thickness and perforation rates in sinus augmentation surgery.
   Poster Presentation, AO Annual Meeting, 2002.

6 Del Fabbro M., Testori T., Francetti L., Weinstein R.
   Systematic review of survival rates for implants placed in the grafted maxillary sinus.
   Int. J. Periodontics Restorative Dent. 2004; 24: 565-77.

7 Elian N., Wallace S., Cho S.C., Jalbout Z.N., Froum S.
   Distribution of the maxillary artery as it relates to sinus floor augmentation.
   Int. J. Oral Maxillofac. Implants 2005; 20: 784-7.

8 Froum S.J., Wallace S.S., Tarnow D.P., Cho S.C.
   Effect of platelet-rich plasma on bone growth and osseointegration in human maxillary sinus grafts: three bilateral case reports.
   Int. J. Periodontics Restorative Dent. 2002; 22: 45-53.

9 Fugazzotto P., Vlassis J.
   A simplified classification and repair system for sinus membrane perforation.
   J. Periodontol. 2003; 74: 1534 41.

10 Jensen O.T., Shulman L.B., Block M.S., Iacono V.J.
   Report of the Sinus Consensus Conference of 1996.
   Int. J. Oral Maxillofac. Implants 1998; 13 Suppl: 11-45.

11 Karabuda C., Arisan V., Hakan O.
   Effects of sinus membrane perforations on the success of dental implants placed in the augmented sinus.
   J. Periodontol. 2006; 77: 1991-7.

12 Kasabah S., Krug J., Siműnek A., Lecaro M.C.
   Can we predict maxillary sinus mucosa perforation?
   Acta Medica (Hradec Kralove) 2003; 46: 19-23.

13 Khoury F.
   Augmentation of the sinus floor with mandibular bone block and simultaneous implantation: a 6-year clinical investigation.
   Int. J. Oral Maxillofac. Implants 1999; 14: 557-64.

14 Kim M.J., Jung U.W., Kim C.S., Kim K.D., Choi S.H., Kim C.K., Cho K.S.
   Maxillary sinus septa: prevalence, height, location, and morphology. A reformatted computed tomography scan analysis.
   J. Periodontol. 2006; 77: 903-8.

15 Kirch A., Ackermann K.L., Hurzeler M.B., Hutmacher D.
   Sinus grafting with porous Hydroxyapatite.
   In: Jensen O.T. The Sinus Bone Graft. Chicago: Quintessence Books 1999: 79-94.

16 Mardinger O., Nissan J., Chaushu G.
   Sinus floor augmentation with simultaneous implant placement in the severely atrophic maxilla: technical problems and complications.
   J. Periodontol. 2007; 78: 1872-7.

17 Peleg M., Chaushu G., Mazor Z., Ardekian L., Bakoon M.
   Radiological findings of the post-sinus lift maxillary sinus: a computerized tomography follow-up.
   J. Periodontol. 1999; 70: 1564-73.

18 Peleg M., Garg AK., Mazor Z.
   Predictability of simultaneous implant placement in the severely atrophic posterior maxilla: a 9-year longitudinal experience study of 2132 implants placed into 731 human sinus grafts.
   Int. J. Oral Maxillofac. Implants 2006; 21: 94-102.

19 Proussaefs P., Lozada J.
   The loma linda Pouch. A technique for repairing the perforated sinus membrane.
   Int. J. Periodontics Restorative Dent. 2003; 23: 593-7.

20 Raghoebar G.M., Timmenga N.M., Reintsema H., Stegenga B., Vissink A.
   Maxillary bone grafting for insertion of endosseous implants: results after 12-124 months.
   Clin. Oral Implants Res. 2001; 12: 279-86.

21 Schwartz-Arad D., Herzberg R., Dolev E.
   The prevalence of surgical complications of the sinus graft procedure and their impact on implant survival.
   J. Periodontol. 2004; 75: 511-6.

22 Shibli J.A., Faveri M., Ferrari D.S., Melo L., Garcia R.V., d'Avila S., Figueiredo L.C., Feres M.
   Prevalence of maxillary sinus septa in 1024 subjects with edentulous upper jaws: a retrospective study.
   J. Oral Implantol. 2007; 33: 293-6.

23 Shlomi B., Horowitz I., Kahn A., Dobriyan A., Chaushu G.
   The effect of sinus membrane perforation and repair with Lambone on the outcome of maxillary sinus floor augmentation: a radiographic assessment.
   Int. J. Oral Maxillofac. Implants 2004; 19: 559-62.

24 Smiler D.G.
   The sinus lift graft: basic technique and variations.
   Pract. Periodontics Aesthet. Dent. 1997; 9: 885-93.

25 Solar P., Geyerhofer U., Traxler H., Windisch A., Ulm C., Watzek G.
   Blood supply to the maxillary sinus relevant to sinus floor elevation procedures.
   Clin. Oral Implants Res. 1999; 10: 34-44.

26 Tarnow D.P., Wallace S.S., Froum S.J., Rohrer M.D., Cho S.-C.
   Histologic and clinical comparison of bilateral sinus floor elevations with and without barrier membrane placement in 12 patients: Part 3 of an ongoing prospective study.
   Int. J. Periodontics Restorative Dent. 2000; 20: 117-25.

27 Tawil G., Mawla M.
   Sinus floor elevation using a bovine bone mineral (Bio-Oss) with or without the concomitant use of a bilayered collagen barrier (Bio-Gide): a clinical report of immediate and delayed implant placement.
   Int. J. Oral Maxillofac. Implants 2001; 16: 713-21.

28 Tepper G., Haas R., Schneider B., Watzak G., Mailath G.,
    Jovanovic S.A., Busenlechner D., Zechner W., Watzek G.
    *Effects of sinus lifting on voice quality. A prospective study
    and risk assessment.*
    Clin. Oral Implants Res. 2003; 14: 767-74.

29 Testori T., Wallace S.S., Del Fabbro M., Taschieri S., Trisi P.,
    Capelli M., Weinstein R.L.
    *Repair of large sinus membrane perforations using stabilized
    collagen barrier membranes: surgical tecniques with
    histological and radiographic evidence of success.*
    Int. J. Periodontics Restorative Dent. 2008; 28: 9-17.

30 Uchida Y., Goto M., Katsuki T., Soejima Y.
    *Measurement of maxillary sinus volume using computerized
    tomographic images.*
    Int. J. Oral Maxillofac. Implants 1998; 13: 811-8.

31 Ulm C.W, Solar P., Krennmair G., Matejka M., Watzek G.
    *Incidence and suggested surgical management of septa in
    sinus-lift procedures.*
    Int. J. Oral Maxillofac. Implants 1995; 10: 462-5.

32 Velasquez-Plata D., Hovey L.R., Peach C.C., Alder M.E.
    *Maxillary sinus septa: a 3-dimensional computerized
    tomographic scan analysis.*
    Int. J. Oral Maxillofac. Implants 2002; 17: 854-60.

33 Vercellotti T., De Paoli S., Nevins M.
    *The piezoelectric bony window osteotomy and sinus membrane
    elevation: introduction of a new technique for simplification of
    the sinus augmentation procedure.*
    Int. J. Periodontics Restorative Dent. 2001; 21: 561-7.

34 Vlassis J.M., Fugazzotto P.A.
    *A classification system for sinus membrane perforations during
    augmentation procedures with options for repair.*
    J. Periodontol. 1999; 70: 692-9.

35 Wallace S.S., Froum S.J., Cho S.C., Elian N., Monteiro D., Kim
    B.S., Tarnow D.P.
    *Sinus augmentation utilizing anorganic bovine bone (Bio-Oss)
    with absorbable and non-absorbable membranes placed over
    the lateral window: histomorphometric and clinical analysis.*
    Int. J. Periodontics Restorative Dent. 2005; 25: 551-9.

36 Wallace S.S., Froum S.J.
    *Effect of maxillary sinus augmentation on the survival of
    endosseous dental implants as compared to the survival of
    implants placed in the non-grafted posterior maxilla: an
    evidence-based literature review.*
    Ann. Periodontol. 2003; 8: 328-43.

37 Wallace S.S., Mazor Z., Froum S.J., Cho S.-C., Tarnow D.P.
    *Schneiderian membrane perforation rate during sinus elevation
    using Piezosurgery®: A report of 100 consecutive cases.*
    Int. J. Periodontics Restorative Dent. 2007; 27: 413-9.

38 Wannfors K., Johansson B., Hallman M., Strandkvist T.
    *A prospective randomized study of 1- and 2-stage sinus inlay
    bone grafts: 1-year follow-up.*
    Int. J. Oral Maxillofac. Implants 2000; 15: 625-32.

39 Ziccardi V.B., Betts N.J.
    Complications of maxillary sinus augmentation.
    In: Jensen OT. The Sinus Bone Graft Chicago: Quintessence
    Books 1999: 201-8.

40 Zijderfeld S.A., van den Bergh J.P., Schulten E.A.,
    ten Bruggenkate C.M.
    *Anatomical and surgical findings and complications in 100
    consecutive maxillary sinus floor elevation procedures.*
    J. Oral Maxillofac. Implants 2008; 66: 1426-38.

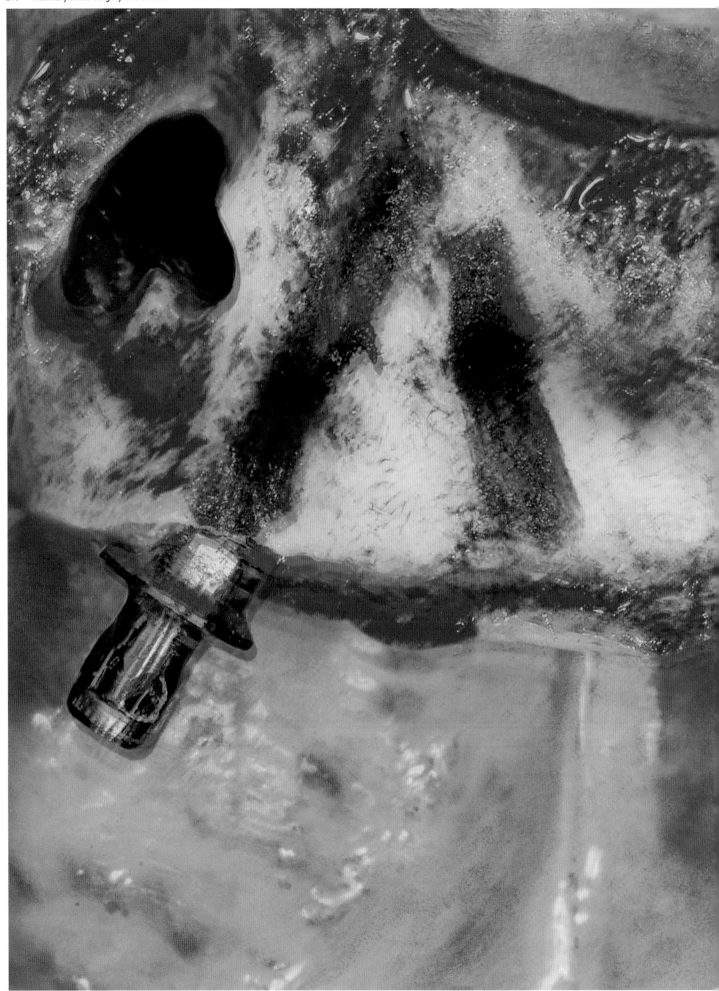

T. TESTORI
F. GALLI
L. FUMAGALLI
A. PARENTI
S.S. WALLACE

Alternatives to sinus floor augmentation

13

13

When reconstructing the maxilla due to monolateral or bilateral atrophy in partly or totally edentulous patients, there are some alternative treatments that should be taken into consideration. Insufficient bone volume in the latero-posterior sectors is not in itself an indication for performing lateral window maxillary sinus augmentation surgery without considering available alternatives.

Careful evaluation of the possible alternatives is mandatory for all patients who, due to general medical problems, pathologies of the maxillary sinus, advanced age or psychological reasons, cannot undergo invasive surgery such as maxillary sinus augmentation.

In patients without molar teeth, it is necessary to assess carefully whether there is a functional and/or esthetic indication that justifies such treatment, also taking into account the patient's requests and expectations.

Another parameter to consider when choosing an alternative treatment is the complexity of the surgical technique. Minimally invasive techniques, which may reduce morbidity, and postsurgical complications as well as accelerate the postoperative healing course, are worthy of consideration.

According to research based on subjective data gathered in a questionnaire filled out by patients (Kayser 1994), it is not possible to establish exactly, from a purely functional point of view, the number of elements required for "normal" functioning of the stomatognathic apparatus (Witter et al. 1997). It is also seen that a reduced number of functional units is not a source of functional deficiency in elderly patients (Meeuwissen et al. 1995) and above all does not cause an increased incidence of temporomandibular disorder (Sarita et al. 2003).

Some authors have assessed the functionality of the stomatognathic apparatus related to the patient's age range (Kayser 1994). This analysis attempted to correlate age with the number of teeth for an optimal, sub-optimal or minimal function level, considering an optimal level (level I) to be 12 pairs of occlusal units for an age range between 20 and 50 years of age, a sub-optimal level (level II) to be 10 occlusal pairs for an age range between 40 and 80 years of age, and a minimal level (level III) to be eight pairs of occlusal units for an age range between 70 and 100 years of age.

The patient's esthetic needs must be analyzed with extreme care by the doctor as they are the result of several individual variables. The surgeon must consider these needs and relate them to the clinical situation.

In addition to the patient's specific requests, the surgeon must evaluate the general health status of the oral cavity, incorporating the implant surgery operation into a global rehabilitation plan.

The patient's future condition in the event of a total failure must also be taken into account. When choosing alternative treatments, it would be advisable to opt for the one that, in the event of total failure, does not create permanent biological damage that will compromise future possibilities for rehabilitation.

With regards to the clinical condition, there are essentially four treatments that have been proposed as alternatives to lateral window sinus augmentation:

- reduced-size implants
- mesio-distally tilted implants
- pre- and post-sinus implants
- prostheses with long distal cantilever
- osteotome sinus elevation (see Chapter 11).

REDUCED-LENGTH IMPLANTS

In the lateroposterior sectors of the maxilla, an insufficient amount of bone is often found for the placement of implants, due to maxillary sinus pneumatization and/or resorption of the alveolar ridge. Under these conditions, a possible alternative treatment to maxillary sinus augmentation may be the use of reduced-length implants (≤8.5 mm long).

The implants must be placed with good primary stability, preparing an implant site that is compliant with the bone quality. Many studies have analyzed the success rate of reduced-length implants, reporting unfavorable values. However, a more in-depth analysis highlights how these clinical studies mainly take analyzed smooth-surface implants, while modern implant surfaces are treated with chemical or physical procedures that increase the surface roughness to different levels depending on the procedure used. The extent to which the implant surface's micromorphology is a decisive factor for implant success, mainly due to its osteoconductive capacity, has been shown (Buser et al. 1991; Trisi et al. 2003).

This variable seems to have an effect in soft bone sites, whereas it has no effect on implant survival in normal or dense bone (Tawil & Younan 2003).

Before evaluating the success of published studies, it is necessary to check the types of implants used and their surfaces.

If we specifically analyze the maxilla, several studies have reported success rates over 94% (Deporter et al. 2000; Testori et al. 2001; Fugazzotto et al. 2004; Nedir et al. 2004; Goené et al. 2005). One study reported a lower success rate of 85.7% (ten Bruggenkate et al. 1998) **TAB. 1**.

Bahat (2000) analyzed the success rate of implants placed in the posterior maxilla, and found that the cumulative survival rate of reduced-size implants in a 12-year follow-up was 93%.

Another multicenter study (Fugazzotto et al. 2004) confirmed these values, showing a cumulative success rate of 94.5% up to 84 months. It specifically evaluated implants of 9 mm or less in length inserted in the first maxillary molar site. It was specified that many implants included in the analysis were 4.1 mm in diameter. Implants with a larger diameter are currently available that, due to the greater surface area available for bone-implant contact, may have a higher implant success rate.

Current evidence allows us to state that implants that are less then 8.5 mm in length do not have a survival rate significantly lower than standard implants (Renouard & Nisand 2005, 2006). However, as in other clinical situations, they must be inserted in an anatomic context that allows correct and easy home oral hygiene **FIG. 1**.

TAB. 1

Survival rate of "short" implants (<10 mm) in the maxilla

STUDY	TYPE OF IMPLANT	INSERTED	FAILED	% FAILED
Quirynen et al. 1991	Brånemark	34	4	11.8%
Naert et al. 1992	Brånemark	30	3	10.0%
Nevins & Langer 1993	Brånemark	55	8	14.5%
Lekholm et al. 1999	Brånemark	22	4	18.2%
Jemt & Lekholm 1993	Brånemark	15	2	13.3%
Friberg et al. 1991	Brånemark	520	37	7.1%
Jemt et al. 1992	Brånemark	300	58	19.3%
Jemt & Lekholm 1995	Brånemark	298	78	26.2%
Friberg et al. 2000	Brånemark	260	17	6.5%
Tawil & Younan 2003	Brånemark	9	1	11.1%
Bahat 1992	Brånemark	6	1	16,7%
SUBTOTAL SMOOTH SURFACE		1549	213	13.7%
Bischof et el. 2006	ITI®	102	2	2.0%
ten Bruggenkate et al. 1998	ITI®	42	6	14.3%
Deporter et al. 2000	Porous-surface	26	0	0.0%
Testori et al. 2001	Osseotite	18	1	5.6%
Nedir et al. 2004	ITI®	47	0	0.0%
Goené et al. 2005	Osseotite	54	3	5.5%
Griffin & Cheung 2004	Ster-Oss Nobel	168	0	0.0%
Fugazzotto et al. 2004	ITI®	979	9	0.9%
Misch et al. 2006	Biorizon HA-coated	745	0	0.0%
Renouard & Nisand 2005	Nobel TiUnite	42	1	2.4%
SUBTOTAL ROUGH SURFACE		2223	22	1.0%
TOTAL		3772	235	6.2%

TAB. 2

Survival rate of mesiodistally tilted implants

	STUDY	TILTED				NON TILTED				
		N. PATIENTS	N. IMPLANTS	IMPLANTS FAILED	RATE OF SURVIVAL	N. IMPLANTS	IMPLANTS FAILED	RATE OF AVERAGE	FOLLOW-UP, MONTHS SURVIVAL (MIN-MAX)	SUCCESS OF PROSTHESIS
DELAYED LOAD	Krekmanov et al. 2000	22	40	1	97.5%	98	6	93.9%	53 (35-60)	100%
	Krekmanov 2000	45	90	6	93.3%	155	1	99.4%	55.2 (18-60)	100%
	Fortin et al. 2002	22	54	4	92.6%	9	0	100%	18 (12-123)	100%
	Aparicio et al. 2001	25	42	2	95.2%	59	5	91.5%	37 (21-87)	100%
	total	114	226	13	94.2%	321	12	96.3%		
IMMEDIATE LOAD	Malo et al. (2005)	38	76	0	100%	132	0	100%	24 / 27	100%
	Testori et al. (2008)	41	82	2	97.5%	164	3	98.2%	37 (18.55)	100%
	total	79	158	2	98.1%	296	3	99.9%		

PRE- AND POST-SINUS IMPLANTS

A further possibility for treatment is the insertion of implants mesially and distally into the maxillary sinus. The possibility of inserting tilted implants so they engage in the frontal wall of the maxillary sinus in partially edentulous patients is excluded if natural teeth are still present, in that the implant site preparation would be affected by the presence of tooth roots. In this case, the implants mesial to the sinus are placed parallel to the adjacent natural teeth. The implants placed in the second molar position can be tilted into the tuberosity area. Success rates for this procedure have been reported in the past as 93% at 21.4 months and 97.6% at 36 months (Bahat 1992; Venturelli 1996).

Another possibility is to place the mesial implant parallel to natural teeth, while the distal implant is mesially tangent to the sinus with the implant head emerging at the second molar level. In some cases it is possible to tilt both the mesial and distal implant without invading the maxillary sinus.

Aparicio et al. (2001) used the two previously described configurations, and the success rate in tilted implants reached 95.2%. In implants placed with an axial load, the success rate was found to be 91.3%.

Pterygomaxillary implants in partially edentulous patients were found to have a slightly higher failure rate (13.7%) (Balshi et al. 1995), although the authors explained that the low bone quality in the area requires a good level of surgical experience by the surgeon in order to obtain optimal primary stability. They also suggest a possible correlation between the operation site, the surgeon's position and the success rate. A further variable to be considered, as previously mentioned, is the implant surface.

MESIODISTALLY TILTED IMPLANTS

Though traditional protocols foresaw a prosthetically guided implant placement, reports have recently emerged that favor the use of tilted implants to overcome anatomically disadvantageous situations.

In cases of totally edentulous subjects, the possible alternative treatment to sinus augmentation for a fixed prosthesis is aimed at exploiting the bone volume in the premaxilla area. The implant configuration has six implants. Four are inserted in a standard axial position from canine to canine. The two distal implants are tilted distally, parallel to the anterior wall of the sinus, exploiting the area between the frontonasal canine mesially, the maxillary sinus floor cranially and the alveolar ridge caudally **FIG. 2**.

An implant survival rate of 93 to 97.5% has been reported in totally edentulous patients (Krekmanov 2000; Fortin et al. 2002). The same implant layout described by Fortin et al. (2002) has been used in cases of total edentulism together with immediate loading, with encouraging success rates, even if these studies still need long-term clinical follow-up (Malo et al. 2005, Capelli et al. 2007; Francetti et al. 2008; Testori et al. 2008) **TAB. 2**. The implant configuration described by Fortin et al. (2002) allows an excellent distribution of implants in the premaxilla.

The case must be studied before surgery using a diagnostic wax model with articulator in order to obtain the correct implant layout that allows a maxillary fixed prosthesis to be constructed with 12 elements and a minimum cantilever **FIG. 3A-I, 4 A-R, 5 A-F**.

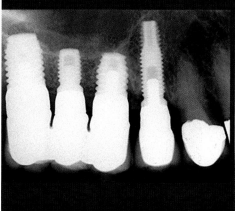

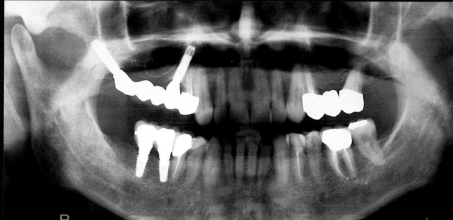

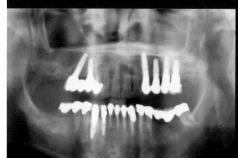

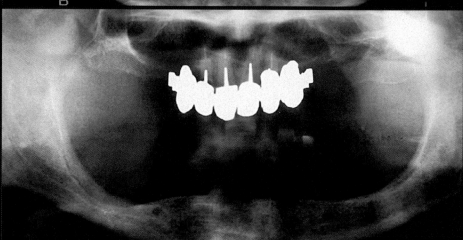

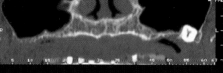

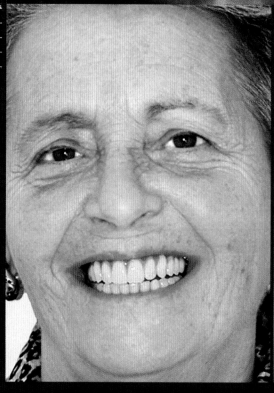

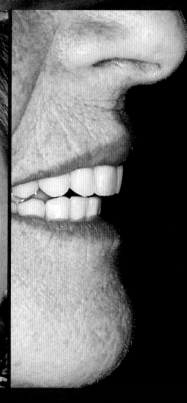

1 → CLINICAL CASE RESOLVED WITH REDUCED-LENGTH IMPLANTS.

2 A→ CLINICAL CASE RESOLVED WITH PRE- AND POST-SINUS TILTED IMPLANTS.

2 B→ CLINICAL CASE RESOLVED ON THE RIGHT SIDE WITH TILTED IMPLANTS, ON THE LEFT SIDE WITH ORTHOGONAL IMPLANTS AND MAXILLARY SINUS AUGMENTATION.

3 A → PRE-OPERATIVE ORTHOPANTOGRAPH.

3 B → PANORAMIC CT SECTION THAT SHOWS ANATOMY OF MAXILLARY EDENTULISM.

3 C → FRONT VIEW OF REHABILITATED PATIENT.

3 D → PROFILE OF REHABILITATED PATIENT.

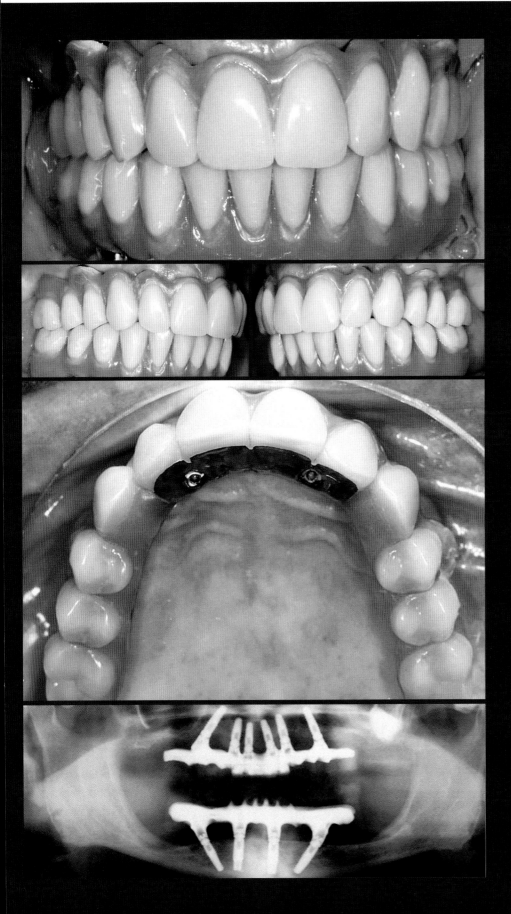

3 E → ANTERIOR VIEW OF SUPERIOR AND INFERIOR IMPLANT PROSTHETIC REHABILITATION.

3 F-G → 45-DEGREE LEFT- AND RIGHT-HAND VIEW OF SUPERIOR AND INFERIOR IMPLANT PROSTHETIC REHABILITATIONS.

3 H → OCCLUSAL VIEW OF SUPERIOR IMPLANT PROSTHETIC REHABILITATION.

3 I → ORTHOPANTOGRAPH OF COMPLETED REHABILITATION. THIS TYPE OF PLANNING ALLOWED TWO FIXED 12-ELEMENT PROSTHESES TO BE CONSTRUCTED WITHOUT OPERATING ON THE MAXILLARY SINUSES.

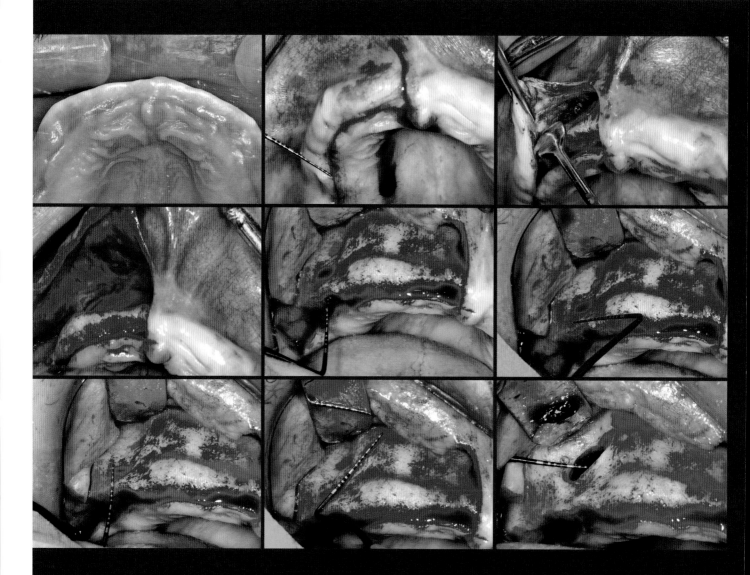

4 A	4 B	4 C
4 D	4 E	4 F
4 G	4 H	4 I

4 A → OCCLUSAL VIEW OF CLINICAL CASE.

4 B → THE MAIN INCISION IS CARRIED OUT ON THE TOTAL THICKNESS OF THE RIDGE. THE INCISION LINE MUST BE MOVED SLIGHTLY TOWARDS THE PALATE TO MOVE A LARGER AMOUNT OF KERATINIZED GUINGIVA TO THE VESTIBULAR AREA. THE CENTRAL FRENULUM INSERTION IS PRESERVED. THE MESIAL VERTICAL INCISION IS PARALLEL TO THE CENTRAL FRENULUM INSERTION. IT IS POSSIBLE TO AVOID THE DISTAL INCISION BY INCREASING THE DISTAL EXTENSION OF THE MAIN INCISION.

4 C-D → THE FLAP IS LIFTED TO ITS TOTAL THICKNESS TO HIGHLIGHT THE ANTERIOR AREA OF THE MAXILLARY SINUS. THE PERIOSTIUM MUST BE KEPT WHOLE TO MAINTAIN THE SURGICAL FIELD AS CLEAR AS POSSIBLE OF BLOOD.

4 E → THE FIRST IMPLANT THAT WILL BE INSERTED IS THE MOST DISTAL, TILTED ONE. THE IMPLANT IS THEN PLACED IN THE INCISOR AREA. THE REMAINING SPACE IS THEREFORE EQUALLY DIVIDED FOR THE PLACEMENT OF THE LAST IMPLANT.

4 F → IN ORDER TO DETERMINE THE AREA FOR PLACEMENT OF THE FIRST IMPLANT, THE MAXILLARY SINUS ANTERIOR WALL IS DETERMINED BY COUNTING THE NUMBER OF CT SECTIONS FROM THE MEDIAN LINE.

4 G → THE RESIDUAL HEIGHT FROM THE SINUS FLOOR TO THE BONE RIDGE IS MEASURED ON THE CT. THIS MEASUREMENT IS THEN USED ON THE RIDGE. IN MANY CASES, SINUS VESTIBULAR COMPACT BONE IS THIN, THE SINUS POSITION CAN BE SEEN AS A GRAY SHADOW.

4 H → A PERIODONTAL PROBE IS SHOWING THE FUTURE IMPLANT LENGTH AND AXIS OF INSERTION ON THE VESTIBULAR WALL.

4 I → TO AVOID UNCONTROLLED INVASION OF THE ANTRAL SPACE, THE AUTHORS SUGGEST OPENING A MODEST ANTROSTOMY ALONG THE ANTERIOR PART OF THE SINUS. THE SINUS MUCOSA IS THEN DETACHED USING THE INSTRUMENTS FOR SINUS ELEVATION.

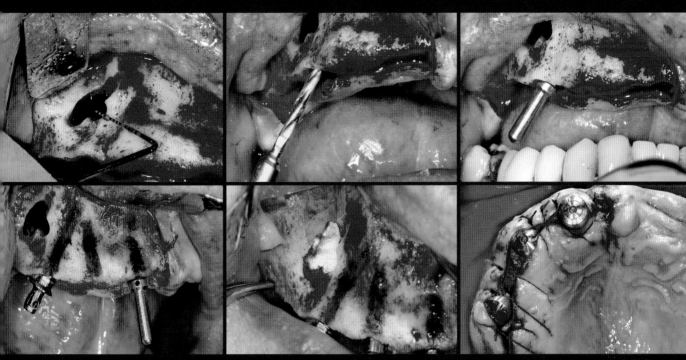

| 4 L | 4 M | 4 N |
| 4 O | 4 P | 4 Q |

4 L → EXTENDING THE ANTROSTOMY MESIALLY IS A RECOMMENDED OPTION FOR BETTER CONTROL OF SINUS ANTERIOR FLOOR PERFORATION.

4 M → THE FIRST TWIST DRILL ENTERS THE PREVIOUSLY SELECTED AREA.

4 N → THE EMERGENCE OF THE FUTURE IMPLANT SITE IS CONTROLLED BY A DIRECTION INDICATOR. CORRECT PREPARATION GUARANTEES EMERGENCE IN THE 5/6 AREA OF THE OPPOSITE ARCH

4 O → THE SECOND IMPLANT IS PLACED IN THE INCISOR SITE ACCORDING TO THE CLASSICAL TECHNIQUE. THE LAST IMPLANT IS CHOSEN IN RELATION TO THE RESIDUAL SPACE AND THE TILT OF THE DISTAL IMPLANT.

4 P → THE SINUS SPACE WHICH HAS BEEN UNCOVERED IS FILLED WITH COLLAGEN SPONGE.

4 Q → SUTURING IS INTERRUPTED ALONG THE VERTICAL INCISION AND BOTH HORIZONTAL MATTRESS AND ALSO ALONG THE CRESTAL INCISION LINE.

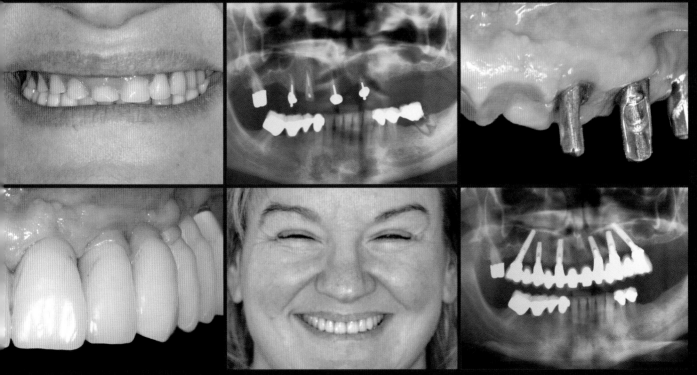

| 5 A | 5 B | 5 C |
| 5 D | 5 E | 5 F |

FIG. 5 A→ CLINICAL CASE OF A PATIENT WITH OVERDENTURE ON NATURAL TEETH, WHICH CANNOT BE RECOVERED, PRESERVING NATURAL ELEMENTS.

FIG. 5 B→ ORTHOPANTOGRAPH OF THE CLINICAL CASE.

FIG. 5 C→ PLACEMENT OF SIX PROSTHETIC ABUTMENTS.

FIG. 5 D→ INTRAORAL VIEW OF FIXED PROSTHESIS IN METAL-CERAMIC COMPRISING 12 TEETH CEMENTED ONTO 6 IMPLANTS.

FIG. 5 E→ EXTRAORAL VIEW WITH PATIENT'S SMILE LINE.

FIG. 5 F→ FINAL RADIOGRAPHIC CONTROL.

IMPLANTS WITH DISTAL CANTILEVER

A different treatment solution may be the placement of implants in the anterior maxillary sinus area, with a distal extension (Shackleton et al. 1994; Becker & Kaiser 2000; Becker 2004).

A prospective study carried out in partially maxillary and mandibular edentulous patients showed how implant-supported prostheses with a distal cantilever can achieve 100% success at 7 years, while those cases with mesial cantilever only achieved a rate of 97.1% (Romeo et al. 2003).

However, it seems that the distal cantilever cases considered were "alternated" i.e. one or more natural teeth were always present. This variation may have a positive effect in the calculation of survival, as a "protected" occlusion tends to reduce functional load on the extension. Although the technique described in this study cannot be applied fully as an alternative to sinus elevation, it may be an alternative if a natural tooth is present distal to the maxillary sinus. The average length of the distal cantilever in treated cases was found to be 6.7 mm (+/- 1.17 mm SD), suited to a prosthetic premolar crown (Romeo et al. 2003).

CONCLUSIONS

A careful evaluation of alternative treatments in the latero-posterior area of the maxilla allows avoidance of more invasive surgery in many cases, without reducing implant success rates.

REFERENCES

1. **Aparicio C., Perales P., Rangert B.**
   Tilted implants as an alternative to maxillary sinus grafting: a clinical, radiologic, and periotest study.
   Clin. Implant. Dent. Relat. Res. 2001; 3: 39-49.

2. **Bahat O.**
   Osseointegrated implants in the maxillary tuberosity: report on 45 consecutive patients.
   Int. J. Oral Maxillofac. Implants 1992; 7: 459-67.

3. **Bahat O.**
   Brånemark system implants in the posterior maxilla: clinical study of 660 implants followed for 5 to 12 years.
   Int. J. Oral Maxillofac. Implants 2000; 15: 646-53.

4. **Balshi T.J., Lee H.Y., Hernandez R.E.**
   The use of pterygomaxillary implants in the partially edentulous patient: a preliminary report.
   Int. J. Oral Maxillofac. Implants 1995; 10: 89-98.

5. **Becker C.M., Kaiser D.A.**
   Implant-retained cantilever fixed prosthesis: where and when.
   J. Prosthet. Dent. 2000 Oct; 84: 432-5.

6. **Becker C.M.**
   Cantilever fixed prostheses utilizing dental implants: a 10-year retrospective analysis.
   Quintessence Int. 2004; 35: 437-41.

7. **Bischof M., Nedir R., Abi Najm S., Szmukler-Moncler S., Samson J.**
   A five-year life-table analysis on wide neck ITI implants with prosthetic evaluation and radiographic analysis: results from a private practice.
   Clin. Oral Implant Res. 2006; 17: 515-20.

8. **Buser D., Schenk R.K., Steinemann S., Fiorellini J.P., Fox C.H., Stich H.**
   Influence of surface characteristics on bone integration of titanium implants. A histomorphometric study in miniature pigs.
   J. Biomed. Mater. Res. 1991; 25: 889-902.

9. **Capelli M, Zuffetti F, Del Fabbro M, Testori T.**
   Immediate rehabilitation of the completely edentulous jaw with fixed prostheses supported by either upright or tilted implants: a multicenter clinical study.
   Int. J. Oral Maxillofac. Implants 2007; 22: 639-44.

10. **Deporter D., Todescan R., Caudry S.**
    Simplifying management of the posterior maxilla using short, porous-surfaced dental implants and simultaneous indirect sinus elevation.
    Int. J. Periodontics Restorative Dent. 2000; 20: 476-85.

11. **Fortin Y., Sullivan R.M., Rangert B.R.**
    The Marius implant bridge: surgical and prosthetic rehabilitation for the completely edentulous upper jaw with moderate to severe resorption: a 5 year retrospective clinical study.
    Clin. Implant. Dent. Relat. Res. 2002; 4: 69-77.

12. **Friberg B., Jemt T., Lekholm U.**
    Early failures in 4,641 consecutively placed Brånemark dental implants: a study from stage 1 surgery to the connection of completed prostheses.
    Int. J. Oral Maxillofac. Implants 1991; 6: 142-6.

13. **Fugazzotto P.A., Beagle J.R., Ganeles J., Jaffin R., Vlassis J., Kumar A.**
    Success and failure rates of 9 mm or shorter implants in the replacement of missing maxillary molars when restored with

individual crowns: preliminary results 0 to 84 months in function. A retrospective study.
J. Periodontol. 2004; 75: 327-32.

14. Goené R., Bianchessi C., Huerzeler M., Del Lupo R., Testori T. Davarpanah M, Jalbout Z. Performance of short implants in partial restorations: 3-year follow-up of Osseotite implants. Implant Dent. 2005; 14: 274-80.

15. Griffin T.J., Cheung W.S.
The use of short, wide implants in posterior areas with reduced bone height: a retrospective investigation.
J. Prosthet. Dent. 2004; 92: 139-44.

16. Jemt T., Lekholm. U.
Oral implant treatment in posterior partially edentulous jaws: a 5-year follow-up report.
Int. J. Oral Maxillofac. Implants 1993; 8: 635-40.

17. Jemt T., Lekholm U.
Implant treatment in edentulous maxillae: a 5-year follow-up report on patients with different degrees of jaw resorption.
Int. J. Oral Maxillofac. Implants 1995; 10: 303-11.

18. Jemt T., Book K., Lindén B., Urde G.
Failures and complications in 92 consecutively inserted overdentures supported by Brånemark implants in severely resorbed edentulous maxillae: a study from prosthetic treatment to first annual check-up.
Int. J. Oral Maxillofac. Implants 1992; 7: 162-7.

19. Kayser A.F.
Limited treatment goals – shortened dental arches.
Periodontol. 2000. 1994; 4: 7-14.

20. Krekmanov L., Kahn M., Rangert B., Lindstrom H.
Tilting of posterior mandibular and maxillary implants for improved prosthesis support.
Int. J. Oral Maxillofac. Implants. 2000; 15: 405-14.

21. Krekmanov L.
Placement of posterior mandibular and maxillary implants in patients with severe bone deficiency: a clinical report of procedure.
Int. J. Oral Maxillofac. Implants 2000; 15: 722-30.

22. Lekholm U., Gunne J., Henry P., Higuchi K.,Linden U., Bergström C., van Steenberghe D.
Survival of the Brånemark implant in partially edentulous jaws: a 10-year prospective multicenter study.
Int. J. Oral Maxillofac. Implants 1999; 14: 639-45.

23. Malo P., Rangert B., Nobre M. All-on-4 immediate-function concept with Branemark System implants for completely edentulous maxillae: a 1-year retrospective clinical study.
Clin Implant Dent Relat Res. 2005;7 Suppl 1:88-94

24. Meeuwissen J.H., van Waas M.A., Meeuwissen R., Kayser A.F., van 't Hof M.A., Kalk W.
Satisfaction with reduced dentitions in elderly people.
J. Oral Rehabil. 1995; 22: 397-401.

25. Misch C.E, Steigenga J., Barboza E., Misch-Dietch F., Cianciola L.J., Kazor C.
Short dental implants in posterior partial edentulism: a multi center retrospective 6-year case series study.
J. Periodontol. 2006; 77: 1340-7.

26. Naert I., Quirynen M., van Steenberghe D., Darius P.
A study of 589 consecutive implants supporting complete fixed prostheses. Part II: Prosthetic aspects.
J. Prosthet. Dent. 1992; 68: 949-56.

25. Nedir R., Bischof M., Briaux J.M., Beyer S., Szmukler-Moncler S., Bernard J.P.
A 7-year life table analysis from a prospective study on ITI implants with special emphasis on the use of short implants.

Results from a private practice.
Clin. Oral Implants Res. 2004; 15: 150-7.

28. Nevins M., Langer B.
The successful application of osseointegrated implants to the posterior jaw: a long-term retrospective study.
Int. J. Oral Maxillofac. Implants 1993; 8: 428-32.

29. Quirynen M., Naert I., van Steenberghe D., Dekeyser C., Callens A.
Periodontal aspects of osseointegrated fixtures supporting a partial bridge. An up to 6-years retrospective study.
J. Clin. Periodontol. 1992; 19: 118-26.

30. Renouard F., Nisand D.
Short implants in the severely resorbed maxilla: a 2-year retrospective clinical study.
Clin. Implant Dent. Relat. Res. 2005; 7: S104-10.

31. Renouard F., Nisand D.
Impact of implant length and diameter on survival rates.
Clin. Oral Implants Res. 2006; 17: S35-51.

32. Romeo E., Lops D., Margutti E., Ghisolfi M., Chiapasco M., Vogel G.
Implant-supported fixed cantilever prostheses in partially edentulous arches. A seven-year prospective study.
Clin. Oral Implants Res. 2003; 14: 303-11.

33. Sarita P.T., Kreulen C.M., Witter D., Creugers N.H.
Signs and symptoms associated with TMD in adults with shortened dental arches.
Int. J. Prosthodont. 2003; 16: 265-70.

34. Shackleton J.L., Carr L., Slabbert J.C., Becker P.J.
Survival of fixed implant-supported prostheses related to cantilever lengths.
J. Prosthet. Dent. 1994; 71: 23-6.

35. Tawil G., Younan R.
Clinical evaluation of short, machined-surface implants followed for 12 to 92 months.
Int. J. Oral Maxillofac. Implants 2003; 18: 894-901.

36. ten Bruggenkate C.M., Asikainen P., Foitzik C., Krekeler G., Sutter F.
Short (6-mm) nonsubmerged dental implants: results of a multicenter clinical trial of 1 to 7 years.
Int. J. Oral Maxillofac. Implants 1998; 13: 791-8.

37. Testori T., Wiseman L., Woolfe S., Porter S.S.
A prospective multicenter clinical study of the Osseotite implant: four-year interim report.
Int. J. Oral Maxillofac. Implants 2001; 16: 193-200.

38. Testori T., Del Fabbro M., Capelli M., Zuffetti F., Francetti L., Weinstein R.L.
Immediate occlusal loading and tilted implants for the rehabilitation of the atrophic edentulous maxilla. One year interim results of a multicenter prospective study.
Clin Oral Implants Res 2008;19:227-232.

39. Trisi P., Lazzara R., Rebaudi A., Rao W., Testori T., Porter S.S.
Bone-implant contact on machined and dual acid-etched surfaces after 2 months of healing in the human maxilla.
J. Periodontol. 2003; 74: 945-56.

40. Venturelli A.
A modified surgical protocol for placing implants in the maxillary tuberosity: clinical results at 36 months after loading with fixed partial dentures.
Int. J. Oral Maxillofac. Implants 1996; 11: 743-9.

41. Witter DJ., Allen P.F., Wilson N.H, Kayser A.F.
Dentists' attitudes to the shortened dental arch concept.
J. Oral Rehabil. 1997; 24: 143-7.

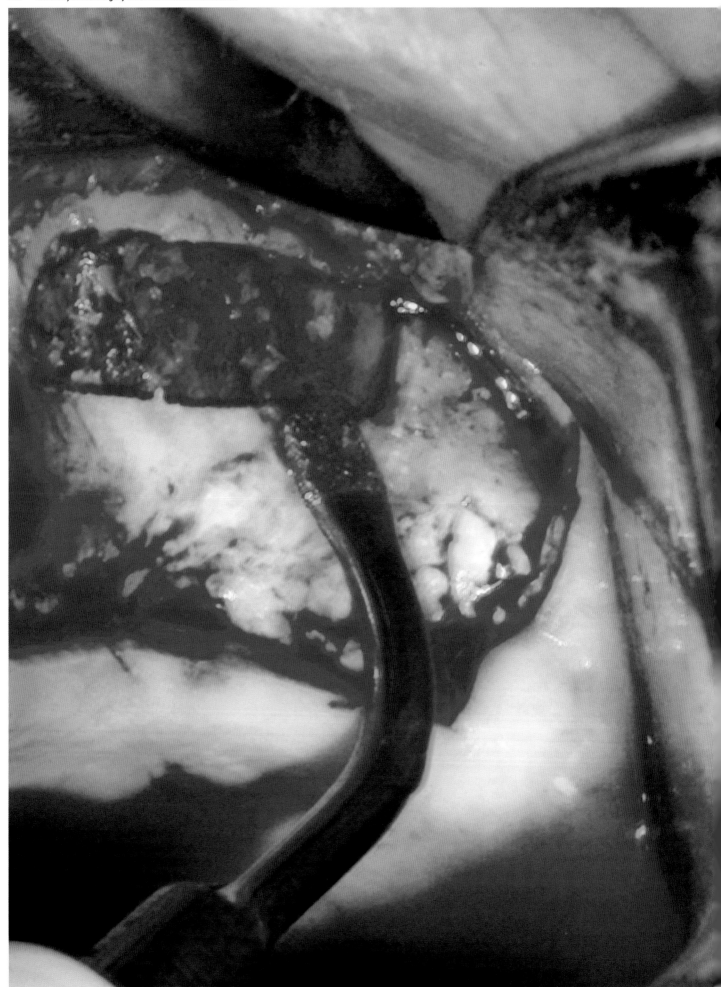

T. VERCELLOTTI

Piezoelectric surgery. Maxillary sinus augmentation techniques

14

14

Bone surgery, in particular maxillary sinus floor augmentation surgery for implantology purposes, has two main objectives. The first is the predictability of long-term results obtained after surgery, in order to achieve a suitable therapeutic goal depending on the clinical needs of the patient. The second is the lowest morbidity possible during the post-operative phase, both in the sinus grafted region where the bone graft has been performed, and in the donor site from where the graft bone has been harvested (Chanavaz 1990; Jensen et al. 1998).

The aim of this chapter is to introduce piezoelectric surgery techniques for sinus lifting, which were developed to improve intra-operative safety for the surgery and reduce morbidity for the patient.

PREOPERATIVE STUDY

After a careful anamnestic analysis and a morpho-functional study of the case, it is advisable to establish the position and number of implants according to prosthetic priorities. This means identifying a correct crown-to-implant ratio compared to the bone quality and function. It is necessary to establish the correct dentogingival relationship in order to satisfy esthetic expectations. For this reason,

we believe it necessary to evaluate the level of the smile line, before planning any type of surgery for maxillary sinus floor augmentation. This helps to avoid the error of lifting the sinus and placing implants in clinical situations that require a further block bone graft to increase the vertical height of the ridge to correct the gingival harmony.

A preoperative investigation should be performed to identify prosthetic goals in relation to the extent of the atrophy. Using a radiopaque diagnostic mask and the corresponding surgical mask, it is possible to learn and therefore exploit the residual anatomy in the best way possible, in order to choose the most suitable, minimally invasive surgical techniques for each case.

The first step is a diagnostic wax model of the missing elements and the subsequent creation of a radiopaque diagnostic mask, which reproduces the future prosthetic crown in the single para-axial sections when placed during the CT exam. Interpretation of the para-axial images allows evaluation of the actual bone volume of the atrophic ridge compared to the planned prosthetic crown for each implant site.

Once this is known, maxillary sinus surgery can be planned for each implant site. Surgical/technical variables include the approach (crestal or vestibular) and the number of operating sessions required, or whether the implant placement can be carried out in the same session as the bone graft, or at a later stage, after the graft has matured inside the sinus cavity.

To simplify the surgical sequence prior to surgery, the classification described takes into consideration the various techniques for augmenting the maxillary sinus for implant purposes.

Atrophy affects the posterior maxilla after loss of natural teeth, and, together with progressive sinus cavity pneumatization, reduces the height of the residual crestal bone.

The bone quantity and quality at the edentulous ridge must be diagnosed carefully for each implant site, using both the radiopaque diagnostic mask and the diagnostic mask for computerized imaging.

The classification proposed for maxillary atrophy can be used for selecting the surgical technique and the number of operating sessions TAB.1.

- **A type atrophy**: the residual bone volume is greater than 70% higher of the ideal implant length, according to a crown-to-implant ratio of 1:1. In this case, primary stability of the implant is guaranteed by the residual crestal bone, and the augmentation technique is also of minimal relevance for implant prognosis, except in the presence of bone quality 4. The recommended surgical technique is a small vestibular window about 6 mm long and 5 mm high. If the sinus has a considerable vestibular-palatal depth, a crestal approach is preferable in order to reduce the volume of graft material needed.

- **B type atrophy**: residual crestal bone is about 30 to 50% of the ideal implant length. As for A type atrophy, primary stability for healing is guaranteed by the residual ridge, but the grafted bone is more important for implant predictability. For this reason, there is a single surgical phase. The recommended approach is via a vestibular window.

- **C type atrophy**: The residual crestal bone is 30 to 50% of the ideal implant length, but the bone quality is type 4. In this case, primary implant stability is not guaranteed and it is therefore necessary in the first stage to graft a suitable amount of bone inside the sinus cavity, so that after maturation (6 to 8 months) it can host the implants. The volume of bone to be grafted is considerable and the approach can only be vestibular.

TYPE OF ATROPHY	RIDGE RESIDUAL	NUMBER OF SURGICAL PHASES	APPROACH CRESTAL	APPROACH VESTIBULAR
TYPE A	› 70%	1	YES	YES
TYPE B	30–50%	1	NO	YES
TYPE C	30–50% QUALITY 4	2	NO	YES
TYPE D	‹ 30%	2	NO	YES

TAB. 1

Preoperative classification of atrophic maxillae according to Vercellotti

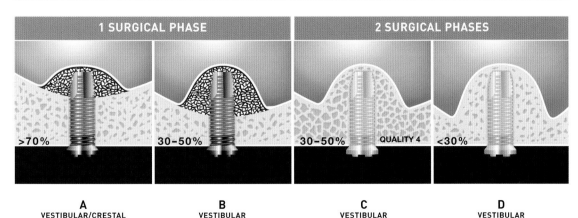

1 SURGICAL PHASE		2 SURGICAL PHASES	
>70%	30–50%	30–50% QUALITY 4	<30%
A VESTIBULAR/CRESTAL APPROACH	**B** VESTIBULAR APPROACH	**C** VESTIBULAR APPROACH	**D** VESTIBULAR APPROACH

- **D type atrophy**: the residual crestal bone is less than 30% of the necessary height and, except in cases with exceptional bone quality, cannot generally guarantee predictable primary stability. It is necessary to plan two surgical sessions: the first operating session consists of the sinus floor augmentation technique using a vestibular approach, the second (6 to 8 months later) consists of placing the implants in the previously grafted bone.

PIEZOELECTRIC BONE SURGERY

Piezoelectric bone surgery, also known as Piezosurgery®, is a new technique for osteotomies and osteoplastic surgery, which uses a special variable modulation ultrasonic surgical device designed by the author to overcome the precision and safety limits of normal manual or motor-powered instruments in bone surgery.

The basic characteristics of piezoelectric cutting are described below.

- Extreme-precision micrometric cutting: the cutting action is generated by the mechanical microvibration action, characterized by a breadth of 20 to 60 μm at a frequency of 29 kHz.
- Selective cutting: the ultrasonic frequency used in Piezosurgery® produces special vibrations that are ideal for cutting mineralized, inactive structures in contact with soft tissue. A much higher frequency would in fact be necessary to cut the latter. The physical incapacity of Piezosurgery® to cut soft tissue represents one of the most interesting surgical advantages. In fact, accidental contact with soft tissues, such as nerve or vascular structures, will not cause clinically significant damage, as shown in orthopedic surgery research (Vercellotti et al. 2001). Selective cutting in maxillary sinus surgery simplifies the access antrostomy techniques, reducing the risk of perforating the Schneiderian membrane when compared with traditional techniques. The membrane perforation rate thus decreases from 25% to 5% (Vercellotti et al. 2001).
- Blood-free operating field: the cavitation of the cooling saline solution produced by sonic and ultrasonic vibration produces tiny particles of water that hit the bone surface, causing an intense cooling action and preventing capillary bleeding at the same time, helping to clean the cutting area with subsequent increase of control and visibility during surgery.
- Piezoelectric osteotomy is carried out as easily as drawing because the pressure needed on the handpiece is extremely low, in contrast to the high pressure needed when using rotary burs and oscillating saws. When cutting bone, the latter use a mechanical action produced by torque and therefore require considerable pressure, which inevitably generates macrovibrations that reduce the operator's sensitivity.
- The absence of macrovibrations increases intra-operative control, aiding cutting safety in the more difficult anatomic areas, for example in the changeover from the compact bone to the lower consistency of cancellous bone. This changeover is usually dangerous with traditional instruments close to delicate anatomic structures, such as the vascular nerve bundle and/or the sinus membrane.
- Any contact that the Piezosurgery® insert may have with soft tissues does not cause histologically relevant damage. A general risk of iatrogenous damage remains, however, if there is excessive hand pressure caused by a lack of surgical skill, due to a non-optimal learning curve for this new technique.
- Piezoelectric bone surgery requires different manual surgical skills.

INTRODUCTION TO PIEZOELECTRIC SURGERY IN MAXILLARY SINUS AUGMENTATION PROCEDURES

Surgical techniques for augmenting the maxillary sinus floor for implant prostheses include the lifting of the integral Schneiderian membrane to accept the bone graft in particles and/or compound graft material. After a period of healing, including incorporation and remodeling, the bone graft transforms to lamellar bone, into which the osseointegratable implants can be placed (Boyne & James 1980; Lozada et al. 1993; Moy et al. 1993; Lundgren & Moy 1996; Halmann et al. 2002; Wallace & Froum 2003).

The reduction of the sinus volume after sinus augmentation does not appear to alter the normal physiology of the paranasal cavities, as long as the respiratory epithelium lining it remains whole. Consequently, all sinus floor augmentation techniques must keep the Schneiderian membrane whole; if it is damaged there can be several sinus and/or bone graft complications.

For example, if the access osteotomy causes a small perforation in the Schneiderian membrane, this could have implications for the success of the surgery, as it may cause serious complications. A small perforation may become a laceration during insertion of the graft material. If displaced through the laceration into an ectopic site above the Schneiderian membrane, the graft material could cause inflammation of the respiratory epithelium, with consequent alteration of the sinus physiology. This would cause damage to the graft itself, the possible loss of implants and the likely need for a further surgical session, with a related increase in patient morbidity.

As briefly stated, the author believes that perforation of the sinus membrane is the main cause of failure and related complications in maxillary sinus surgery. Therefore, in the event of perforation, it is wise to evaluate whether to perform the graft or whether to postpone this phase to another surgical session for each case individually (Vlassis & Fugazzotto 1999). Obviously, in this case it will be necessary to wait for the regeneration of the membrane. The author is therefore surprised that the problem of sinus membrane perforation in maxillary sinus floor augmentation techniques is not given sufficient attention in the literature. This contrasts with the author's personal experience, in which perforation has been the only cause for increased morbidity during his learning curve. Indeed, evaluations carried out on the predictability of maxillary sinus floor augmentation techniques have only been focused on the residual ridge and the type of graft material used (Jensen et al. 1998).

No authors refer to possible complications deriving from a poorly managed perforation. The author believes that, in order to be predictable, maxillary sinus augmentation surgery must be carried out in the absence of any untreated perforation. Such complications could be specifically ascribed to the technique itself, and the risk of sinus membrane perforation may persist, although decreasing, at the end of the learning curve. Indeed, success does not depend on the surgeon, but on the surgical instruments used. In an attempt to overcome this obstacle, in 1998 Torrella proposed using a normal ultrasonic curette to carry out access osteotomy to the paranasal cavity (Torrella et al. 1998). In the same period, the author carried out similar tests with ultrasound, reaching the same conclusions: access osteotomy with normal ultrasonic equipment could only be carried out in the presence of a bone wall with a maximum thickness of 1 mm, and cutting could only be carried out with extremely sharp inserts, with a concomitant risk of perforation.

After searching the literature for the use of ultrasound in bone surgery, in addition to the study by Torelli only a few articles were found, which had negative and contradictory results (Horton et al. 1975, 1981).

Horton et al. (1975, 1981) concluded that the limits of this method were insurmountable. Therefore, they decided to abandon the ultrasonic surgery techniques used up to that point, and designed an innovative variable modulation, ultrasonic piezoelectric instrument that, having overcome the limits described above, allowed a new surgical method to be developed, called piezoelectric bone surgery.

If at the end of the learning curve, the surgical technique produces one perforation for every four cases treated, it cannot be considered a predictable technique and as such, cannot be offered to patients. The present author published a study in response to this problem (Vercellotti et al. 2000) in which all the phases of maxillary sinus surgery were carried out using piezoelectric instruments. A perforation rate of 5% was reported, which became a 100% success rate in later years in his hands. The study focused on window access osteotomies (95%), including all surgical phases. Surgical perforations have mostly (80%) been observed at the point of adhesion of the membrane to the sinus floor, in correspondence with previous sinus tracts, due to the persistence of granulation tissue. The remaining 20% of lesions were found at the site of bone septa characterized by particularly difficult anatomy for separating the membrane from the bone planes.

The results obtained using piezoelectric surgery not only significantly modified the success rates, but also simplified surgical techniques, making them accessible to an increasing number of surgeons, all to the advantage of prosthetic rehabilitation on implants of posterior maxillary atrophy.

Piezoelectric bone surgery allows all osteotomy and osteoplastic surgery techniques to be carried out in all anatomic conditions, and when applied to maxillary sinus floor augmentation, it has simplified techniques, considerably reducing the possible risk of membrane perforation.

The surgical technique involves four phases FIG. 1 -I:

- access antrostomy
- membrane separation
- membrane lifting
- harvesting of bone graft.

ACCESS ANTROSTOMY

Access antrostomy can be performed on the vestibular wall of the sinus or through the floor using the crestal route.

VESTIBULAR APPROACH

The vestibular approach can be performed using two different surgical techniques: piezoelectric osteotomy of the bony window and piezoelectric osteoplastic surgery of the bony window.

PIEZOELECTRIC OSTEOTOMY OF THE BONY WINDOW

This technique requires the use of a diamond-point piezoelectric insert for osteotomy, which allows the frame of the bony window to be drawn without perforating the Schneiderian membrane, even if touched. This method is recommended when the sinus vestibular wall is extremely thin.

PIEZOELECTRIC OSTEOPLASTIC SURGERY OF THE BONY WINDOW

This technique requires the use of a sharp osteoplastic piezoelectric insert, which thins the bone wall and at the same time collects the bone fragments. These will later be grafted into the sinus cavity, after the elevation phase. This technique is recommended when the sinus vestibular wall is thicker than 1 mm. Once osteoplastic surgery has been carried out, a film of bone sometimes remains stuck to the membrane. The frame can be drawn with diamond-point inserts as in the above-described osteotomy technique.

When carrying out the osteotome technique, it is preferable to cut starting from a corner of the diamond-coated insert tip, and then continue by gripping in the initial portion of the vertical part of the insert and not by wearing down as normally happens with rotary burs. One solution is to fully complete the osteotomy, especially in the frame corners, and to refine the walls so that they are not sharp, before proceeding with the next phase.

MEMBRANE SEPARATION

When performed with traditional techniques using sinus detachers, this phase may be critical when the membrane is very thin (clinically recognizable by a bluish color rather than white, typical of a eutrophic endosteum). The membrane begins to be separated from the interior sinus cavity walls when the cavity is adhered to the window edges.

With a sharp manual elevator, a lack of elasticity may cause a laceration or enlarge a small perforation caused by using rotary burs. In contrast, when using piezoelectric surgery, this phase is extremely safe, not only due to the fact that no perforations are made during osteotomy, but also because an inverted-cone shape, atraumatic insert is used. This is inserted about 2 mm into the window edge, detaching the sinus membrane easily.

MEMBRANE LIFTING

Membrane lifting can be carried out easily at the end of separation, using manual or piezoelectric detachers, used manually without the application of vibrational energy. This is useful in the event of membrane adherence to the sinus floor, at extraction points with previous orosinus communications and sites of connective repair tissue.

In these cases, it is advisable not to persist with manual detachers, to avoid laceration. Rather, a piezoelectric detacher can be used with caution. If this maneuver is not sufficient, it is advisable to use a diamond-point or ball-tip piezoelectric insert, going over the residual alveolar via the crestal route to lift the membrane next to the adherence. The membrane must

always be lifted up to the point where it touches the mesial wall, the nasal wall and until all internal pull has been removed, to avoid laceration in the graft compacting phase.

BONE GRAFT HARVESTING

Harvesting autogenous bone particulate using the piezoelectric technique is performed using an osteoplastic instrument and with traction movement. The most suitable donor site is chosen according to the amount of bone volume needed for each operation. The body of the mandible is the ideal locaton for harvesting large volumes of bone. Piezoelectic osteoplastic surgery performed on the mandible's vestibular compact bone from the premolar area to the mandibular corner allows sufficient bone to be harvested for sinus augmentation for two or three implants.

Less autogenous bone may sometimes be required for the graft. Clinical rationality suggests using compound grafts made of a reduced percentage of autogenous bone (20 to 30%) mixed with resorbable minerals for osteoconduction. Using a graft compound reduces morbidity by avoiding surgery on the donor site, and also has a better clinical result. At the end of the incorporation period, biomaterial mixed with autogenous bone does not contract consistently, unlike bone particles alone.

In maxillary sinus surgery using the piezoelectric technique, the chosen site for small amounts for harvesting autogenous bone (0.5 to 1 cm3) is the maxillary zygomatic process. In fact, the bone segments are immediately displaced from the donor sites inside the sinus cavity by the very action of piezoelectric osteoplastic procedure. This technique is extremely simple and effective as it is not necessary to elevate a further flap to expose the donor site next to the bony window.

The patient should be informed of the probable appearance of a small facial bruise with no pain.

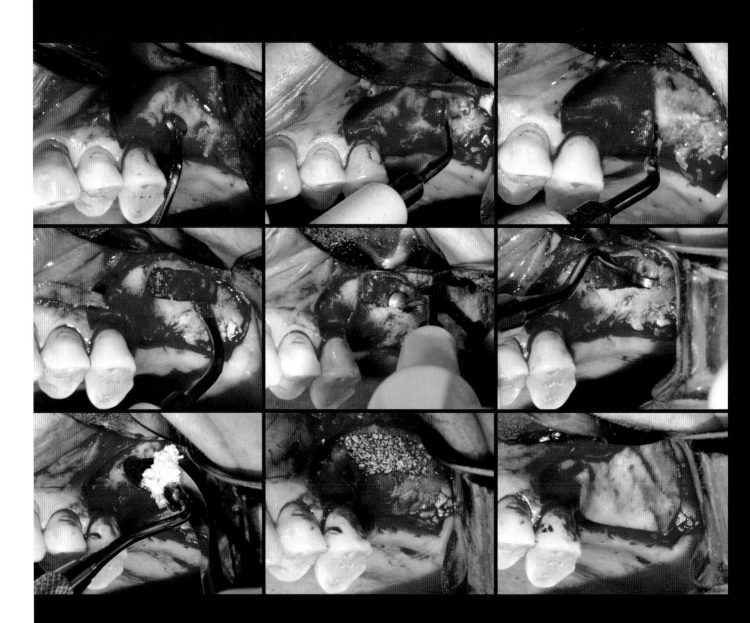

1 A	1 B	1 C
1 D	1 E	1 F
1 G	1 H	1 I

1 A → PIEZOELECTRIC ANTROSTOMY ALLOWS MEMBRANE INTEGRITY EVEN IN THE EVENT OF ACCIDENTAL CONTACT.

1 B-D → COLLECTION OF BONE FRAGMENTS FROM THE SINUS VESTIBULAR CORTEX.

1 E-F → INITIAL PHASE OF MEMBRANE DETACHMENT.

1 G-I → FINALIZATION OF GRAFT AND COMPACTING.

CONCLUSIONS

The micrometric cutting precision of piezoelectric bone surgery, or Piezosurgery®, allows maximum control of surgical action during the operation.

The frequency of the ultrasound microvibrations, which is specific for mineralized tissues, allows the Schneiderian membrane to be respected. All these special characteristics have simplified the sinus floor augmentation techniques for implant or therapeutic purposes.

Predictability of the surgery is now close to 100%.

Piezosurgery® is also extremely useful for collecting intraoral bone fragments needed for graft compounds.

The bone withdrawal technique consists of osteoplastic surgery that creates a bony window with maximum saving of the patient's tissue. It is often not necessary to elevate another flap for the donor site, for example in the posterior mandibular region.

Finally, Piezosurgery® is a bone microsurgery technique that, by using microvibrations for cutting, produces surgical microprecision and tissue micro-traumas, which aid the healing mechanisms, as has been found in scientific studies carried out in several universities in Italy and beyond.

REFERENCES

1. Boyne P.J., James R.A.
Grafting of the maxillary sinus floor with autogenous marrow and bone.
J. Oral Surg. 1980; 38: 613-6.

2. Chavanaz M.
Maxillary sinus: anatomy, physiology, surgery and bone grafting related to implantology. Eleven years of experience (1979–1990).
J. Oral Implantol. 1990; 16: 199-209.

3. Hallman M., Sennerby L., Lundgren S.
A clinical and histologic evaluation of implant integration in the posterior maxilla after sinus floor augmentation with autogenous bone, bovine hydroxyapatite, or a 20:80 mixture.
Int. J. Oral Maxillofac. Implants 2002; 17: 635-43.

4. Horton J.E., Tarpley T.M. Jr, Jacoway J.R.
Clinical applications of ultrasonic instrumentation in the surgical removal of bone.
Oral Surg. Oral Med. Oral Pathol. 1981; 51: 236-42.

5. Horton J.E., Tarpley T.M. Jr, Wood L.D.
The healing of surgical defects in alveolar bone produced with ultraonic instrumentation, chisel and rotary bur.
Oral Surg. Oral Med. Oral Pathol. 1975; 39: 536-46.

6. Jensen O.T., Shulman L.B., Block M.S., Iacono V.J.
Report of the sinus consensus conference of 1996.
Int. J. Oral Maxillofac. Implants 1998: 13 (Suppl); 11-45.

7. Lozada J.L., Emanuelli S., James R.A., Boskovic M., Lindsted K.
Root-form implants placed in subantral grafted sites.
J. Calif. Dent. Assoc. 1993; 21: 31-5.

8. Lundgren S., Moy P.
Augmentation of the maxillary sinus floor with particulate mandible: A histologic and histomorphometric study.
Int. J. Oral Maxillofac. Implants 1996; 11: 760-6.

9. Moy P.K., Lundgren S., Holmes R.E.
Maxillary sinus augmentation: Histomorphometric analysis of graft materials for maxillary sinus floor augmentation.
J. Oral Maxillofac. Surg. 1993; 51: 857-62.

10. Torella F., Pitarch J., Cabanes G., Anitua E.
Ultrasonic osteotomy for the surgical approach of the mzaxillary sinus: a technical note.
Int. J. Oral Maxillofac. Implants 1998; 13: 697-700.

11. Vercellotti T., De Paoli S., Nevins M.
The piezoelectric bony window osteotomy and sinus membrane elevation: introduction of a new technique for simplification of the sinus augmentation procedure.
Int. J. Periodontics Restorative Dent. 2001; 21: 561-7.

12. Vercellotti T., Russo C., Gianotti S.
A New Piezoelectric Ridge Expansion Technique in the Lower Arch—A Case Report (online article).
World Dent. 2000; 1(2)

13. Vlassis J.M., Fugazzotti P.A.
A classification system for sinus membrane perforations during augmentation procedures with options for repair.
J. Periodontol. 1999; 70: 692-9.

14. Wallace S.S., Froum S.J.
Effect of maxillary sinus augmentation on the survival of endosseous dental implants. A systematic review.
Ann. Periodontol. 2003; 8: 328-43.

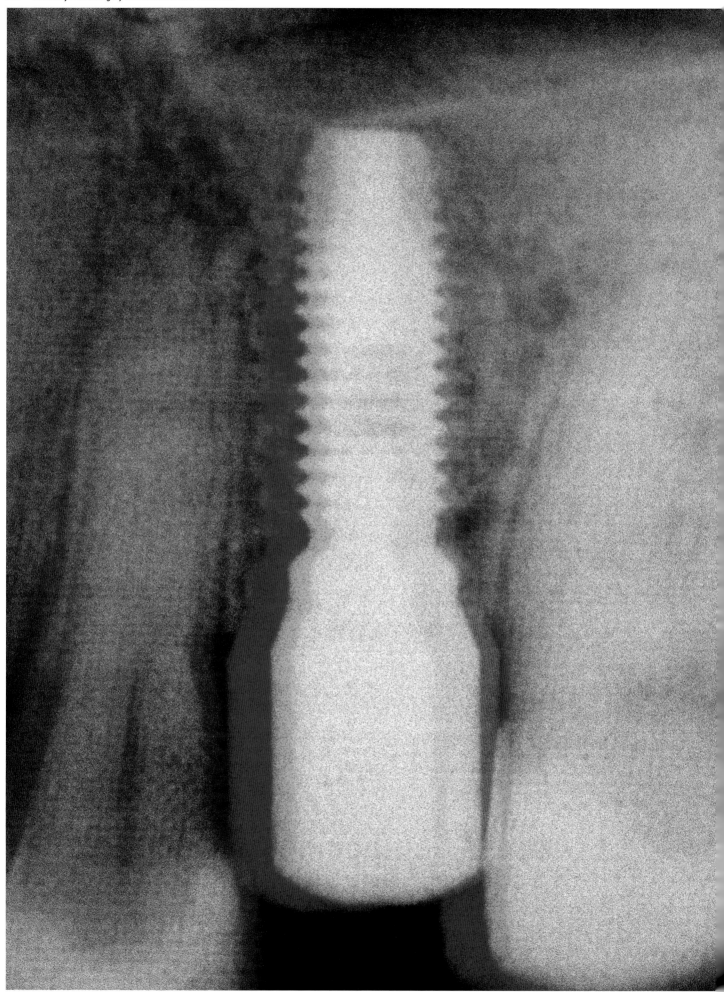

G. CORDIOLI
Z. MAJZOUB

Maxillary sinus augmentation crestal techniques

15

15

INTRODUCTION

The insertion of implants in the posterior maxilla is often complicated by the inadequate quantity and quality of bone tissue. Among the surgical procedures proposed for resolving the above-stated anatomical limitations of this area, sinus augmentation using autogenous bone or bone substitutes has proven to be a safe method with high predictability of success (Hirsch & Ericsson 1991; Smiler et al. 1992; Raghoebar et al. 1993; Wheeler et al. 1996; Fugazzotto & Vlassis 1998; Froum et al. 1998; Peleg et al. 1999; Kahnberg et al. 2001; Stricker et al. 2003). A less invasive surgical approach for lifting the sinus, using a crestal access, was proposed in 1986 by Tatum and then perfected by Summers in 1994 (Summers 1994a, 1994b).

The osteotome sinus floor elevation (OSFE) technique aims to lift the sinus floor using the bone obtained from preparing the osteotomic site, while the bone-added osteotome sinus floor elevation (BAOSFE) technique obtains the same result using graft material, which is pushed into the osteotomic site using a set of osteotomes (Summers 1994a). Both techniques can be used for a single implant as well as for multiple implants and are considered more predictable when the residual bone ridge height is at least

5 to 6 mm (Summers 1994a). The crestal or indirect augmentation of the maxillary sinus allows the simultaneous insertion of implants in all cases where there is residual bone ridge that allows primary implant stability. Otherwise, a crestal elevation of the sinus can be performed using a deferred approach (future site development, FSD) (Summers 1995) to create a suitable bone volume, in order to proceed with the delayed placement of implants. Several modifications to the crestal approach for maxillary sinus augmentation were introduced by various authors, after the original description made by Summers (Coatoam 1997; Bruschi et al. 1998; Fugazzotto 1999, 2001; Cosci & Luccioli 2000; Cavicchia et al. 2001; Nkenke et al. 2002b).

TECHNIQUES AND MATERIALS

CRESTAL ELEVATION OF THE SINUS WITH DELAYED IMPLANT PLACEMENT

FUTURE SITE DEVELOPMENT – SUMMERS 1995

This technique is used when the ridge bone height is less than 5 mm and implants will be inserted in a later phase. Using a trephine bur with a 5 mm internal diameter, an osteotomy is carried out up to the sinus floor. Later, the bone cylinder taken with a trephine bur is pushed using an osteotome n. 5 with concave point, and pressure or small strikes with the surgical mallet. The sinus membrane is then lifted by the bone cylinder, which acts as a hydraulic piston. Autogenous bone and/or bone substitutes are progressively added until the osteotomic site is completely filled. The future site (FS) osteotome is used with graft material to determine further apical movement of the bone cylinder, thus aiding a more extensive detachment of the Schneiderian membrane. This latter phase is repeated until the sinus is lifted to the volume required FIG. 1 A-D. The osteotomes must not penetrate the sinus space during the FS procedure. Using this technique, the lifted bone cylinders remain adherent to the Schneiderian membrane and remain vital in order to supply osteoprogenitor cells and blood to the grafted site. Also, the osteotomy site created in the residual bone ridge has better healing potential than the grafted site inside the maxillary sinus (Summers 1995). In 2001, Fugazzotto introduced a modification to this technique, limiting the apical displacement of the bone cylinder to a depth 1 mm less than the height of the preparation made with the trephine bur; the possibility of displacing the bone cylinder inside the sinus is thus reduced and at the same time better mechanical stability is obtained (Fugazzotto 2001) **FIG. 2**.

MODIFIED TREPHINE/OSTEOTOME TECHNIQUE – FUGAZZOTTO 2001

Fugazzotto made a change to Summers' FSD technique for the cases in which a maxillary tooth is extracted, in order to preserve the buccopalatal dimensions and increase the apicocoronal height of the subantral area. Immediately after a traumatic molar extraction, a bone cylinder is prepared in the maxilla using a trephine bur suitably sized to include the intraradicular septum and at least 50% of the postextraction alveolus. The site is prepared up to 1 to 2 mm from the sinus floor. The bone cylinder, with corresponding sinus membrane, is then pushed apically by a calibrated osteotome with gentle strikes of a mallet, to a depth at least corresponding to the apicocoronal height of the bone cylinder. The residual crestal bone deficiency is filled with deproteinized bovine bone, and can be protected with a resorbable membrane, according to the principles of guided bone regeneration (GBR). The flaps are sutured, to obtain primary flap closure, if possible. The implants are inserted at a later stage, depending on the healing period, the morphology and initial size of the deficiency and the desired regeneration results. Using this simultaneous combination of dental extraction and GBR sinus augmentation procedure, three-

dimensional ridge resorption is avoided. The apicocoronal volume of the bone is increased for the future insertion of implants at least 10 mm long and 4.8 mm in diameter in the molar region of the maxilla. The limitation of this technique is the limited elevation of the sinus floor, and therefore the potential need for further sinus augmentation when the implants are inserted. Another limitation is the potential complication connected with the non-primary closure of the flap, or the onset of postoperative dehiscences, which could cause an infection in the underlying membrane, with possible loss of grafted material.

CRESTAL ELEVATION OF THE SINUS WITH IMMEDIATE INSERTION OF IMPLANTS

WITHOUT MATERIAL GRAFTING

• OSTEOTOME SINUS FLOOR ELEVATION – SUMMERS 1994B, 1994C

This procedure is usually used in marrow bone tissue and its main aim is to maintain all the bone harvested from the walls of the osteotomy site and then push it apically to elevate the sinus floor.

The height of the residual crestal bone ridge is measured on preoperative radiographs. The site is prepared by the first osteotome, which is pushed below the sinus floor. The site is later expanded with a series of osteotomes. Ideally, the tip of the instruments should not penetrate inside the sinus space, and the Schneiderian membrane should not be touched. The apical displacement of the bone collected by the instruments should cause the lifting of the sinus floor and the membrane, without using other dissection instruments. If the compact bone is dense, burs may be necessary; this will cause partial or total loss of the bone collected in the osteotomic site. Graft material should then be used to elevate the sinus floor and the sinus membrane.

In addition to the original osteotomes developed by Summers, many others are now available. These osteotomes are shaped to adapt to the profile and size of the implants used. They are designed to allow the tip of the next instrument to penetrate the site created by the previous one and have a concave tip that cuts the bone in the osteotomic site and allows it to be collected in the concavity. Summers has stated that, using this technique, it is possible to obtain an increase in the maxillary sinus of more than 5 mm **FIG. 3A-C**.

Malchiodi (2003) proposed a modification to the Summers technique: a sequential series of osteotomes of increasing length (3.5, 5, 6.5, 8 and 9.5 mm) with a crestal stop. The 3.5, 6.5 and 9.5 mm osteotomes have a concave tip while the 5, 8 and 10 mm osteotomes have a convex tip. According to the author, the advantages of this approach are:

- a gradual, controlled increase in the depth of the implant site that reduces the possibility of membrane perforation
- the alternate use of concave and convex tip osteotomes allows the collected bone to be compacted better both vertically and laterally **FIG. 4A-E**.

• LOCALIZED MANAGEMENT OF SINUS FLOOR (LMSF) – BRUSCHI ET AL. 1998

Bruschi described a technique that combines maxillary sinus augmentation, alveolar ridge expansion and implant insertion (Bruschi et al. 1998). After elevating a partial thickness flap buccally and and a full thickness flap palatally, a long groove is made across the bone ridge using a scalpel no. 64 Beaver Blade (Becton Dickinson Acute Care, Franklin Lakes, NJ, USA), to the depth of the sinus floor. The buccal bone ridge is then gently displaced in a vestibular direction, using a Heidbrink radicular elevator (Hu-Friedy, Chicago, IL, USA) to deepen the initial groove by 0.5 to 1 mm below the sinus floor. The implant site is then prepared using a series of osteotomes with a rounded tip and an increasing diameter (2.5, 3.3 and 4 mm). Initial site preparation is carried out using a 2.5 mm osteotome, which is malleted to compress the remaining 1 to 1.5 mm of bone against the sinus floor cortex. The procedure is repeated with 3.3 and 4 mm osteotomes, until

the sinus floor is fractured, without displacing bone into the sinus. The sinus floor and Schneiderian membrane is moved apically using osteotomes. A collagen membrane is adapted in the implant sites, with the later insertion of implants in the newly created sites **FIG. 5A-D**.

• MODIFIED TREPHINE/OSTEOTOME TECHNIQUE – FUGAZZOTTO 2002

The trephine bur/osteotomes technique described in 1999 was modified by the simultaneous insertion of implants. The implant site is prepared using a 3-mm exterior diameter trephine bur at a distance of 1 to 2 mm from the sinus floor. The bone cylinder is then pushed apically to a depth of 1 mm less than the one made with the bur, using an osteotome of the same diameter as the trephine bur. The final preparation of the implant site is carried out using osteotomes of increasing diameters, always inserting them to the same depth if self-threading implants are not used. The implants are inserted at a speed of 30 rpm, causing controlled lateral movement of the bone cylinder inside the space created by the movement of the sinus membrane. The author suggests using the formula 2x -2 to calculate the maximum height of the implant to be inserted using this technique, where x is equal to the apicocoronal height of the residual bone ridge.

WITH MATERIAL GRAFTING

• OSTEOTOME SINUS FLOOR ELEVATION – SUMMERS 1994B, 1994C

In this technique, initial preparation is carried out using an osteotome, which is gently pushed with a surgical mallet, until it reaches 1 to 2 mm from the sinus floor. It is sometimes necessary to use a bur if the compact bone is dense. Resistance is felt when the sinus floor is reached and a change can be noted in the sound of the osteotome. At this point, a periapical radiograph is taken to correctly evaluate the depth to which the osteotome has penetrated. When the instrument is 1 to 2 mm from the

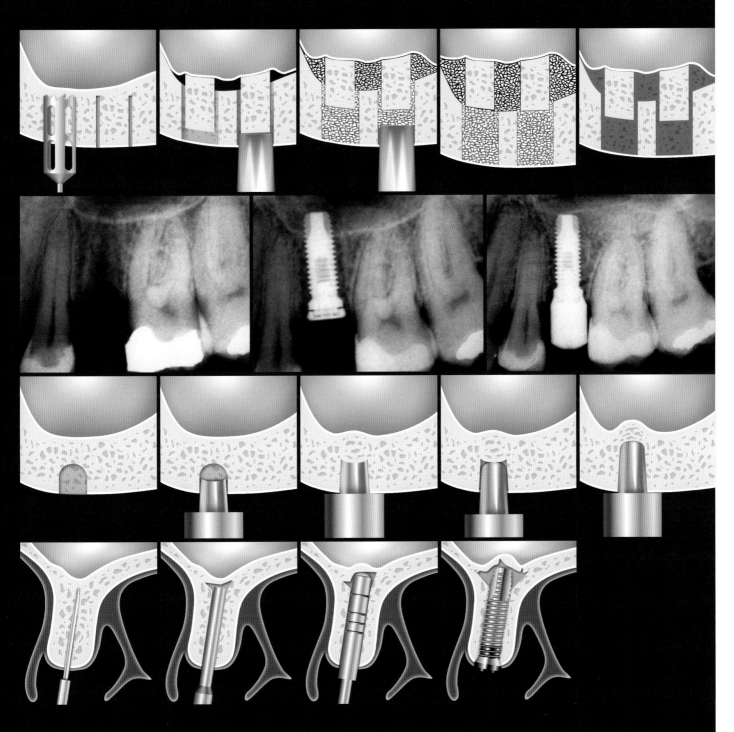

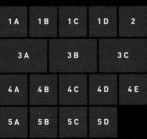

1 A → A BONE CYLINDER IS MADE BELOW THE SINUS FLOOR USING A BUR WITH INTERNAL DIAMETER 5 MM.

1 B → THE BONE CYLINDER IS PUSHED APICALLY WITH SMALL STRIKES OR PRESSURE WITH THE OSTEOTOME N. 5. LIFTING OF THE MEMBRANE AT THIS STAGE IS MINIMAL.

1 C-D → GRAFT MATERIAL IS INSERTED TO OBTAIN FURTHER ELEVATION OF THE BONE CYLINDER AND TO FILL THE CRESTAL DEFICIENCY.

2 → THE TECHNIQUE PROPOSED BY FUGAZZOTTO IN 2001 IS SIMILAR TO THE FSD TECHNIQUE INTRODUCED BY SUMMERS, WITH THE EXCEPTION THAT THE BONE CYLINDER OBTAINED WITH THE TREPHINE BUR IS PUSHED TO A DEPTH OF 1 MM LESS THAN THE ONE MADE WITH THE BUR.

3 A → PREOPERATIVE RAGIOGRAPH SHOWING AN EDENTULOUS RIDGE IN THE PREMOLAR SITE, 2 MONTHS AFTER EXTRACTIONS.

3 B → A 13-MM IMPLANT WAS PLACED WITHOUT A BONE GRAFT. NOTE THE PRESENCE OF A RADIOPAQUE MASS AT THE IMPLANT APEX, ADJACENT TO THE BONE CORTEX FRAGMENT, A RESULT OF THE SINUS FLOOR FRACTURE IN COMBINATION WITH AUTOGENOUS BONE COLLECTED DURING IMPLANT SITE PREPARATION AND PUSHED APICALLY WITH THE TIP OF THE INSTRUMENTS.

3 C → RADIOGRAPHIC CONTROL 6 MONTHS AFTER THE SUGERY, WHICH HIGHLIGHTS THE SUCCESS OF SINUS ELEVATION AND THE APICAL POSITION OF THE NEW SINUS FLOOR.

4 A-E → THE MALCHIODI OSTEOTOMES WITH CRESTAL STOPS AND CONCAVE TIPS FOR CUTTING AND COMPACTING VERTICALLY, AND THE CONVEX POINT FOR HORIZONTAL COMPRESSION.

5A → AN INTRAOSSEOUS GROOVE IS CREATED WITH A NO. 64 BEAVER SCALPEL UNDER THE SINUS FLOOR.

5 B → A RADICULAR ELEVATOR IS USED TO WIDEN THE OSTEOTOMY AND BEGIN THEBUCCAL EXPANSION OF THE RIDGE.

5 C → THE FINAL PREPARATION OF THE IMPLANT SITE AND THE INITIAL SINUS FLOOR FRACTURE ARE PERFORMED USING A SET OF ROUNDED-TIP PROBES WITH INCREASING DIAMETERS.

5 D → IMPLANT PLACED IN THE SITE.

sinus floor, the osteotome site is widened using osteotomes of increasing diameter, always maintaining the same working depth. The graft material is inserted in the osteotome site, before making any attempt to raise the floor. According to the author, the volume of graft material should not exceed 3 mm in height before starting the sinus floor elevation. At this point, the last osteotome is inserted, the sinus compact bone is infractured using small mallet strikes and the sinus floor is lifted. The later sequences of adding graft material are constantly repeated, always pushing the osteotome to the previously defined depth. The osteotome tip should not, or only slightly, exceed the original limit of the maxillary sinus. According to the author, the membrane is lifted due to the hydraulic force produced by the osteotome pushing the graft material and liquid in the osteotome site and not due to the direct effect of the instruments' tips. The sinus augmentation procedure is continued until the desired elevation is achieved, without exceeding the Schneiderian membrane stretching limit.

Care must be taken when selecting the length of the implant that is to be inserted **FIG. 6A–E**. Inserting the implant in an osteotomic site involves displacing the graft material more apically and laterally, with a further consequent stretching of the membrane in a more apical position. Among the other factors, the final size of the implant should be selected in relation to the sinus membrane's stretching capacity (Winter et al. 2002). Taking into account the 1 to 2 mm shrinkage of graft material during the healing phase of the grafted area, we recommend using shorter implants than the height of the grafted site. Cosci & Luccioli (2000) suggest that there should be at least 2 to 3 mm of graft material above the implant apex. Coatoam (1997) recommends avoiding the use of implants that are more than 4 mm longer than the apex of adjacent teeth.

Preparing the implant site with osteotomes should be avoided when a force of more than 20 MPa is required (Nkenke et al. 2002a), as the integrity of the osteocytes and angiogenesis would be affected negatively by excessive compression forces exceeding this limit (Müller et al. 1985). Consequently, the use of osteotomes must be applied if bone quality is 3 or 4, in order to avoid excessive compression and displacement of the marrow space trabecular bone, an eventuality that would alter blood flow. Using the osteotomy technique on dense bone may cause excessive compression on intraosseous vessels, with subsequent damage to the osseointegration processes (Strietzel et al. 2002).

With the technique proposed by Summers (1994a, 1994b), the initial access to the sinus cavity is the most crucial part of the sinus augmentation procedure, especially when the sinus floor is thick and compact (compact bone). Infracturing the sinus floor with osteotomes is difficult to control and may be a risky maneuver. If excessive malleting is required to perforate the sinus floor, it may be advisable to use the bur to perforate the bone. Coatoam (1997) suggests infracturing the sinus floor directly with a convex-tip osteotome before proceeding with adding graft material. Cavicchia et al. (2001) used a similar approach, fracturing the sinus floor directly with osteotomes or with a cylindrical probe. Some authors have recommended inserting one or more resorbable collagen sponges in the implant site after infracturing the sinus floor; this material acts as a buffer for the Schneiderian membrane and helps to lift the membrane prior to initiating the grafting procedure.

Unlike the Summers protocol, the surgical technique used by Deporter involves penetrating the sinus with the osteotome tip, although it remains separated from the sinus membrane by the layer of graft material and the bone cylinder obtained from fracturing the sinus floor (Deporter et al. 2000).

• COSCI & LUCCIOLI 2000

To avoid a greenstick fracture of the sinus floor when using osteotomes, Cosci and Luccioli (2000) proposed a new surgical technique, using a specific bur to perforate the sinus floor. The authors suggest that laceration of the Schneiderian membrane while perforating the sinus floor with rotating instruments is a less frequent occurrence than that of fracturing the floor with osteotomes. Initially, a trephine bur is used to prepare the implant site and harvest a small amount of autogenous bone. The trephine bur is inserted up to the sinus floor floor. Metal markers are then placed in the prepared site, in order to take periapical radiographs for confirmation that the sinus floor has been reached. The first bur must be 1 mm longer than the height established radiographically. The specific bur system (Fresissima, Turin, Italy) has a cutting angle of 30 degrees and also has an irrigation system; the burs also have a safety system that stops them at the bone ridge. If the sinus floor compact bone is not perforated (control with a rounded-tip probe), the next bur can be used, which is 1 mm longer. The autogenous bone collected previously can be used together with other types of graft material. Graft material is pressed into the implant site using a "body lifting" instrument, which is pushed up to 4 mm inside the site using a surgical mallet **FIG. 7A-C**. The graft material is inserted until the sinus is lifted to the level required, which is also checked by radiograph. Finally, a traditional bur that is slightly longer than the height of the residual bone ridge is used to give the final shape to the implant site.

• ENDOSCOPICALLY CONTROLLED OSTEOTOME SINUS FLOOR ELEVATION (ECOSFE) - NKENKE ET AL. 2002B

Nkenke hypothesized that Schneiderian membrane perforation can occur if sharp bone fragments are used directly to lift the membrane (Nkenke et al. 2002b). The authors propose an alternative technique by which the sinus bone floor is directly fractured by the osteotome tip and not by the force of the graft material pushed using a concave tip osteotome. After initial preparation to a depth of 2 mm using the pilot bur, the implant site is prepared using osteotomes with increasing diameters. After using the final osteotome with the widest concave tip, the sinus bone floor is infractured under endoscopic control, lifted with the adherent sinus membrane and later lifted with an osteotome, until it detaches spontaneously at the sinus floor/sinus membrane interface. Further lifting of the sinus membrane from the sinus floor is then carried out using a specific detacher. Graft material is then added, using the widest osteotome inserted into the site **FIG. 8A-C**. During all these operating phases, the wide osteotome tip is inserted above the sinus floor, but the osteotome is always separated from the sinus membrane by the interposition of a thin layer of compact bone, which was lifted at the beginning of the procedure.

SINOSCOPIC FINDINGS

Performing endoscopy during maxillary sinus augmentation surgery has been proposed to exclude sinus pathologies, to check the graft position and to reduce membrane perforation risks, and therefore to avoid postoperative complications (Engelke & Deckwer 1997; Wiltfang et al. 2000; Aimetti et al. 2001; Nkenke et al. 2002b; Timmenga et al. 2003). When the BAOSFE technique is used, the endoscopic control to check the Schneiderian membrane's integrity allows the surgeon to check the elastic deformation of the membrane, and thus permits better lifting of the sinus, in order to insert the longest implants possible (Baumann & Ewers 1999; Nkenke et al. 2002b).

A review of data published on sinus lifting under endoscopic control showed a low frequency of membrane laceration, both when the membrane is lifted using the mass of graft material that acts as a hydraulic force (Summers 1994b; Baumann & Ewers 1999; Reiser et al. 2001; Berengo et al. 2004), and when the sinus bone floor is fractured and lifted (Nkenke et al. 2002b). Data on the incidence of complications from sinus augmentation procedures in both clinical practice and on cadavers have been summarized **TAB. 1-2**.

Lacerations of the sinus membrane can be caused by:

- the presence of thin membranes, the inadequate use of osteotomes pushed too far apically, the overly rapid insertion of large volumes of graft material (Summers 1994a)
- presence of septa (Reiser et al. 2001)
- the use of burs more than 2 mm from the sinus floor, which may require greater force for lifting the compact bone with osteotomes (Reiser et al. 2001)
- preparation of implant sites to a depth of more than 4 mm than the level of the apices of the adjacent teeth (Coatoam 1997)
- Lifting of membrane more than 5 mm (Cavicchia et al. 2001).

It has been hypothesized that oblique sinus floors allow the sinus to be lifted more than flat sinus floors; in fact, the stress applied to the membrane is lower as it is already stretched apically and laterally (Cavicchia et al. 2001). This hypothesis must still be confirmed with endoscopic findings and/or with radiographic control studies.

Sinus conditions are not altered in the short and long term by accidental small perforations that occur during sinus lifting procedures. Baumann & Ewers (1999) reported the complete healing of small membrane perforations further to endoscopic control carried out 6 weeks after the BAOSFE, with simultaneous implant inser-

tion. Similarly, the absence of sinus pathologies and complete healing of the perforation, despite the displacement of the graft material into the sinus, were found on the endoscopy control 6 months after the sinus augmentation procedure in a patient in whom one of the two implants inserted showed obvious laceration of the membrane (Nkenke et al. 2002b). In the same clinical study, a second patient had antral poliposis after the sinus augmentation surgery, although perforations were not found during the procedure; this patient showed no sign of sinus suffering. Similar post-surgical endoscopic findings were reported by Aimetti et al. (2001), who showed that small sinus membrane lacerations occurring during sinus augmentation procedures using lateral osteotomy were associated with normal maxillary sinus conditions 31 months after surgery.

Two types of morphological behavior of sinus membrane lifting have been reported regarding the membrane stretch (Reiser et al. 2001; Berengo et al. 2003). In the first, lifting is limited to the implant apex and has a localized vertical and slightly lateral projection. In the second, lifting is dome-shaped, which involves several implants, with a large lifting area that is lateral to the implants. In the BAOSFE technique, where direct surgical elevation of the sinus membrane cannot be performed, lifting the membrane between the implants in multiple sites adjacent to or distant from the perimeter of a single implant is not predictable. The extent of the new subantral space after lifting the Schneiderian membrane is related to the inter-implant distance, the elastic characteristics of the membrane and the membrane's quality of adhesion to the underlying bone plane. The clinical importance of the behavior of membrane lifting using the BAOSFE technique must still be investigated **FIG. 9A-D**.

CLINICAL RESULTS

The short- and long-term results of sinus augmentation using the crestal route are shown in several studies (Summers 1994; Coatoam & Krieger 1997; Horowitz 1997; Fugazzotto & Vlassis 1998; Bruschi et al. 1998; Komarnyckyj & London 1998; Zitzmann & Schärer 1998; Yildirim et al. 1998; Fugazzotto 1999, 2001, 2002; Rosen et al. 1999; Cosci & Luccioli 2000; Cavicchia et al. 2000; Ioannidou & Dean 2000; Leonetti et al. 2000; Cavicchia et al. 2001; Fugazzotto & De Paoli 2002; Nkenke et al. 2002b; Winter et al. 2002; Artzi et al. 2003). These studies show a high success rate with various implant morphologies and lengths, with multiple surgical techniques and various types of graft material (osteotome-based crestal elevation procedure TAB. 3) (FSD technique TAB. 4). Previous studies that used burs in quality 4 bone for implant site preparation showed much lower success rates than the ones obtained in denser quality bone (van Steenberghe et al. 1987; Adell et al. 1990; Jaffin & Berman 1991; Friberg et al. 1995). In spite of the lack of controlled studies to compare the preparation of the implant site with osteotomes or with burs, it seems that the osteotome technique significantly improves the success rate of implants in the posterior maxilla compared to the use of burs (Glauser et al. 1998; Zitzmann & Schärer 1998). One common note concerning the single stage sinus augmentation technique reported by several authors is that the majority of implant failures occur early, during the healing period, at the implant–abutment connection or at the latest within the

Review of published data concerning results of control endoscopy carried out after sinus augmentation procedures using osteotomes

TAB. 1

AUTHORS	NUMBER OF PATIENTS (NUMBER OF SINUSES)	ENDOSCOPIC CONTROL INTRA-SURGERY	BLEEDING	PERFORATIONS	ENDOSCOPIC CONTROL POST-SURGERY	PATHOLOGICAL FINDINGS INTRA-SINUS	CLINICAL SYMPTOMS POST-SURGERY
Baumann & Ewers 1999	7 (7)	Yes	0	1	In the site perforated	None	None
Nkenke et al. 2002b	14 (18)	Yes	1 (patient #10)	1 (patient #1) (Valsalva negative)	Yes	Migration of the material grafted into sinus, perforation no longer visible Mucosal polyp (patient #11)	None
Berengo et al. 2003	8 (8)	Yes	0	2 (Valsalva negative)	No	–	None

AUTHORS	NUMBER OF CADAVERS (NUMBER OF IMPLANTS)	ENDOSCOPIC CONTROL INTRA-SURGERY	INCREASE VERTICAL OF HEIGHT BONE	PERFORATIONS
Baumann & Ewers 1999	10 (not specified)	Yes	13 mm implants used	0
Reiser et al. 2001	14 (25)	No	4-8 mm	6/25

TAB. 2

Review of published data concerning results of sinus augmentation with osteotomy on cadavers

first 12 months (Coatoam & Krieger 1997; Komarnyckyj & London 1998; Rosen et al. 1999; Fugazzotto 2002). Failures are connected with smoking (Rosen et al. 1999; Cavicchia et al. 2001), occlusal overload (Cavicchia et al. 2001), a lack of primary stability (Cavicchia et al. 2001), the presence of a residual crestal bone height less than 50% of the final height of the implant (Cavicchia et al. 2001), or with a bone ridge of less than 4 mm high (Rosen et al. 1999). This latter factor is probably the decisive cause of failure. We therefore recommend that this procedure is used in clinical cases where there is at least 5 mm of residual crestal bone, as primary stability is mainly linked to the original ridge height.

High functional loads, reduced bone volume and low bone quality have a negative effect on the success of smooth surface implants in the posterior maxilla. Short implants that are used to overcome anatomical limitations of height in the posterior maxillary regions have a higher failure rate than longer implants (Quirynen et al. 1992; Bahat 1993; Lazzara et al. 1996; Jendersen et al. 1998; Weng et al. 2003). This behavior occurs less when rough surface implants are used (Buser et al. 1997; Khang et al. 2001; Testori et al. 2001) and in good bone quality (van Steenberghe et al. 1990). Although no direct comparison is available, the results of a recent long-term randomized controlled study between short and long implants inserted using the sinus crestal elevation technique showed that short, wide-diameter implants have similar success rates those obtained with long implants. In a prospective clinical study, Deporter et al. (2000) used porous surface implants that were shorter than 10 mm (average length of implants 6.9 mm) and were 4.0 and 5.0 mm in diameter, inserted at the second maxillary premolar and the first and second maxillary molar levels, and reported a 100% success rate for the follow-up period of 11.1 months. Similar high success rates were found with the modified trephine bur/osteotome technique, using ITI

implants that were 7 and 12 mm long and 3.75 and 4.8 mm in diameter, in the posterior maxillary regions and with prosthetic post-load follow-up after 4 years (Fugazzotto 2002). A success rate of 93.75% was achieved when using 8 and 10 mm implants (4.1 mm diameter) covered with titanium plasma-spray, in a single-stage osteotome technique (Komarnyckyj & London 1998). These good results for the posterior maxilla using short implants may be attributed to improved osseointegration after using the osteotome technique (Zitzmann & Schärer 1998; Nkenke et al. 2002a) and the use of rough surface implants that optimize primary stability and bone healing (Deporter et al. 2000; Cavicchia et al. 2001; Davarpanah et al. 2001; Fugazzotto 2002).

RADIOGRAPHIC RESULTS

Results regarding the increase of bone height, achieved through the sinus crestal elevation technique, are summarized **TAB. 3**.

At present, a limited number of longitudinal studies on the changes in the size of bone grafts in sinus augmentation procedures have been reported (Block et al. 1998; Froum et al. 1998; Shulman et al. 1999; Geurs et al. 2001; Johansson et al. 2001; Ozyuvaci et al. 2003). In an observation period of 5 and 10 years, Block et al. (1998) observed a reduction in height of mineralized tissue in single-stage sinus lifts, using autogenous iliac bone particulate or bone taken from the maxillary as graft material. In a recent retrospective radiographic study on lateral approach sinus augmentation, a loss of graft height (between 0.82 and 2.09 mm on average) was found with a large variety of graft materials, including intraoral or extraoral autogenous bone, heterologous or alloplastic materials or a combination of both (Geurs et al. 2001). In a clinical study concerning the changes in volume of bone grafts in atrophic maxillae, the DentaScan performed in the first few weeks and at 7 months

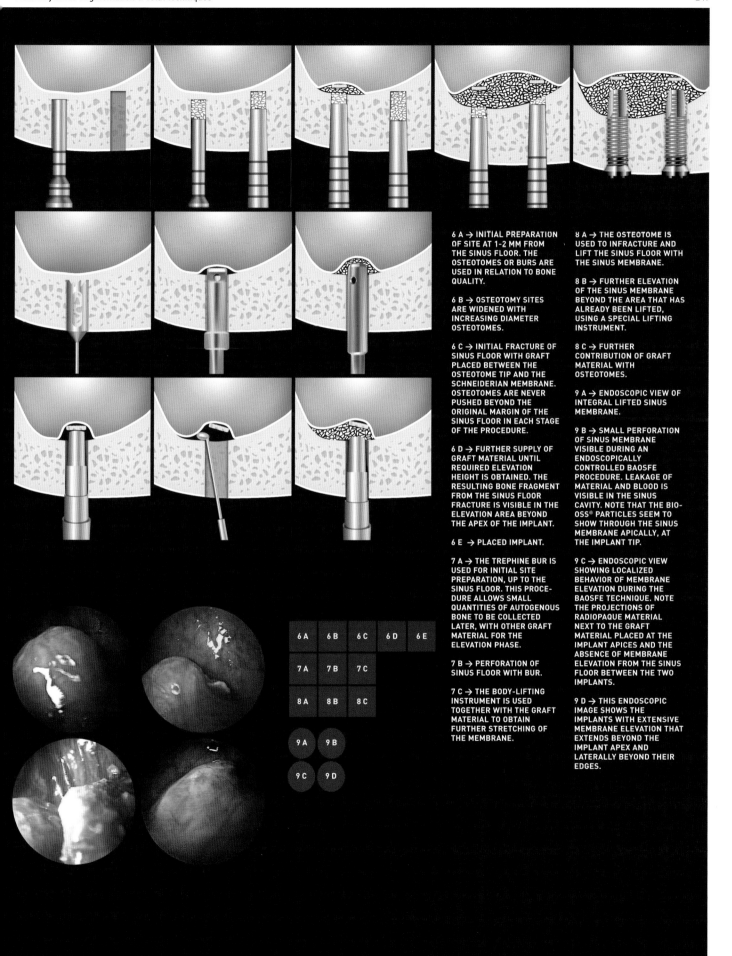

6 A → INITIAL PREPARATION OF SITE AT 1-2 MM FROM THE SINUS FLOOR. THE OSTEOTOMES OR BURS ARE USED IN RELATION TO BONE QUALITY.

6 B → OSTEOTOMY SITES ARE WIDENED WITH INCREASING DIAMETER OSTEOTOMES.

6 C → INITIAL FRACTURE OF SINUS FLOOR WITH GRAFT PLACED BETWEEN THE OSTEOTOME TIP AND THE SCHNEIDERIAN MEMBRANE. OSTEOTOMES ARE NEVER PUSHED BEYOND THE ORIGINAL MARGIN OF THE SINUS FLOOR IN EACH STAGE OF THE PROCEDURE.

6 D → FURTHER SUPPLY OF GRAFT MATERIAL UNTIL REQUIRED ELEVATION HEIGHT IS OBTAINED. THE RESULTING BONE FRAGMENT FROM THE SINUS FLOOR FRACTURE IS VISIBLE IN THE ELEVATION AREA BEYOND THE APEX OF THE IMPLANT.

6 E → PLACED IMPLANT.

7 A → THE TREPHINE BUR IS USED FOR INITIAL SITE PREPARATION, UP TO THE SINUS FLOOR. THIS PROCE-DURE ALLOWS SMALL QUANTITIES OF AUTOGENOUS BONE TO BE COLLECTED LATER, WITH OTHER GRAFT MATERIAL FOR THE ELEVATION PHASE.

7 B → PERFORATION OF SINUS FLOOR WITH BUR.

7 C → THE BODY-LIFTING INSTRUMENT IS USED TOGETHER WITH THE GRAFT MATERIAL TO OBTAIN FURTHER STRETCHING OF THE MEMBRANE.

8 A → THE OSTEOTOME IS USED TO INFRACTURE AND LIFT THE SINUS FLOOR WITH THE SINUS MEMBRANE.

8 B → FURTHER ELEVATION OF THE SINUS MEMBRANE BEYOND THE AREA THAT HAS ALREADY BEEN LIFTED, USING A SPECIAL LIFTING INSTRUMENT.

8 C → FURTHER CONTRIBUTION OF GRAFT MATERIAL WITH OSTEOTOMES.

9 A → ENDOSCOPIC VIEW OF INTEGRAL LIFTED SINUS MEMBRANE.

9 B → SMALL PERFORATION OF SINUS MEMBRANE VISIBLE DURING AN ENDOSCOPICALLY CONTROLLED BAOSFE PROCEDURE. LEAKAGE OF MATERIAL AND BLOOD IS VISIBLE IN THE SINUS CAVITY. NOTE THAT THE BIO-OSS® PARTICLES SEEM TO SHOW THROUGH THE SINUS MEMBRANE APICALLY, AT THE IMPLANT TIP.

9 C → ENDOSCOPIC VIEW SHOWING LOCALIZED BEHAVIOR OF MEMBRANE ELEVATION DURING THE BAOSFE TECHNIQUE. NOTE THE PROJECTIONS OF RADIOPAQUE MATERIAL NEXT TO THE GRAFT MATERIAL PLACED AT THE IMPLANT APICES AND THE ABSENCE OF MEMBRANE ELEVATION FROM THE SINUS FLOOR BETWEEN THE TWO IMPLANTS.

9 D → THIS ENDOSCOPIC IMAGE SHOWS THE IMPLANTS WITH EXTENSIVE MEMBRANE ELEVATION THAT EXTENDS BEYOND THE IMPLANT APEX AND LATERALLY BEYOND THEIR EDGES.

6 A	6 B	6 C	6 D	6 E
7 A	7 B	7 C		
8 A	8 B	8 C		

| 9 A | 9 B |
| 9 C | 9 D |

TAB. 3

Review of published data concerning the results of sinus augmentation using osteotomes with various surgical techniques, with different types of graft materials and with different implants

AUTHORS	NUMBER OF PATIENTS (IMPLANTS)	TYPE OF IMPLANTS	RESIDUAL BONE HEIGHT	IMPLANT SITES	GRAFT MATERIAL	FOLLOW-UP IN MONTHS (AVERAGE)	AVERAGE HEIGHT OF SINUS ELEVATION	AVERAGE GRAFT HEIGHT	IMPLANT SUCCESS
Summers 1994b	55 (143)	Press-Fit (Microvent®, Integral®, Hexcylinder)	≥5 mm	Bone type IV (anterior areas, premolar, molar and tuberosity)	Autogenous bone + DFDB + HA resorbable	11-27	—	—	96%
Coatoam & Krieger 1997	77 (89)	Screw-Vent, Bio-Vent, Steri-Oss, PACE	—		Autogenous bone + FDB + tetracycline powder	6-48	—	—	92.1%
Horowitz 1997	18 (34)	ITI	—	—	—	2-15 (5.9)	—	3 mm	97%
Bruschi et al. 1998	303 (499)	IMZ, Frialit	5-7 mm	Posterior maxilla	None (LMSF technique)	24-60	—	About 3-7 mm	97.5%
Komarnyckyj & London 1998	(16)	TPS (ITI)	3-9 mm	Posterio maxilla, bone type III and IV	Autogengous bone	3-38	—	2-7 mm (3.25 mm)	93.75%
Ziztmann & Schärer 1998	20 (59)	MKII Nobel Biocare	> 6 mm (8.8 mm)	Posterior maxilla	Bio-Oss®	6-24 (16.5)	12.3 mm	(3.5 mm)	95%
Rosen et al. 1999	101 (174)	ITI TPS Screws, Interpore + 3i TPS Cylinders, Nobel Biocare Screws, 3i + Implamed + Dentsply Screws	≥ 3 mm	—	Autogenous bone, DFDB, Osteograf-N, Bio-Oss®	6-66 (20.2)	—	—	95.4%
Baumann & Ewers 1999	5	IMZ	6-8 mm	Posterior maxilla	Autogenous bone + Algipore®	—	Implants 13 mm		—
Cosci & Luccioli 2000	237 (265)	Cylindrical (Integral)	2-10 mm	1st and 2nd premolar, 1st and 2nd molar	Autogenous bone + DFDBA + TCP	72	Implants 13/15 mm	—	96.9%
Deporter et al. 2000	16 (26)	Endopore	Minimum of 3 mm	2nd premolar, 1st and 2nd molar	Bio-Oss®	6-36 (11.1)	Implants 7/9.7 mm	—	100%
Cavicchia et al. 2001	(97)	IMZ Frialit	≥ 5 mm	—	Autogenous bone + not specified	35	—	1-6 mm (2.9 mm)	88.6%
Winter et al. 2002	34 (58)	Frialit-2, Osseotite	0.6-4 mm (2.87 mm)	Posterior maxilla	None (LMSF Technique)	22	9.12 mm	—	91.4%
Nkenke et al. 2002b	14 (22)	Brånemark Mk II, ITI, Ankylos, Frialit-2	4-9 mm (6.8 mm)	1st and 2nd premolar, and 1st molar	Autogenous bone + tricalcium phosphate	6	—	2-5 mm (3 mm)	90.90%
Artzi et al. 2003	(10)	—	6-9 mm (7.8 mm)	1st and 2nd molar (post-extraction immediate)	—	—	—	2.5-6 mm (4.3 mm)	100%

after the surgery showed an average reduction of 49.5% of the initial bone graft volume in 10 patients who underwent bilateral sinus augmentation using bone graft particulate (Johansson et al. 2001). More recently, Ozyuvaci et al. (2003) observed losses in graft height of 0.94, 1.49 and 1.5 mm, using DFDBA, bovine hydroxyapatite, hydroxyapatite and beta tricalcium phosphate, 6 months after maxillary sinus augmentation.

Using the maxillary sinus crestal elevation technique, a slight contraction of grafted material was noted compared with the healing of implants inserted at the same time with the BAOSFE technique (Summers 1994b; Coatoam 1997; Deporter et al. 2000). However, a quantitative evelution was not carried out. In a retrospective study on 72 implants inserted using the BAOSFE technique and BioOss® grafts, the authors found a 1.14-mm reduction in mineralized tissue height in a clinical follow-up at 37.3 months. The contraction in the mineralized tissue height may be linked to the lateral movement of the grafted material and/or to the volume retraction of the mass of grafted material in the postoperative phase (Summers 1994; Coatoam 1997) FIG. 10A–C.

There is a clear demarcation between grafted material and the sinus floor in the post-surgery phase in sites treated with sinus crestal elevation. As the healing process continues, the limits of the original sinus floor become more difficult to distinguish and later a new sinus floor can be seen on radiographs in a more apical position (Summers 1994; Coatoam & Krieger 1997; Fugazzotto 2002; Bruschi et al. 1998; Komarnyckyj & London 1998; Cosci & Luccioli 2000; Ioannidou & Dean 2000; Deporter et al. 2000; Cavicchia et al. 2001; Winter et al. 2002).

Review of published data concerning the results obtained with the modified trephine/osteotome technique with immediate or deferred insertion of implants   TAB. 4

AUTHORS	TECHNIQUE	SITES	NUMBER OF PATIENTS (IMPLANTS)	HEIGHT OF RIDGE RESIDUAL BONE (AVERAGE)	GRAFT MATERIAL	TYPES OF IMPLANTS (LENGTH)	SITES REQUIRING FURTHER ELEVATION	FOLLOW-UP (MONTHS)	IMPLANT SUCCESS
Fugazzotto 2001	Modified trephine/ osteotome technique with deferred implant insertion	Post-extraction sites healed in posterior maxilla	(51)	4-5 mm	Bio-Oss®	ITI	2	0-36	100%
Fugazzotto & De Paoli 2002	Modified trephine/ osteotome technique with deferred implant insertion	Immediate implants in post-extraction sites of 1st and 2nd molar	(137)	—	Bio-Oss®	ITI, Osseotite (8-11.5 mm)	—	0-36	97.8%
Fugazzotto 2002	Modified trephine/ osteotome technique with simultaneous implant insertion	Healed post-extraction sites in posterior maxilla	103 (116)	4-5 mm	None	ITI, 3i (7-11 mm)	—	0-48	98.3%

No data are yet available regarding the radiographic morphology of the sinus floor after inserting single or multiple implants combined with the BAOSFE technique. A retrospective study carried out at the University of Padua found two types of radiographic behavior. In one, the radiographic profile of the new sinus floor showed an increase in mineralized tissue at the top of the implant, while the other showed a more linear behavior with the new sinus floor profile. These radiographic aspects respect the various membrane configurations found during endoscopic controls (Reiser et al. 2001; Berengo et al. 2003) **FIG. 11A–B**.

HISTOLOGIC RESULTS

It has been suggested that using osteotomes can improve the osseointegration of endosseous implants by the lateral compression of bone trabeculae and by compacting the bone layer around the osteotomy (Summers 1994a). The difference in bone healing at the interface of rough surface cylindrical implants inserted using the osteotome technique, compared to preparation using burs, was evaluated in the distal part of the femur condyles of New Zealand rabbits (Nkenke et al. 2002a). The implant sites prepared using the osteotome technique showed a statistically significant greater bone-implant contact compared with sites prepared using burs at 2 weeks (55.0±7.1% for osteotomes vs. 29.2±4.8% for burs) and at 4 weeks (71.1±7.2% for osteotomes vs. 59.0±6.3% for burs). The statistical difference was no longer present at 8 weeks. The authors concluded that by using osteotomes to prepare implant sites, better bone-implant contact is created in the early healing phases after implant insertion.

Limited histologic data concerning bone-implant contact or bone density in sinus crestal elevation procedures are available for humans. In a series of human biopsies collected after 6 to 8 months from sites treated with the BAOSFE technique, a bone density between 38 and 52% was reported, with better results obtained by combining autogenous bone and DFDBA (Coatoam & Krieger 1997). The authors suggested that the formation of fibrous tissue in the augmented sites is less likely with sinus crestal elevation, as long as the endoantral periosteum is preserved whole. The space created by lifting the Schneiderian membrane is completely closed and therefore favors selective cell recruitment of osteoprogenitor cells. This hypothesis can be corroborated by recent studies that indicate that the exclusion of soft tissue from a bone healing site is a crucial factor for preventing the growth of connective tissue in the bone regeneration site adjacent to the bone wall, and to allow a predictable level of bone increase in spaces far from the bone plane (Yamada et al. 2003).

ADVANTAGES OF THE SINUS CRESTAL ELEVATION TECHNIQUE

When the sinus is lifted using the osteotome technique, an increase in volume of about 0.5 cm^3 is necessary (Nkenke et al. 2002b), compared to a volume of 3.5±1.33 cm^3 which is required for a lateral sinus elevation, when the residual bone ridge is 5 mm and it is necessary to place a 13 mm implant (Uchida et al. 1998).

The reduced volume increase using the BAOSFE technique causes minor changes to the sinus morphology and function (Nkenke et al. 2002b). Moreover, when using the osteotome technique for augmenting the sinus, the elevation of the mucoperiosteal flap is often limited to the crestal area, therefore limiting damage to the blood flow in the lateral wall of the sinus (Nkenke et al. 2002b).

Complications after sinus augmentation using the osteotome technique, such as intra-operative bleeding, membrane perforation and postoperative sinus pathologies, have been described in a limited number of clinical studies (Baumann & Ewers 1999; Nkenke et al. 2002b;

Berengo et al. 2003) and in studies on cadavers (Baumann & Ewers 1999; Reiser et al. 2001). The results of these studies **TAB. 1–2** show a low incidence of membrane perforations, pathological alterations to the sinus mucosa and sinusitis compared to those carried out with lateral sinus access (Tidwell et al. 1992; Small et al. 1993; Jensen et al. 1994; Block & Kent 1997; Raghoebar et al. 1997; Wiltfang et al. 2000; Doud Galli et al. 2001; Kahnberg et al. 2001; Aimetti et al. 2001; Wilkert Walter et al. 2002; Kasabah et al. 2003; Stricker et al. 2003). Slight nose bleeding, which disappears within 24 to 48 hours, was observed in some cases (Bruschi et al. 1998), although this complication has never been reported in other studies (Cavicchia et al. 2001). Coatoam and Krieger (1997) reported another complication, the displacement of a cylindrical implant into the sinus cavity while tightening the coverage screw in the fourth week after surgery. They also highlighted periapical radiotransparency, which the authors attributed to contamination during surgery.

DISADVANTAGES OF THE SINUS CRESTAL ELEVATION TECHNIQUE

One of the main negative aspects of the sinus augmentation technique using osteotomes is using a surgical mallet to compact the bone trabeculae with the osteotome. A greater force is also required to infracture the sinus floor using an osteotome, with or without the presence of graft material. These repeated strikes can be traumatic and uncomfortable for the patient. Using burs significantly reduces the need to use the surgical mallet, but this approach also brings about a considerable loss of bone tissue, which is instead preserved when preparing the implant site with osteotomes. Without direct endoscopy, it is difficult to evaluate whether the membrane has been perforated while the sinus was being lifted. The Valsava maneuver has low clinical reliability and may indeed be

negative if membrane perforations are found using the endoscope during the surgery (Nkenke et al. 2002b). Another limitation of the sinus crestal elevation technique is the reduced height of sinus elevation using the BAOSFE technique compared to that obtained with a lateral approach (Zitzmann & Schärer 1998), as the elevation involves a reduced area of the sinus membrane. The increase in the vertical height obtained using the BAOSFE technique, performed at the same time as implants are inserted, varies from 3 to 5 mm as reported by various authors (Summers 1994b; Komarnyckyj & London 1998; Zitzmann & Schärer 1998; Deporter et al. 2000). These average sinus lift values, obtained using the osteotome technique, remain much lower than the averages of 10 mm obtained using the lateral approach (Komarnyckyj & London 1998). There is a lack of information regarding the biomechanical effect of localized peri-implant elevation using the crestal approach. In a study analyzing three-dimensional finite elements, concerning the geometric shape obtained further to lateral sinus elevation **FIG. 12A–C**, Tepper et al. (2002) concluded that:

- a large amount of peri-implant tissue significantly reduces implant displacement
- the stress on the implant and on the tissue-implant interface was less than that found in cases where there was a thin 1 mm layer of bone around the implants, in the middle third and the top third.

The authors concluded that a considerable amount of bone, obtained with a large insertion of material around the implants, is advisable in sinus elevations, in order to provide rigidity and good mechanical support to the entire implant-bone system for long-term success. The clinical implications of these results must be investigated further with long-term, randomized controlled clinical studies (Tepper et al. 2002).

10 A → PREOPERATIVE RADIOGRAPH.

10 B → RADIOGRAPH TAKEN IMMEDIATELY AFTER IMPLANT PLACEMENT. NOTE THE DOME-SHAPED RADIOPAQUE AREA NEXT TO THE GRAFT MATERIAL INSERTED AT THE IMPLANT TIP.

10 C → 20 MONTHS AFTER THE SURGERY, THE RADIOGRAPH SHOWS A VERTICAL INCREASE IN THE SIZE OF ALVEOLAR BONE AND A NEW SINUS FLOOR LEVEL. NOTE ALSO THE REDUCTION IN THE HEIGHT OF THE GRAFTED MATERIAL BETWEEN THE RADIOGRAPH TAKEN AFTER SURGERY AND 20 MONTHS LATER.

11 A → TWO DISTINCT SINUS CRESTAL ELEVATIONS CAN BE SEEN. DIFFERENT CLINICAL BEHAVIOR OF TWO IMPLANTS PLACED AT THE SAME TIME.

11 B → NOTE THE SINGLE SINUS CRESTAL ELEVATION THAT INCLUDES TWO IMPLANTS.

12 A-B → PARTIAL OR FULL FILLING OF MATERIAL WHEN SINUS ELEVATION IS CARRIED OUT USING A LATERAL APPROACH.

12 C → CONFIGURATION OF PERI-IMPLANT MATERIAL THAT IS OBTAINED WITH THE MAXILLARY SINUS CRESTAL ELEVATION PROCEDURE.

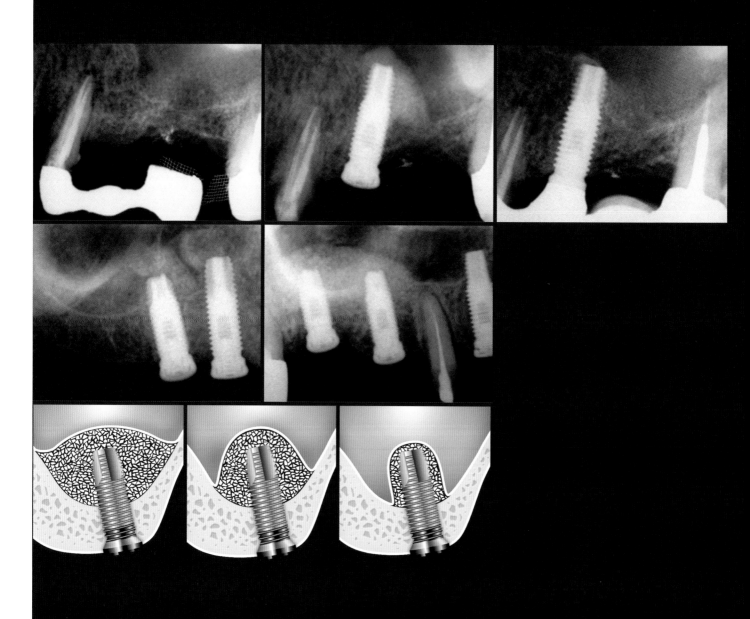

CONCLUSIONS

The crestal approach in maxillary sinus augmentation, with its several variations, including different osteotome techniques, different types of implants and graft materials, is a highly predictable procedure, especially when the residual crestal bone is at least 5 mm in height. Using a simple, non-invasive procedure, this technique allows a significant increase in the implant success rate in the posterior maxillary areas, it has a low incidence of intra- and post-surgical complications and does not cause clinical alterations to the sinus membrane.

REFERENCES

1 Adell R., Eriksson B., Lekholm U., Brånemark P.I., Jemt T.A.
A long-term folow-up study of osseointegrated implants in the treatment of the totally edentulous jaw.
Int. J. Oral Maxillofac. Implants 1990; 5: 347-59.

2 Aimetti M., Romagnoli R., Ricci G., Massei G.
Maxillary sinus: The effect of macrolacerations and microlacerations of the sinus membrane as determined by endoscopy.
Int. J. Periodontics Restorative Dent. 2001; 21: 581-9.

3 Artzi Z., Parson A., Nemcovsky C.E.
Wide-diameter implant placement and internal sinus elevation in the immediate postextraction phase: clinical and radiographic observations in 12 consecutive molar sites.
Int. J. Oral Maxillofac. Implants 2003; 18: 242-9.

4 Bahat O.
Treatment planning and placement of implants in the posterior maxilla: Report of 732 consecutive Nobelpharma implants.
Int. J. Oral Maxillofac. Implants 1993; 8: 151-61.

5 Baumann A., Ewers R.
Minimal invasive sinus lift. Grenzen und Möglichkeiten im atrophen Oberkiefer.
Mund Kiefer Gesichts Chir. 1999; 3: S70-3.

6 Berengo M., Sivolella S., Majzoub Z., Cordioli G.P.
Endoscopic evaluation of the bone-added osteotome sinus floor elevation procedure.
Int. J. Oral Maxillofac. Surg. 2004; 33: 189-94.

7 Block M.S., Kent J.N.
Sinus augmentation for dental implants: The use of autogenous bone.
J Oral Maxillofac Surg. 1997: 55: 1281-6.

8 Block M.S., Kent J.N., Kallukaran F.U., Thunthy K., Weinberg R.
Bone maintenance 5 to 10 years after sinus grafting.
J. Oral Maxillofac. Surg. 1998; 56: 706-14.

9 Bruschi G.B., Scipioni A., Calesini G., Bruschi E.
Localized management of sinus floor with simultaneous implant placement: A clinical report.
Int. J. Oral Maxillofac. Implants. 1998; 13: 219-26.

10 Buser D., Mericske-Stern R., Bernard J.P., Behneke A., Behneke N., Hirt H.P., Belser U.C., Lang N.P.
Long-term evaluation of non-submerged ITI implants. Part 1: 8-year life table analysis of a prospective multi-center study with 2359 implants.
Clin. Oral Implants Res. 1997; 8: 161-72.

11 Cavicchia F., Bravi F., Petrelli G.
Localized augmentation of the maxillary sinus floor through a coronal approach for the placement of implants.
Int. J. Periodontics Restorative Dent. 2001; 21: 475-85.

12 Coatoam G.W.
Indirect sinus augmentation procedures using one-stage anatomically shaped root-form implants.
J. Oral Implant. 1997; 23: 25-42.

13 Coatoam G.W., Krieger J.T.
A four-year study examining the results of indirect sinus augmentation procedures. J. Oral Implant. 1997; 23: 117-27.

14 Cosci F., Luccioli M.
A new sinus lift technique in conjunction with placement of 265 implants: A 6-year retrospective study.
Implant Dent. 2000; 9: 363-68.

15 Davarpanah M., Marinez H., Tecucianu J.F., Hage G., Lazzara R.
The modified osteotome technique.
Int. J. Periodontics Restorative Dent. 2001; 21: 599-607.

16 Deporter D., Todescan R., Caudry S.
Simplifying management of the posterior maxilla using short, porous-surfaced dental implants and simultaneous indirect sinus elevation.
Int. J. Periodontics Restorative Dent. 2000; 20: 477-85.

17 Doud Galli S.K., Lebowitz R.A., Giacchi R.J., Glickman R., Jacobs J.B.
Chronic sinusitis complicating sinus lift surgery.
Am. J. Rhinol. 2001; 15: 181-6.

18 Engelke W., Deckwer I.
Endoscopically controlled sinus floor augmentation. A preliminary report.
Clin. Oral Implants Res. 1997; 8: 527-31.

19 Friberg B., Sennerby L., Roos J., Lekholm U.
Identification of bone quality in conjunction with insertion of titanium implants. A pilot study in jaw autopsy specimens.
Clin. Oral Implants Res. 1995; 6: 213-9.

20 Froum S.J., Tarnow D.P., Wallace S.S., Rohrer M.D., Cho S-C.
Sinus floor elevation using anorganic bovine bone matrix (OsteoGraf/N) with and without autogenous bone: A clinical, histologic, radiographic, and histomorphometric analysis- Part 2 of an ongoing prospective study.
Int. J. Periodontics Restorative Dent. 1998; 18: 529-43.

21 Fugazzotto P.A.
Sinus floor augmentation at the time of maxillary molar extraction: Technique and report of preliminary results.
Int. J. Oral Maxillofac. Implants 1999; 14: 536-42.

22 Fugazzotto P.A.
The modified trephine/osteotome sinus augmentation technique: Technical considerations and discussion of indications.
Implant Dent. 2001; 110: 259-64.

23 Fugazzotto P.A.
Immediate implant placement following a modified trephine/ osteotome approach: Success rates of 116 implants to 4 years of function.
Int. J. Oral Maxillofac. Implants 2002; 17: 113-20.

24 Fugazzotto P.A., De Paoli S.
Sinus floor augmentation at the time of maxillary molar extraction: Success and failure rates of 137 implants in function for up to 3 years.
J. Periodontol. 2002; 73: 39-44.

25 Fugazzotto P.A., Vlassis J.
Long-term success of sinus augmentation using various surgical approaches and grafting materials.
Int. J. Oral Maxillofac. Implants 1998; 13: 52-8.

26 Geurs N.C., Wang I.C., Shulman L.B., Jeffcoat M.K.
Retrospective radiographic analysis of sinus graft and implant placement procedures from the Academy of Osseointegration Consensus Conference on Sinus Grafts.
Int. J. Periodontics Restorative Dent. 2001; 21: 517-23.

27 Glauser G., Naef R., Schärer P.
The osteotome technique- a different method of implant placement in the posterior maxilla.
Implantologie 1998; 2: 103-20.

28 Hirsch J.M., Ericsson I.
Maxillary sinus augmentation using mandibular bone grafts and simultaneous installations of implants: a surgical technique.
Clin. Oral Implants Res. 1991; 2: 91-6.

29 Horowitz R.A.
The use of osteotomes for sinus augmentation at the time of implant placement.
Compend. Contin. Educ. Dent. 1997; 18: 441-7.

30 Ioannidou E., Dean J.W.
Osteotome sinus floor elevation and simultaneous, non-submerged implant placement: Case report and literature review.
J. Periodontol. 2000; 71: 1613-9.

31 Jaffin R.A., Berman C.L.
The excessive loss of Brånemark fixtures in type IV bone: A 5-year analysis.
J. Periodontol. 1991; 62: 2-4.

32 Jendersen M.D., Allen E.O., Bayne S.C., Donovan T.E., Goldman S., Hume R., Kois J.C.
Annual review of selected dental literature: Report of the committee on scientific investigation of the American Academy of Restorative Dentistry.
J. Prosthet. Dent. 1998; 80: 81 120.

33 Jensen J., Sindet-Pedersen S., Oliver A.J.
Varying treatment strategies for reconstruction of maxillary atrophy with implants: Results in 98 patients.
Int. J. Oral Maxillofac. Surg. 1994; 52: 210-6.

34 Johansson B., Grepe A., Wannfors K., Hirsch J.M.
A clinical study of changes in the volume of bone grafts in the atrophic maxilla.
Dentomaxillofac. Radiol. 2001; 30: 157-61.

35 Kahnberg K.E., Ekestubbe A., Gröndahl K., Nilsson P., Hirsch J.M.
Sinus lifting procedure. I. One-stage surgery with bone transplant and implants.
Clin. Oral Implants Res. 2001; 12: 479-87.

36 Khang W., Feldman S., Hawley C.E., Gunsolley J.
A multi-center study comparing dual acid-etched and machined-surfaced implants in various bone qualities.
J. Periodontol. 2001; 72: 1384-90.

37 Kasabah S., Krug J., Simunek A., Lecaro M.C.
Can we predict maxillary sinus mucosa perforation?
Acta Medica (Hradec Kralove). 2003; 46: 19-23.

38 Komarnyckyj O.G., London R.M.
Osteotome single-stage dental implant placement with and without sinus elevation: A clinical report.
Int. J. Oral Maxillofac. Implants 1998; 13: 799-804.

39 Lazzara R.J., Siddiqui A.A., Binon P., Feldman S.A., Weiner R., Philipps R., Gonshor A.
A retrospective multicenter analysis of 3i endosseous dental implants placed over a 5-year period.
Clin. Oral Implants Res. 1996; 7: 73-83.

40 Leonetti J.A, Rambo H.M., Throndson R.R.
Osteotome sinus elevation and implant placement with narrow size bioactive glass.
Implant Dent. 2000; 9: 177-82.

41 Malchiodi L.
Chirurgia Implantare.
Edizioni Martina Bologna. 2003; 219-25.

42 Müller W., Löwicke G., Naumann H.
Reconstruction of the alveolar process using molded and compressed spongiosa. A clinical and experimental study.
Zahn Mund Kieferheilkd. Zentralbl. 1985; 73: 464-70.

43 Nkenke E., Kloss F., Wiltfang J., Schultze-Mosgau S., Radespiel-Tröger M., Loos K., Neukam F.W.
Histomorphometric and fluorescence microscopic analysis of bone remodelling after installation of implants using an osteotome technique. Clin. Oral Implants Res. 2002a; 13: 595-602.

44 Nkenke E., Schlegel A., Schultze-Mosgau S., Neukam F.W., Wiltfang J.
The endoscopically controlled osteotome sinus floor elevation: A preliminary prospective study.
Int. J. Oral Maxillofac. Implants 2002b; 17: 557-66.

45 Ozyuvaci H., Bilgiç B., Firatli E.
Radiologic and histomorphometric evaluation of maxillary sinus grafting with alloplastic graft materials.
J. Periodontol. 2003; 74: 909-15.

46 Peleg M., Mazor Z., Garg A.K.
Augmentation grafting of the maxillary sinus and simultaneous implant placement in patients with 3 to 5 mm of residual alveolar bone height.
Int. J. Oral Maxillofac. Implants 1999; 14: 549-56.

47 Quirynen M., Naert I., van Steenberghe D.
Fixture design and overload influence marginal bone loss and fixture success in the Brånemark system.
Clin. Oral Implants Res. 1992; 3: 104-11.

48 Raghoebar G.M., Brouwer T.J., Reintsema H., van Oort R.P.
Augmentation of the maxillary sinus floor with autogenous bone for the placement of endosseous implants: a preliminary report.
J. Oral Maxillofac. Surg. 1993; 51: 1198-203.

49 Raghoebar G.M., Vissink A., Reintsema H., Batenburg R.H.K.
Bone grafting of the floor of the maxillary sinus for the placement of endosteal implants.
Br. J. Oral Maxillofac. Surg. 1997; 35: 119-25.

50 Reiser G.M., Rabinovitz Z., Bruno J., Damoulis P.D., Griffin T.J.
Evaluation of maxillary sinus membrane response following elevation with the crestal osteotome technique in human cadavers.
Int. J. Oral Maxillofac. Implants 2001; 16: 833-40.

51 Rosen P.S., Summers R., Mellado J.R, Salkin L.M, Shanaman R.H., Marks M.H., Fugazzotto P.A.
The bone-added osteotome sinus floor elevation procedure: Multicenter retrospective report of consecutively treated patients.
Int. J. Oral Maxillofac. Implants 1999; 14: 853-8.

52 Shulman L.B., Jensen O..T, Block M.S., Iacono V.J.
A consensus conference on the sinus graft.
In: The Sinus Bone Graft, Jensen OT (ed). Chicago:
Quintessence Publishing 1999: 209-27.

53 Small S.A., Zinner I.D., Panno F.V., Shapiro H.J., Stein J.I.
Augmenting the maxillary sinus for implants: Report of 27 patients.
Int. J. Oral Maxillofac. Implants 1993; 8: 523-8.

54 Smiler D.G., Johnson P.W, Lozada J.L., Misch C., Rosenlicht J.L.,
Tatum O.H., Wagner J.R.
*Sinus lift grafts and endosseous implants. Treatment of the
atrophic posterior maxilla.*
Dent. Clin. North Am. 1992; 36: 151-86.

55 Stricker A., Voss P.J., Gutwald R., Schramm A., Schmelzeisen R.
*Maxillary sinus floor augmentation with autogenous bone grafts
to enable placement of SLA-surfaced implants: preliminary
results after 15-40 months.*
Clin. Oral Implants Res. 2003; 14: 207-12.

56 Strietzel F.P., Nowak A., Küchler I., Friedmann A.
*Peri-implant alveolar bone loss with respect to bone quality
after use of the osteotome technique. Results of a retrospective study.*
Clin. Oral Implants Res. 2002; 13: 508-13.

57 Summers R.B.
*A new concept in maxillary implant surgery: The osteotome
technique.*
Compendium 1994a; 15: 152-60.

58 Summers R.B.
*The osteotome technique. Part 3- Less invasive methods of
elevating the sinus floor.*
Compendium 1994b; 15: 698-708.

59 Summers R.B.
The osteotome technique. Part 4- Future site Development.
Compendium 1995; 16: 1090-9.

60 Tatum O.H Jr.
Maxillary and sinus implant reconstructions.
Dent. Clin. North Am. 1986; 30: 207-29.

61 Tepper G., Haas R., Zechner W., Krach W., Watzek G.
*Three-dimensional finite element analysis of implant stability
in the atrophic posterior maxilla. A mathematical study of the
sinus floor augmentation.*
Clin. Oral Implants Res. 2002; 13: 657-65.

62 Testori T., Wiseman L., Woolft S., Porter S.
*A prospective multicenter clinical study of the Osseotite
implant: Four-year interim report.*
Int. J. Oral Maxillofac. Implants. 2001; 16: 193-200.

63 Tidwell J.K., Blijdorp P.A., Stoelinga P.J.W., Brouns J.B.,
Hinderks F.
*Composite grafting of the maxillary sinus for placement of
endosteal implants.*
Int. J. Oral Maxillofac. Surg. 1992; 21: 204-9.

64 Timmenga N.M., Raghoebar G.M., van Weissenbruch R., Vissink A.
*Maxillary sinus floor elevation surgery. A clinical, radiographic
and endoscopic evaluation.*
Clin. Oral Implants Res. 2003; 14: 322-8.

65 Uchida Y., Goto M., Katsuki T., Akiyoshi T.
*A cadaveric study of maxillary sinus size as an aid in bone
grafting of the maxillary sinus floor.*
J. Oral Maxillofac. Surg. 1998; 56: 1158-63.

66 van Steenberghe D., Quirynen M., Calberson L., Demanet L.
*A prospective evaluation of the fate of 697 consecutive
intraoral fixtures ad modum Brånemark in the rehabilitation of
edentulism.*
J. Head Neck Pathol. 1987; 6: 53-8.

67 van Steenberghe D., Lekholm U., Bolender C., Folmer T., Henry
P., Herrmann I., Higuchi K., Laney W., Linden U., Åstrand P.
*Applicability of osseointegrated oral implants in the
rehabilitation of partial edentulism: A prospective multicenter
study on 558 fixtures.*
Int. J. Oral Maxillofac. Implants 1990; 5: 272-81.

68 Weng D., Jacobson Z., Tarnow D., Hürzeler M.B., Faehn O.,
Sanavi F., Barkvoll P., Stach R.M.
*A prospective multicenter clinical trial of 3i machined-surface
implants: Results after 6 years of follow-up.*
Int. J. Oral Maxillofac. Implants 2003; 18: 417-23.

69 Wheeler S.L., Holmes R.E., Calhoun, C.J.
Six-year clinical and histologic study of sinus-lift grafts.
Int. J. Oral Maxillofac. Implants 1996; 11: 26-34.

70 Wilkert-Walter C., Janicke S., Spuntrup E., Laurin T.
*Maxillary sinus examination after sinus floor elevation
combined with autologous onlay osteoplasty.*
Mund Kiefer Gesichtschirurgie. 2002; 6: 336-40.

71 Wiltfang J., Schultze-Mosgau S., Merten H.A., Kessler P.,
Ludwig A., Engelke W.
*Endoscopic and ultrasonographic evaluation of the maxillary
sinus after combined sinus floor augmentation and implant
insertion.*
Oral Surg. Oral Med. Oral Pathol. Oral Radiol. Endod.
2000; 89: 288-91.

72 Winter A.A., Pollak A.S., Odrich R.B.
*Placement of implants in the severely atrophic posterior
maxilla using localized management of the sinus floor: a
preliminary report.*
Int. J. Oral Maxillofac. Implants 2002; 17: 687-95.

73 Yamada Y., Nanba K., Ito K.
*Effects of occlusiveness of a titanium cap on bone generation
beyond the skeletal envelope in the rabbit calvarium.*
Clin. Oral Implants Res. 2003; 14: 455-63.

74 Yildirim M., Edelhoff D., Hanisch O., Spiekermann H.
*Internal sinus elevation – an adequate alternative to sinus floor
elevation? (In German)*
Zahnärztl Implantol. 1998; 14: 124-135.

75 Zitzmann N.U., Schärer P.
*Sinus elevation procedures in the resorbed posterior maxilla.
Comparison of the crestal and lateral approaches.*
Oral Surg. Oral Med. Oral Pathol. Oral Radiol. Endod.
1998; 85: 8-17.

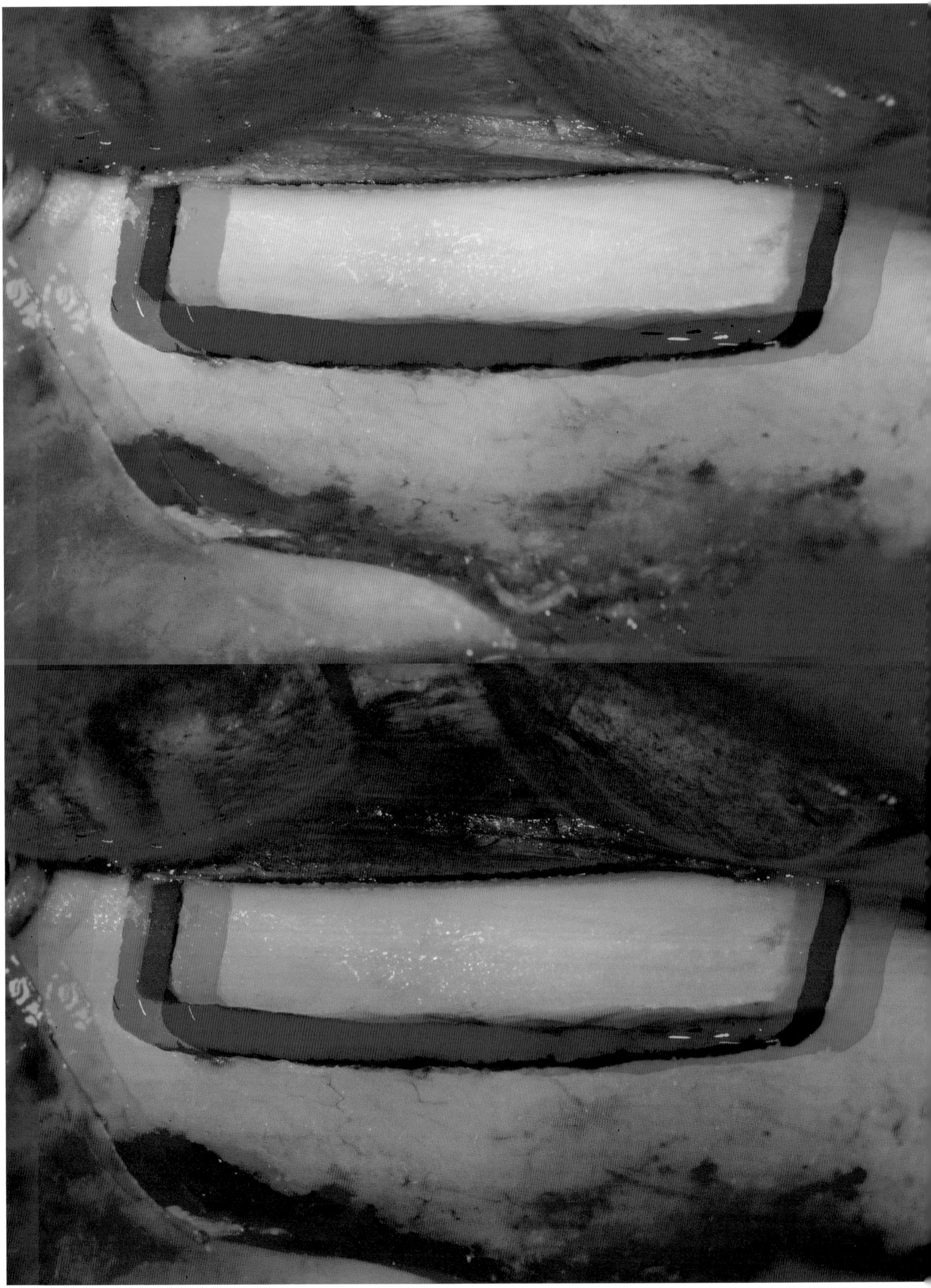

M. CAPELLI
T. TESTORI

Autogenous bone harvesting techniques from intraoral sites

16

16

The high implant predictability for both substitution of a single tooth and substitution of several teeth has allowed modern osseointegrated implantology to evolve, which leads to treatment of clinical cases with severe bone atrophy. Following tooth extraction, the residual bone ridge is resorbed on the three spatial planes, and prosthetically correct implant placement may be precluded.

The ideal solution is to restore the missing bone volume using bone grafts, in order to allow implants to be placed in an ideal prosthetic position.

Regeneration via the membrane with bone particulate or the use of appositional bone grafts are both predictable techniques for the vertical and horizontal restoration of atrophic ridges (Buser et al. 1994), in addition to allowing maxillary sinus elevation techniques.

If the amount of bone to be grafted is only minimal, an intraoral harvest – especially from the menton (lowest point of the mandibular symphysis) and the ascending ramus of the mandible – is the best option in terms of bone quantity supplied by the donor site.

MANDIBULAR RAMUS/BODY

TOPOGRAPHIC ANATOMY

The ascending mandibular ramus or branches of the mandible originate from the posterior area of the body on both sides. They are a flat rectangular shape, and with the mandibular body, or horizontal ramus, form an obtuse angle (115° to 120°) that decreases in adulthood and varies in extent, depending on gender and race.

Each ramus has two faces (lateral and medial), an anterior and posterior margin and ends with two processes: condyloid and coronoid. These processes are separated by the sigmoid notch, with a superior concavity, through which the nerve and masseter vessels pass.

At the mandibular angle, the lateral face has rough bumps that are the insertion of the masseter muscle.

Also at the mandibular angle, the medial face also has a rough surface, the insertion of the internal pterygoid muscle.

The antero-lateral face has an external oblique line, an oblique protruberence in a posterior-anterior and craniocaudal direction that starts anteriorly from the chin and continues on the front edge of each ascending ramus, forming the external border. This line becomes evident at the point of the last two molars and externally borders the buccinator sulcus, the insertion of the buccinator muscle. The thickness of the alveolar process is extremely pronounced at the vestibular end in the molar region, due to the insertion of the buccinator muscle. Lingually, the mandible is thicker in the incisor, canine and premolar areas, due to the insertion of the mylohyoid muscle, and then becomes thinner near to the molars.

The mandibular canal is often a true canal with different walls, which contains vessels and the inferior alveolar nerves. However, sometimes it is a simple passage in the spongy tissue that is hard to find. The neuro-vascular bundles destined for teeth arise from here. The direction of the inferior alveolar nerve in the mandible remains on a rather straight line, while its relations with the external and internal table and the dental apices change due to an upper concave curve that it follows in the horizontal branch. The canal is higher next to the third molar and the first premolar and lower at the second and first molar (Lloyd 1982). The vertical medical distance between the upper part of the canal and the cortex surface next to the external oblique line is about 7 mm at the second molar, 11 mm at the third molar and 14 mm at the base of the coronoid process (Hendy et al. 1996). The greatest distance of the mandibular canal from the vestibular cortex in a vestibular-lingual direction is in the distal half of the first molar (4.05 mm) (Rajchel et al. 1986).

The vascular system of the latero-posterior mandibular area is basically that of the cheek area and the system found in the mandibular canal.

In the cheek region there are: ramifications of the lacrymal artery; the infraorbital artery, which comes out of the infraorbital foramen, and the buccal artery that sends rami to the buccinator muscle; the transverse facial artery that starts on the buccinator fascia, parallel to the parotid duct; the facial artery that surrounds the horizontal mandibular ramus in the area in front of the anteroinferior angle of the masseter muscle and heads obliquely upwards and forwards towards the labial commissure.

In the cheek area are the motor nerves for the temporo-facial and cervical-facial ramus, which are distributed to the smooth muscles. The sensory nerves are the buccal nerve; the infraorbital nerve; and the zygomatofacial nerve, a ramus of the zygomatic nerve (Brizzi 1983). The surgical incision to access the mandibular latero-posterior area to carry out bone harvesting involves a posterior extension parallel to the external oblique line that may involve the buccal nerve. Damage to this nerve can rarely alter internal cheek sensitivity, but this is often not felt by the patient (Hendy et al. 1996).

PREOPERATIVE CONSIDERATIONS

A full general medical history must be evaluated and an intraoral evaluation must be carried out for the patient due to undergo bone harvesting from the mandibular ramus. Special attention must be paid to systemic illnesses that may cause surgical complications.

Uncontrolled diabetes mellitus, heavy smoking and conditions or therapies that can alter immune defenses preclude the patient from this type of surgery.

The intraoral exam involves a dental and periodontal evaluation, in addition to identifying any changes to soft and hard tissues.

Radiography must be performed on the mandible, with the aid of an orthopantograph and a CT exam of the latero-posterior portion of the mandible and the ascending ramus. This exam is aimed at identifying the position of the inferior alveolar nerve related to the external cortex, and therefore the volume of bone available in order to carry out harvesting.

SURGICAL PROCEDURE

Surgical access to the mandibular ramus must be preceded by careful palpation, in order to identify the external oblique line.

There are three different surgical techniques. The differences lie in the location of the vestibular incision:
- intrasulcular
- paramarginal
- crestal.

INTRASULCULAR INCISION

This type of incision is made when natural periodontally healthy teeth are present. The incision begins in the distal corner of the second premolar and extends distally, passing laterally to the retromolar trigone, staying mesially to the external oblique line.

To aid suturing, the incision can be made while preserving the coronal portion of the papilla. This incision may be advisable if there is a thin, scalloped gingival biotype, in order to

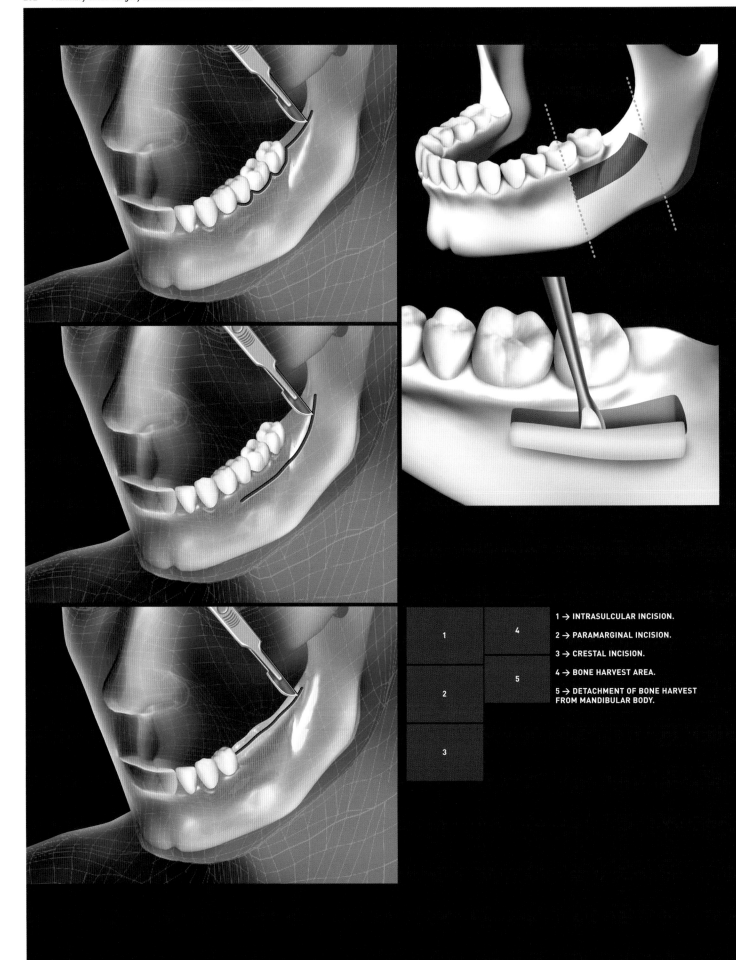

1 → INTRASULCULAR INCISION.

2 → PARAMARGINAL INCISION.

3 → CRESTAL INCISION.

4 → BONE HARVEST AREA.

5 → DETACHMENT OF BONE HARVEST FROM MANDIBULAR BODY.

reduce the risk of postoperative recession between teeth **FIG. 1**.

The distal extension of the incision must use the occlusal plane of the mandibular teeth as a coronal reference, in order to prevent damage to the buccal artery and to avoid exposure of Bichat's adipose body.

PARAMARGINAL INCISION

The paramarginal incision is recommended if there are premolar and molar prostheses and if there are natural teeth with slight periodontal defects. The incision is made along the mucogingival line, in order to minimize the formation of scars and to aid the repositioning of flaps during suturing. As the incision is not made directly in the muscle, postoperational sequelae are reduced.

This type of incision avoids the risk of recession next to the prosthetic teeth.

The distal extension of the incision is made with the same characteristics as the previous technique **FIG. 2**.

CRESTAL INCISION

This type of incision is recommended if the ridge is edentulous. The incision may be marginal or paramarginal next to residual teeth located mesially to the edentulous ridge, and then continues distally towards the mandibular ramus at the center of the residual keratinized gingiva.

If the crestal incision is made solely to harvest bone from the mandibular ramus without the simultaneous placement of implants or to graft the harvest as a homolateral host site, the crestal incision is made without marginal or paramarginal extension to the teeth. This incision is sufficient to allow bone harvest procedures **FIG. 3**.

Once the incision has been made, a total thickness flap is reflected to expose the latero-posterior part of the mandibular body, up to the base of the coronoid process.

A rectangular harvest 4 mm thick can be sculpted from the mandibular ramus (Misch 1997). The length of the bone harvest may be up to 3.5 cm, while it cannot be more than 1 cm in height **FIG. 4**.

The ostectomy begins at the base of the coronoid process and remains 4 to 5 mm medially of the external oblique line, continuing mesially up to the distal portion of the first molar, even if there is a second molar.

Anterior and posterior vertical ostectomies are carried out adjacent to the end of the horizontal ostectomy and continue 1 cm downwards in a craniocaudal direction.

Bones are cut using a fissure bur mounted on a straight handpiece or using an oscillating saw, with copious irrigation. Recently, this type of procedure has been carried out using ultrasonic piezoelectric inserts. Together with the oscillating saw, the latter allows for much more conservative ostectomies compared to the fissure bur. The cut is deepened progressively up to the marrow, which can be recognized by the softer bone consistency and greater bleeding than the cortical bone.

The lower ostectomy that connects the two vertical ostectomies is made using a round bur mounted on a straight handpiece insert. Given the difficult access and the low visibility found in the posterior area of the mandible, only one groove is made on the bone cortex, to create an area of lower resistance and allow easy separation of the bone harvest from the mandibular base. While the bone groove is being created, attention must be paid to avoid lacerating the periosteum next to the harvest area and to avoid causing damage to the facial artery, which passes over the periosteum on its route from the mandibular angle towards the lower lip. To solve this problem, the flap must be protected by the interposition of a periosteum detacher between the mandibular base and the flap.

With the angled piezoelectric inserts, this maneuver can be performed more easily and without any risk of damaging the cheek's periosteum, as they can only cut mineralized tissues.

To check the full mobility of the compact bone from the underlying marrow portion, a small chisel is used at first, followed by a larger chisel that is inserted into the horizontal ostectomy and used slowly with leverage until the harvest is separated from the portion of the mandibular ramus **FIG. 5**.

After removal the bone harvest is placed in saline solution. At the same time, bleeding in the surgical area is controlled. Bleeding does not generally last long and is easily managed by placing collagen material or by replacing the buccal flap above the bone harvest area.

MANAGING THE BONE HARVEST

The bone segment can be used in two ways:

- monocortical
- particulate.

The first is used for appositional or interpositional grafts of bone deficiencies in the alveolar process or in maxillary sinus augmentation procedures, with or without the simultaneous placement of implants (Hirsch & Ericsson 1991).

The second is used in regenerative techniques with membranes, as graft material in maxillary sinus augmentation techniques because it improves the adaptation of the graft to maxillary sinus bone walls, or by mixing it with heterologous materials (Moy & Palacci 2001).

MANAGING THE HOST AREA

The host site must be prepared before harvesting the bone. The site is measured and thus a correctly sized harvest can be taken to graft into the host area. In this way, the time spent from the harvest to the placement of the graft in the host area is reduced to a minimum.

The graft must be placed on the host site with the endosteal side against the previously prepared bone plane, as precisely as possible, reducing the space between the graft and the underlying bone plane. To aid the graft integration phases, the compact bone must be perforated using a fissure bur together with ample irrigation, to aid bleeding from the underlying marrow tissue (Buser et al. 1994). It has been proposed (Zeiter et al. 2000) that compact bone should be removed from the host area, to guarantee more rapid access from the marrow to the bone graft for vessel and cell activity.

Once the graft has been adapted, it is rounded off at the corners and edges in order to prevent any perforation of the flap during placement and the healing stage.

To guarantee total graft immobility, titanium fixation screws fixed to the underlying bone are used; they will be removed once graft integration is complete.

To avoid graft fractures while the screws are being fixed, we advise the use of small countersinks on the bone cortex using a diamond round bur, in order to house the fixation screw head and reduce surface stress, which may cause a graft fracture in thin grafts while the screws are being tightened.

Graft mobility promotes the formation of fibrous tissue between the host site and the graft, preventing the migration of osteoclasts and even graft integration (Buser et al. 1994).

If the graft does not adapt corectly to the host site, we recommend adding autogenous bone particulate harvested from the donor site using a rongeurs. If a large volume of bone fragments is needed, a small bone harvest can be made from the same donor site, which is then transformed into particulate and inserted below and laterally to the graft, to fill all the empty space. In this case, it is advisable to apply a nonresorbable membrane to prevent gingival connective tissue migration inside the grafted bone particulate.

To aid healing of the overlying gingival tissue, it is necessary to create flaps without tension. It is therefore advisable to make angled incisions to the side of the vertical cut-back incisions, and if these are not sufficient to passively release the flaps, it is possible to carry out a horizontal periosteal incision (Tinti et al. 1996) **FIG. 6-16**.

SUTURE TECHNIQUES

The suture technique used depends on the type of incision made.

If an intrasulcular incision is made, without papilla preservation, interrupted or suspended sutures can be used on the teeth. If an intrasulcular incision is made with papilla preservation, interrupted sutures are sewn between the flap and the center of the papilla base.

Continuous sutures are recommended in the case of a paramarginal incision, to obtain perfect adaptation in the flap edges. This suture is from the mesial to the distal end.

In the event of an edentulous ridge, single or continuous sutures can be used.

If regeneration techniques are carried out at the same time as bone harvesting, it is advisable to associate the above sutures with horizontal mattress sutures to adapt the internal portion of the flaps better and thus favor healing of the wound edges (Zeiter et al. 2000), in order to prevent dehiscences and therefore exposure of any membranes.

MENTAL SYMPHYSIS

Given the easy surgical access, the mandibular symphysis is one of the most frequently used intraoral harvest sites (Raghoebar et al. 2001; Nkenke et al. 2001) The area available for carrying out bone harvesting is the intra-foramen area above the inferior incisor apex. In particular, the ostectomy must be carried out 5 mm mesially of the most mesial portion of the mental foramen, 5 mm apically of the inferior incisor apex and 5 mm coronally of the lower edge of the mandible.

Bone harvesting is mainly carried out on the vestibular cortex, marginally involving the underlying marrow bone, while the lingual cortical bone is never involved in the bone harvesting procedure. The lingual cortical bone must never be involved in order to avoid vascular damage on the sub-menton and sub-lingual vessels. Removing marrow bone means increasing the paresthesia on the inferior incisors, therefore this procedure is not at all recommended for edentulous patients.

TOPOGRAPHIC ANATOMY

From an anatomic point of view, the mental symphysis has a convex bone formation in an antero-posterior direction and a concave shape in the vestibular, in an apicocoronal and posterior-anterior direction.

The muscles present are the two mental muscles that have a distribution of muscular bundles that run in the direction of the skin; they converge and intersect with those of the controlateral muscle. Only the most lateral bundles meet a homolateral insertion.

Vessels are the labial artery, a branch of the facial artery that starts between the muscular subgingival layers; the mental artery, a ramus of the inferior alveolar artery that can be found beneath the mentolabial groove, which comes out of the inferior alveolar foramen; and the submental artery, a ramus of the facial artery and which runs along the lower edge of the mandible. The veins run with the arteries and into the facial, submental and lower jugular veins. The nerves of the mental symphysis area are branches of the facial nerve for motor purposes, while sensory nerves arise from the mental nerve. The incisor nerve is present in the marrow bone, which is responsible for the altered sensitivity of the mandibular incisors if deep bone removal is carried out on the marrow bone.

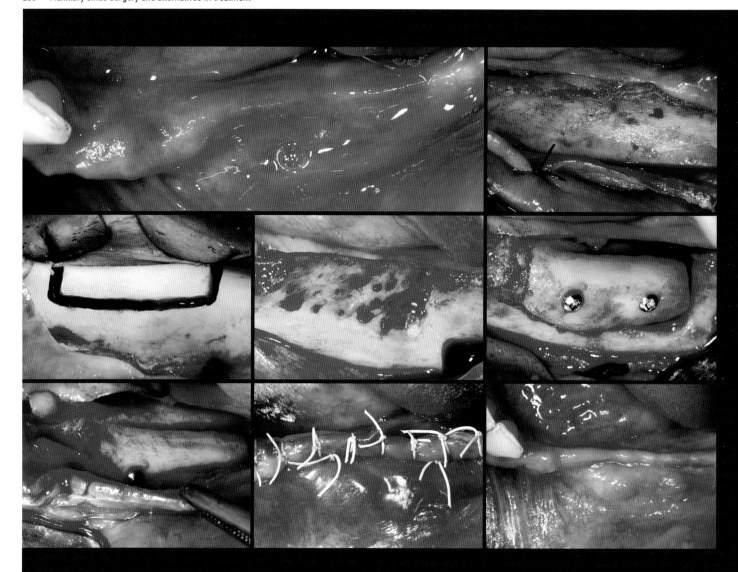

	6	7
8	9	10
11	12	13

6 → LEFT-HAND HEMIMANDIBULAR ATROPHY IN VESTIBULAR-LINGUAL AND APICOCORONAL DIRECTION.

7 → CRESTAL INCISION FROM DISTAL SURFACE OF LATERAL INCISOR TO BASE OF CORONOID PROCESS.

8 → BONE HARVEST FROM MANDIBULAR RAMUS USING FISSURE BUR MOUNTED ON STRAIGHT HANDPIECE.

9 → PREPARATION OF HOST SITE THROUGH OSTEOPLASTIC SURGERY, TO ALLOW ACCEPTABLE GRAFT ADAPTATION.

10 → FIXATION OF BONE GRAFT WITH TWO FIXATION SCREWS.

11 → VERIFICATION OF FLAP PASSIVATION.

12 → SUTURE WITH HORIZONTAL MATTRESS SUTURES AND INTERRUPTED SUTURES.

13 → APPEARANCE OF SOFT TISSUES AFTER 4 MONTHS OF HEALING.

SURGICAL TECHNIQUE

Surgical incisions that may be carried out to access the underlying bone base are as follows:

- marginal incision
- paramarginal incision
- crestal incision in edentulous patients
- labial incision.

MARGINAL INCISION

This type of incision is made by running the scalpel blade inside the periodontal sulcus of teeth, starting with the mandibular, right premolar and moving to the controlateral premolar. To carry out this incision it is necessary that teeth do not present prosthetic crowns and that there is no periodontal disease. The risk of causing esthetic damage further to periodontal damage on several teeth is sufficient not to recommend this type of incision.

PARAMARGINAL INCISION

The paramarginal incision is not used frequently as its performance requires a sufficient amount of keratinized gingiva. The incision is made next to the space between the alveolar and the keratinized gingiva. The keratinized gingiva is usually not present around mandibular incisors, which most often only have a minimum band of keratinized gum, making sutures more difficult due to the low consistency of the gum and less favorable healing.

CRESTAL INCISION

Crestal incisions are used in mandibular edentulous patients. They are carried out at total depth to the centre of the residual keratinized gingiva, stretching from the premolar to the controlateral area. Vertical release incisions are not necessary if the crestal incision stretches posteriorly.

LABIAL INCISION

This incision is chosen to access the bone base and is the same technique adopted for mentoplasty.

Avoiding the lower lip, an incision is made on the gingival and subgingival plane from the canine-premolar area, keeping the scalpel perpendicular to the lip. Once this phase has been carried out, the scalpel changes direction, proceeding perpendicularly to the underlying bone plane until the periosteal plane is cut in one session.

The flap can be elevated in a traditional way, using an elevator. This procedure consists of detaching the flap using wet, rolled-up gauzes that are applied to the gingival incision area, compressing the bone and pushing it downwards. In this way, detachment is achieved rapidly and without trauma to the soft tissues.

Once the bone plane has been reached, it is advisable to delimit the area in which the ostectomy will be carried out, highlighting the mental foramen, the lower edge of the mandible and the radicular length of the inferior incisors. Once these anatomic markers have been found, it is advisable to limit the ostectomy to 5 mm, protecting the mental foramen with periosteum detachers and lip soft tissues by spreading them well.

The ostectomy can be carried out using:

- fissure bur
- oscillating and reciprocal saws
- cylindrical coring burs
- diamond-tip disks
- piezoelectric inserts.

Ostectomies using fissure burs is the most rapid technique compared to all the others, giving rise to a larger cut with more irregular edges. The use of saws, diamond-tip disks and piezoelectric inserts results in a more precise, thinner cut, but takes more time. The use of cylindrical trephine burs is advisable each time a bone harvest is planned

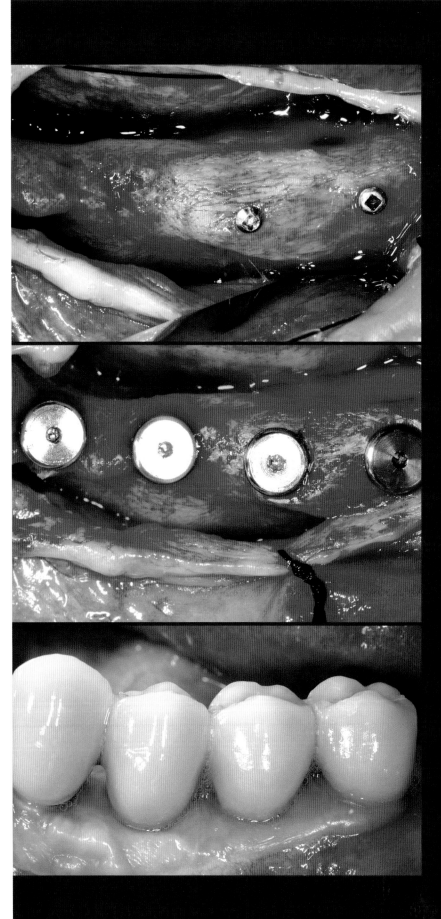

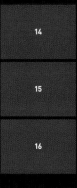

14 → THE GRAFT AFTER MATURATION.

15 → IMPLANT PLACEMENT WITH COVERAGE SCREWS.

16 → COMPLETION OF CASE WITH METAL-CERAMIC CROWNS.

for a particulate graft, as adapting it to a bone deficiency is difficult. As mentioned previously, the ostectomy must be limited to the vestibular cortex and it is not advisable to remove the marrow bone portion, in order to avoid causing damage to the incisor nerve. Once the ostectomy has been carried out, the bone segment or segments are separated from the bone base using chisels or levers. The bone segments are placed in a container with sterile physiologic solution and hemorrhage from the endosteal vessels is then checked. It is usually sufficient to place resorbable material in the donor site and compress the area with wet gauze. The use of electrosurgery is not recommended as it could create bone necrosis damage (Hunt & Jovanovic 1999).

SUTURES

Suturing of the surgical area involves a dual layer of sutures. The first layer is carried out to accurately replace the muscle-periosteum layer that is represented by the two mental muscles. This first suture must be made using resorbable suture thread in horizontal mattress running stitches. The second layer of sutures is carried out to replace the gingival layer and in this case a non-resorbable, small diameter thread is preferred, with detached surgical stitches or with running stitches **FIG. 17-21**.

POSTSURGICAL COURSE

From a strictly surgical point of view, the postsurgery course is generally favorable, with symptoms that are easily managed with suitable pharmacologic treatment.

Contrary to bone harvesting from the mandibular ramus, harvesting from the mental symphysis frequently causes paresthesia to the lower lip and the chin. This complication is caused simply by the stretching of the lip and the the mental nerve. This type of paresthesia can generally be reversed over a period of 2 to 3 months. A frequent complication that can

also be irreversible is the paresthesia of the inferior incisors, caused by damage to the incisor nerve. This event is inevitable and cannot be foreseen. It is linked to normal bone harvesting procedures, and can be made more serious by harvesting from the marrow bone component.

CONCLUSIONS

Bone harvests from the ascending ramus of the mandible and from the mental symphysis can be used to restore atrophic ridges, in order to allow prosthetically correct implant placement and for monolateral maxillary sinus augmentation procedures.

In both cases, the graft requires an integration period of about 4 months, for both the appositional graft and for maxillary sinus elevations, with minimal resorption of the graft, offering a type 1 or 2 bone density (Trisi & Rao 1999).

The ascending ramus also has low morbidity, and an excellent postsurgery course for the patient.

Due to the lateral-posterior site of the harvest area, visibility is difficult in some patients, consequently limiting the amount of bone harvested **TAB. 1**.

Unlike the ascending ramus of the mandible, the mental symphysis offers easy surgical access for the surgeon, while offering a similar amount of bone. As the harvest is mainly of compact bone, it causes type 1 and 2 bone density, whether single-block appositional or particulate is used.

The substantial difference compared to the mandibular ascending ramus is the postsurgery course for the patient, which is more bothersome, increasing morbidity and limiting its use (Clavero & Lundgren 2003).

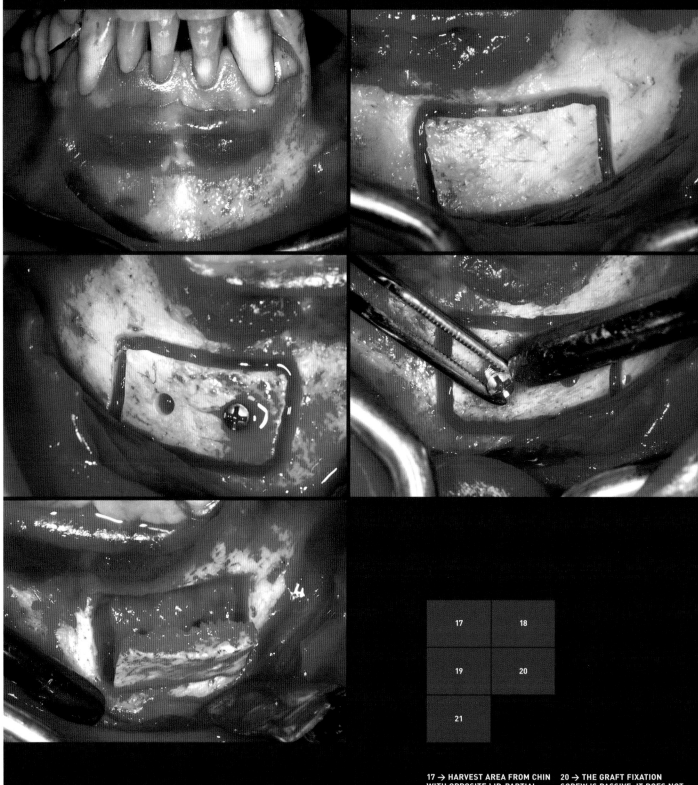

17 → HARVEST AREA FROM CHIN WITH OPPOSITE LIP. PARTIAL THICKNESS GINGIVAL INCISION, AND DETACHMENT OF MUSCULAR PLANES, REACHING THE BONE PLANE.

18 → OSTECTOMY FOR BLOCK GRAFT USING FISSURE BUR.

19 → PREPARATION OF FIXATION SITES AND GRAFT NOT YET HARVESTED.

20 → THE GRAFT FIXATION SCREW IS PASSIVE. IT DOES NOT TOUCH THE WALLS OF THE GRAFT.

21 → BONE HARVEST WITHOUT REMOVAL OF DEEP MARROW COMPONENT.

HARVESTING FROM MANDIBULAR RAMUS	
ADVANTAGES	**DISADVANTAGES**
Low patient morbidity	Difficult surgical access
Same embryogenetic origin of host site	Mainly compact bone quality
Low resorption in healing stage	Low bone quantity compared to extraoral harvests
Bone quality after healing: I, II	

TAB. I

Summary table of advantages and disadvantages of bone harvesting from mandibular ramus

REFERENCES

1   Brizzi E., Casini M., Castorina S., Franzi T., Levi C., Lucheroni A., et al.
    Anatomia Topografica; Generalità-Testa- Collo.
    Milano; Edi-Ermes 1983; 112-6.

2   Buser D., Dahlin C., Shenk R.K.
    Guided tissue regeneration in implant dentistry.
    Chicago: Quintessence Publishing 1994.

3   Clavero J., Lundgren S.
    Ramus or chin grafts for maxillary sinus inlay and local onlay augmentation: comparison of donor site morbidity and complications.
    Clin. Implant Dent. Relat. Res. 2003; 5: 154-60.

4   Hendy C.W., Smith K.G., Robinson P.P.
    Surgical anatomy of the buccal nerve.
    Br. J. Oral Maxillofac. Surg. 1996; 43: 457-60.

5   Hirsch J.M., Ericsson I.
    Maxillary sinus augmentation using mandibular bone grafts and simultaneous installation of implants: a surgical technique.
    Clin. Oral Impl. Res. 1991; 2: 91-6.

6   Hunt D.R, Jovanovic S.A.
    Autogenous bone harvesting: a chin graft tecnique for particulate and mocortical bone blocks.
    Int. J. Periodontics Restorative Dent. 1999; 19: 165-73.

7   Lloyd D.B.
    Anatomia orale di Sicher.
    Milano: Edizione Ermes 1982; 54-61.

8   Misch C.M.
    Comparison of the intraoral donor sites for onlay grafting prior to implant placement.
    Int. J. Oral Maxillofac. Implants 1997; 12: 767-76.

9   Moy P., Palacci P.
    Minor bone augmentation procedure.
    Esthetic. Implant Dent. 2001; 137-58.

10 Nkenke E., Schultze-Mosgau S., Radespiel-Troger M., Kloss F., Neukam F.W.
    Morbidity of harvesting of chin grafts: a prospective study.
    Clin. Oral Implants Res. 2001; 12: 495-502.

11 Raghoebar G.M., Louwerse C., Kalk W.W.I., Vissink A.
    Morbidity of chin bone harvesting.
    Clin. Oral Implants Res. 2001; 12: 503-7.

12 Rajchel J., Ellis E., Fonseca R.J.
    The anatomical location of the mandibular canal: its relationship to the sagittal ramus osteotomy.
    Int. J. Adult Orthodon. Orthognath. Surg. 1986; 1: 37.

13 Tinti C., Benfenati S.P., Polizzi G.
    Vertical ridge augmentation: what is the limit?
    Int. J. Periodontics Restorative Dent. 1996; 16: 619-27.

14 Trisi P., Rao W.
    Bone classification: clinical-histomorphometric comparison.
    Clin. Oral Implants Res. 1999; 10: 1-7.

15 Zeiter D.J., Reis W.L., Sanders J.J.
    The use of a bone block graft from the chin for alveolar ridge augmentation.
    Int. J. Periodontics Restorative Dent. 2000; 20: 619-27.

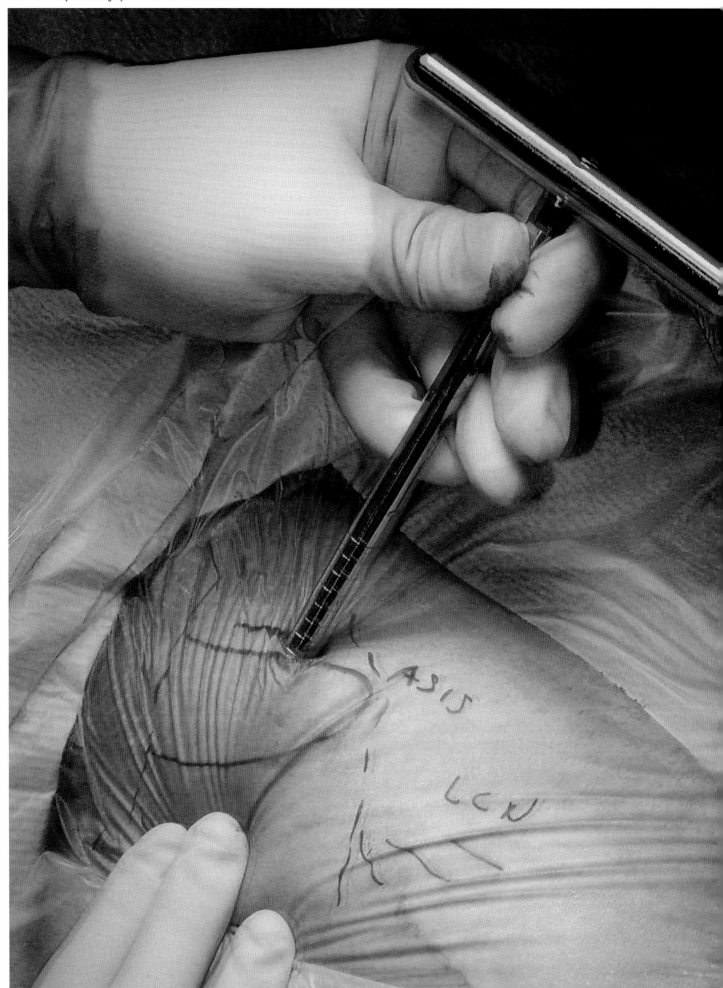

A. BAJ
A.B. GIANNI
R. MONTEVERDI
T. TESTORI

Autogenous bone harvesting techniques from extraoral sites: iliac crest, calvaria, fibula and tibia

17

17

Bone grafting and the transposition of free flaps containing bone are important reconstructive techniques.

Bone reconstruction surgery could be necessary for several pathologic or physiopathologic conditions, caused by trauma, malformations, neoplastic pathologies, or pre-prosthetic surgery deficiencies.

Implant-suported rehabilitation of the atrophic maxilla has increased considerably in the last 10 years, and consequently there has been an increase in surgeries aimed at the correction of alveolar bone atrophies. Some of the foundations underlying the success of prosthetic rehabilitation on implants are adequate bone height and volume, in order to receive a suitably sized (length and diameter) implant, with a correct relationship between the bone's vertical and sagittal dimensions and sufficient quality and quantity of keratinized peri-impant tissue.

These conditions, however, are not always found in patients who have been edentulous for a long period, due to the loss of trophic action in the roots, adjacent to the alveolar bone. To address these needs, a branch of maxillofacial surgery known as pre-implant reconstructive surgery has been developed.

The correct conditions for a successful implant rehabilitation is effectively carried out using autogenous bone grafts with or without osteotomies. Bone osteotomies correct any alterations in the maxillomandibular relationaship, and in extreme atrophies the transposition of revascularized bone tissue free flaps is used. The rationale behind resorting to major preventive surgery for implant rehabilitation lies in the high success rate of the various techniques, which exceeds 90%. In this chapter we will illustrate the extraoral bone donor sites that are most commonly used in pre-implant reconstructive surgery.

BONE GRAFT AND TRANSPOSITION OF REVASCULARIZED BONE

Autogenous bone grafts are the transplant of free flaps taken from a donor site and placed in a host site in the same person **FIG. 1**. Bone grafts are successful when they are later revascularized through angiogenesis, originating from the nearby tissue or when resorption and substitution have been completed.

On the other hand, in free revascularized flaps, the bone is harvested from the donor site together with the vascular bundle and it is immediately revascularized by microvascular anastomoses between the vascular bundle and the host vessels, usually from the neck **FIG. 2**.

The most commonly used extraoral harvesting sites are the iliac crest, the calvaria bone and the tibia for bone grafts, whereas the fibula is used more commonly for revascularized transplants.

THE ILIAC CREST

The iliac crest is a remarkable source of compact and cancellous bone, and is therefore one of the main sites used when bone grafts are required (Wolfe & Kawamoto 1978). Iliac ossification is enchondral, and it provides a sizeable amount of cancellous bone contained in an extremely thin cortex structure. Iliac crest can supply a considerable amount of bone rich in cells that allows rapid graft revascularization (Canady et al. 1993). Owing to its ability to be shaped it can be easily adapted and is therefore suitable for three-dimensional reconstructions, especially in the maxilla.

Iliac crest provides both cancellous marrow grafts and cortico-cancellous block grafts.

CANCELLOUS BONE GRAFT

Cancellous bone can be harvested under local anesthesia, and preferably associated with conscious sedation. The cutaneous incision (1 cm) is made 2 cm posterior to the anterior superior iliac spine (ASIS), centered and as deep as the bone crest edge.

Using specific instruments (Shepard & Dierberg 1987), it is possible to obtain cancellous bone harvests that guarantee a sufficient amount of bone for effective grafts, for example for major grafting of maxillary sinuses or for treating palatal clefts (McGurk et al. 1993) **FIG. 3-5**.

This type of harvest reduces morbidity in the donor site (Boustred et al. 1997).

CORTICAL CANCELLOUS GRAFT

Harvesting can be carried out on the iliac crest anteriorly or posteriorly, close to the sacroiliac joint. There are various cutaneous incisions and approaches to the donor site, which can be divided into medial and lateral, for the anterior harvest (Kurz et al. 1989). Both allow monocortical and bicortical harvesting. Given the use of iliac bone for pre-implant reconstruction, this chapter will describe in detail only the technique that the authors prefer to use in this type of surgery, because of the sufficient quantity of bone tissue and the minimal invasiveness due to the minimum detachment of deambulatory muscle insertions to the iliac bone, which reduces patient morbidity.

The patient is placed in a supine position: it is advisable to place a special silicone bedsore protector behind the hip to allow better exposure of the hemipelvis that will be used for harvesting (Mrazik et al. 1980). A dermographic pen is used to outline the iliac crest, with special care in defining the ASIS. It

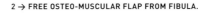

1 → MONOCORTICAL BONE HARVEST FROM ILIAC CREST.

2 → FREE OSTEO-MUSCULAR FLAP FROM FIBULA.

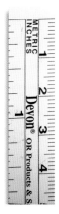 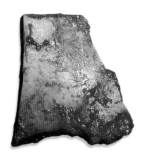

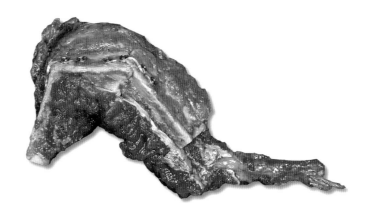

is also advisable to draw the approximate line of the cutaneous lateral femoral nerve in the thigh, the lateral cutaneous branch of the subcostal nerve and the lateral cutaneous branch of the iliohypogastric nerve that must be carefully avoided during dissection to avoid permanent anesthesia of the lateral area of the thigh and the buttock (Marx & Morales 1988).

The surgical field must be prepared carefully, taking care to leave exposed the navel, superiorly the last rib, medially the median line of the abdomen, inferiorly the upper part of the pubic area and laterally a sufficient amount of the buttock; the wide field will allow the surgeon to change technique, operating strategy or type of harvest if necessary, without needing to reprepare the operating field. The cutaneous incision is 4 to 5 cm: it must be minimal since the different plane of the dissection can slide along the bone plane, exposing the bony area for harvesting. The incision is normally made laterally of the crest, about 2 cm above the ASIS. This prevents damage to the cutaneous lateral nerve in the thigh, and in most cases, hides the remaining scar, which will be in an unseen area **FIG. 6**.

We suggest placing the cutaneous incision medially of the crest, 2 cm behind the ASIS, for several reasons: the harvest that we carry out for pre-prosthetic reasons is a partial thickness graft with no superior osteotomy that does not involve the crest border **FIG. 7–8**. In this situation, a medial cutaneous approach allows more efficient access to the internal pelvis area, with improved visibility; the

3-4-5 → HARVESTING OF CANCELLOUS BONE ONLY.

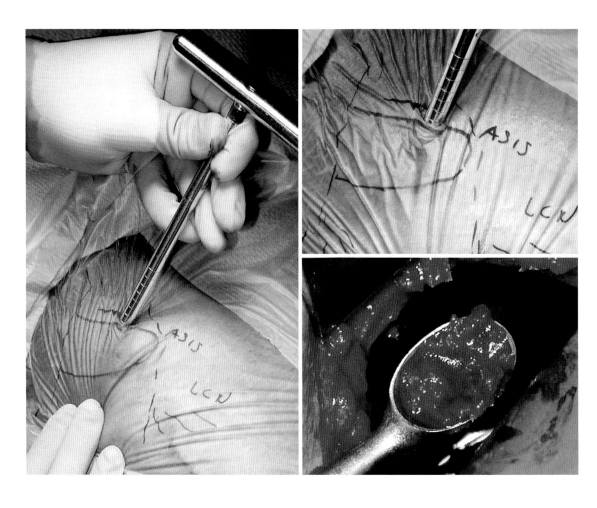

medial approach allows for a smaller cutaneous incision as there is no need to separate the cutaneous gap medially to achieve good surgical access. Finally, when working on the medial area, the cutaneous nerves mentioned above are in a deeper layer, collected in a single bundle, and therefore more difficult to damage. The advantage of a medial approach without osteotomy lies in the fact that it completely avoids the disinsertion of the gluteus muscles and the tensor muscle of the fascia lata, which play an important role in the extrarotational movement of the leg and in knee stability.

Once the position of the cutaneous incision has been decided, the incision is made up to the subcutaneous fat tissue in a single stroke. Hemostasis is controlled and then electroscalpels are used until the externa oblique muscle fascia is encountered. The incision is then continued laterally on this plane, until the top of the crest is reached **FIG. 9–10**.

At this point, the tensor fascia – now fused together – of the abdominal and gluteus area muscles, which form an anchored sling at the edge of the crest, are dissected up to the bone plane. By making a medial incision, the surgeon minimizes the risk of injury to the lateral muscle insertions **FIG. 11–12**. After detaching the medial attachment of the abdominal muscles, the iliac muscle is separated from the internal cortical bone of the pelvis, for the length required for harvesting **FIG.13**.

The osteotomies are performed using a reciprocating and oscillating saw at 90 degrees, directing the convergent vertical osteotomies

6 → REPRESENTATION OF THE MAIN ANATOMICAL MARKERS IN THE ILIAC REGION.

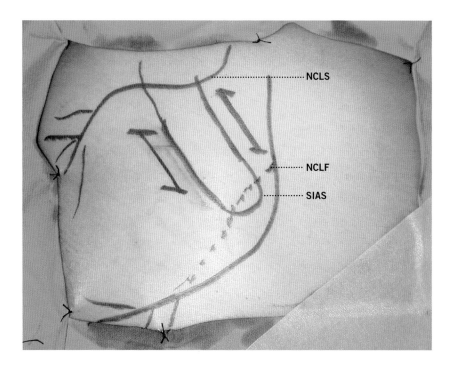

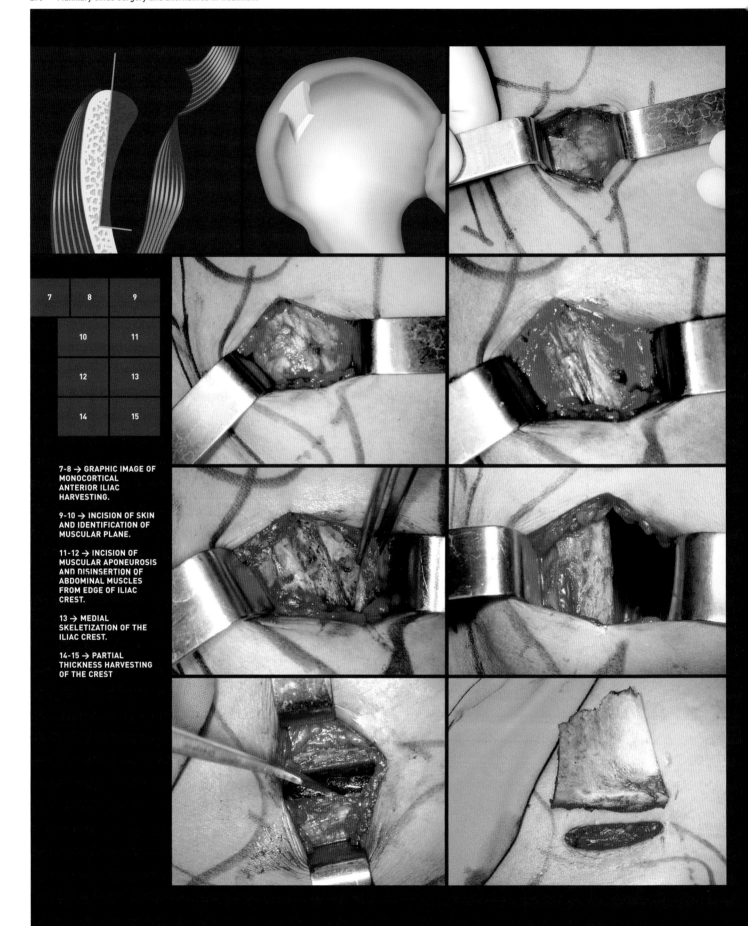

7	8	9
	10	11
	12	13
	14	15

7-8 → GRAPHIC IMAGE OF MONOCORTICAL ANTERIOR ILIAC HARVESTING.

9-10 → INCISION OF SKIN AND IDENTIFICATION OF MUSCULAR PLANE.

11-12 → INCISION OF MUSCULAR APONEUROSIS AND DISINSERTION OF ABDOMINAL MUSCLES FROM EDGE OF ILIAC CREST.

13 → MEDIAL SKELETIZATION OF THE ILIAC CREST.

14-15 → PARTIAL THICKNESS HARVESTING OF THE CREST

downwards to aid bone removal. Once the bone has been harvested, bone chips can be added by simply removing them between the cortical plates posteriorly, an area in which the cancellous bone is prevalent **FIG. 14–15**.

The harvest site is then closed after careful hemostasis, first the bone, using bone wax if necessary, and then the soft tissues, paying special attention to the periosteal surface of the iliac muscle. It is advisable to place blocks of hemostatic material in the bone gap, which, in addition to acting as a coagulant, will also maintain the space and promote bone healing.

A drain can be placed depending on the extent of the harvest. This should always be placed above the level of the transverse muscles in order to avoid continuous drainage next to the bone gap, which would otherwise continue to bleed. Suturing is performed on each layer up to the skin, where intra-dermal sutures ensure optimal esthetic results.

If a bicortical harvest is to be carried out, we use the technique with a lateral vascularized osteotomy, in which the initial phases of the surgery are identical.

Once the crest has been uncovered, however, a 1 cm horizontal osteotomy is carried out below the crest edge, followed by vertical osteotomies that allows a small lid to be lifted, attached to the lateral muscles **FIG. 16–19**. The next full-thickness harvest is smaller than the length of the superior lid so that a support is created on which to replace the upper bone portion, which will be fixed by two small plates or steel wires (Grillon & Gunther 1984) **FIG. 20–24**.

In major reconstructions, requiring a considerable amount of bone, we harvest bone from the posterior region of the crest. As previously mentioned, the posterior harvest is more complicated, as we need to place the patient in a prone position with consequent impossibility of working simultaneously with two teams. However, this allows postsurgical sequelae to be drastically reduced.

POSTERIOR ILIAC HARVEST

Preparing the patient is crucial: the patient is placed prone (lying face down) on a 210-degree split operating table, which allows the posterior iliac area to be positioned as high as possible, reducing vein pressure and therefore also preoperative bleeding). Two silicone bedsore protector cushions are normally placed, one near the pubic bone and the other on the chest, so that the abdomen is free, to avoid diaphragm or vena cava compression. Cutaneous nerves that must be saved are also present if posterior access is carried out: these are the branches for cutaneous sensitivity originating from L_1, L_2 and L_3, and those concerning the dorsal ramus of the sacrum, S_1, S_2 and S_3.

Cutaneous access is carried out by an incision parallel to the median line, next to the sacroiliac joint. Once the insertion of the gluteus medius has been located on the edge of the posterior iliac crest, it may be detached when a direct approach is to be used, while detachment may be avoided if only small amounts of bone or only cancellous bone are being harvested (Ahlmann & Patzakis 2002) **FIG. 25**.

ADVANTAGES

The advantages of harvesting bone from the iliac crest are the considerable amount of bone available and the good quality of the bone. The harvest can be bicortical if required, as for interpositional grafts after Le Fort I osteotomies or monocortical grafts, which owing to the adaptability offered by the cancellous side, can be used in three-dimensional reconstructions of the maxilla when a vertical increase is also required (LaRossa et al. 1995).

Bone harvesting is easy and can be carried out simultaneously to the preparation of the receptor site.

Rapid revascularization of the graft ensures rapid integration and higher resistance to bacterial attack.

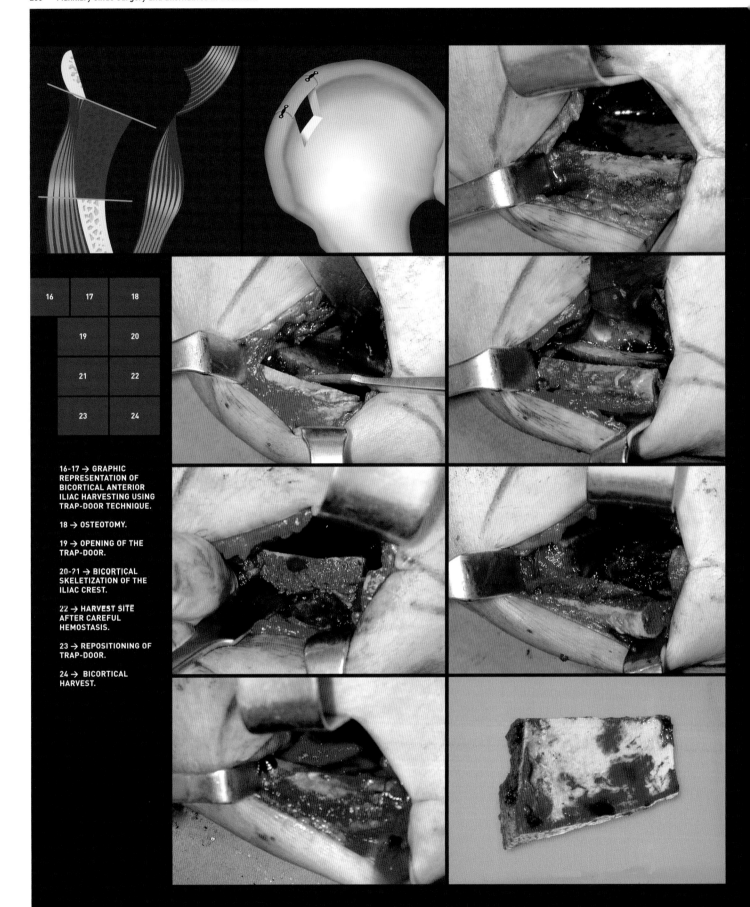

16-17 → GRAPHIC REPRESENTATION OF BICORTICAL ANTERIOR ILIAC HARVESTING USING TRAP-DOOR TECHNIQUE.

18 → OSTEOTOMY.

19 → OPENING OF THE TRAP-DOOR.

20-21 → BICORTICAL SKELETIZATION OF THE ILIAC CREST.

22 → HARVEST SITE AFTER CAREFUL HEMOSTASIS.

23 → REPOSITIONING OF TRAP-DOOR.

24 → BICORTICAL HARVEST.

DISADVANTAGES

The disadvantages of this harvest site are mainly the extent of enchondral bone resorption (50 to 70%).

One of the consequences for the enchondral origin of the iliac crest is its extremely thin cortex, with less cortical bone and a large amount of richly cellular cancellous bone, that aids rapid revascularization but also promotes osteoclastic activity.

In fact, a bone graft left in position and not suitably stimulated by implant load would be almost completely resorbed. This problem can be solved in the maxilla by placing large amounts of bone, and stimulating it by placing implants 3 months post-surgery (McCarthy et al. 2003), and loading them at 6 months. This cannot be performed, for example, in the mandible, where it is more difficult to cover the excess grafted bone with soft tissue.
Fortunately there are alternatives that are chosen depending on the clinical case, such as for interpositional grafts or alveolar distraction.

One disadvantage is the complications that may occur at the harvest site. The patient may complain of claudication (limping) and pain in the iliac region for 5 to 15 days (Laurie et al. 1984); the harvest site is also prone to the formation of seromas or small hematomas, especially when a bicortical harvest is carried out, that heal spontaneously within 1 month (Beirne et al. 1996); hernias (Bosworth 1955) and visceral lesions have also been reported.

It is advisable to use local anesthesia, as many authors describe (Puri et al. 2000) in the harvest site to reduce postoperative pain (Wilson 1995). Claudication can be reduced by avoiding the disinsertion of the genteal muscles, but to a certain extent it cannot be eliminated completely. However the sensation is limited to a maximum period of 15 days. The above-described technique pays special attention to the muscle (minimus and medius) tendon insertions and fully respects the tensor fasciae latae, in order to reduce the discomfort when walking after surgery.

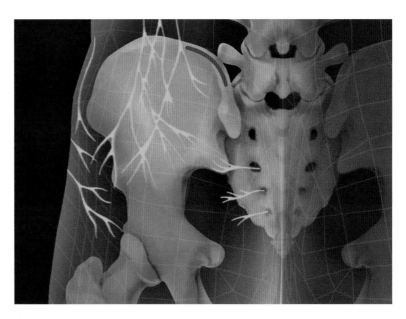

25 → OUTLINE OF POSTERIOR ILIAC HARVESTING.

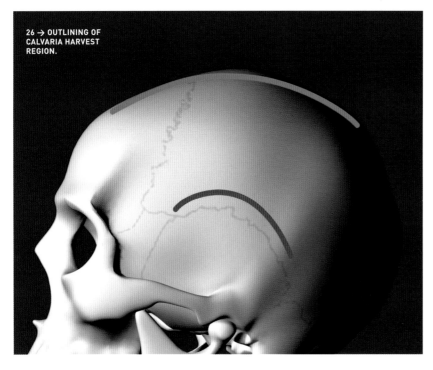

26 → OUTLINING OF CALVARIA HARVEST REGION.

CALVARIA BONE HARVEST

The calvaria is a bone with membranous ossification, made up of two thick cortexes that enclose a very thick cancellous layer, the diploe. The calvaria has been used as a bone harvest site since the 1970s; membranous ossification makes the calvaria identical to the maxilla and a large part of the mandible, so it has become a reference site for bone reconstruction of these areas.

This type of graft has optimal load-bearing capacity because it is very dense and resorbs slowly compared to other commonly used grafts. However, it is harder to revascularize.

HARVEST TECHNIQUES

We advise that computerized tomography (CT) of the cranium is performed beforehand to assess the thickness of the temporal bone. This makes the harvesting technique safer as monocortical bone graft is removed in most cases. Bicortical harvesting must always be carried out with the aid of a specialist in neurosurgery.

Usually, parietal bone is harvested and it is vital to know the areas to avoid, i.e. medially of the sagittal sinus and below the temporal line (Frodel et al. 1993) **FIG. 26**.

The bone must therefore be harvested at a suitable distance from these areas, to avoid the risk of large hemorrhages or even lacerating the dura mater cranialis due to the thinness of the area below the temporal line.

The patient must be prepared the evening prior to surgery. A povidone-iodine shampoo must be used, and once the incision point has been determined the hair around it should be parted.

Generally speaking, the median region provides bone that is curved to a certain extent, while occipital harvesting provides straighter bone. In the surgical site, once the head has been positioned and the harvest area identified, an incision is made in the scalp, long enough to precisely identify the danger zones. The scalpel must be angled to the same angle as the hair, in order to save hair bulbs that will allow hair to grow through the scar. The incision must reach the pericranium in a single stroke. Hemostasis must not be performed by bipolar cauterization, to avoid creating areas of alopecia. It is better to use gauze, applied to hemostatic forceps, or gauze alone on the edges of the scalp flaps. The pericranium is cut and detached **FIG. 27**. A dermographic pen is used to drawn the outline of the bone harvest. This cannot be longer than 5 cm or thicker than 2 cm in order to avoid the risk of fragmenting the internal cortex. It is possible to harvest more bone but the pieces must be separated from each other (Frodel 1996) **FIG. 28**.

The outline of the graft is cut through the whole thickness of the external cortex using a fissure bur with copious irrigation. With a large pear-shaped bur, a notch is created around the previous incision to insert the osteotomes in a

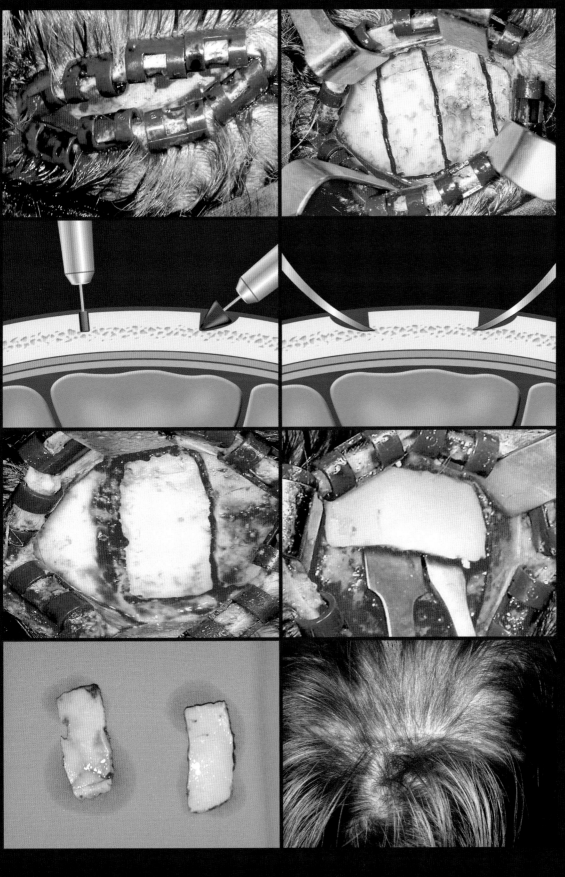

27 → SKELETIZATION OF CRANIAL THECA.

28 → PREPARATION OF OSTEOTOMY SITE.

29-30 → CORRECT OSTEOTOMY SITE PREPARATION.

31 → CALVARIA PREPARED FOR HARVESTING.

32 → INSERTION OF OSTEOTOMES.

33 → MONOCORTICAL CALVARIA BONE.

34 → RESULTING SCAR.

parallel direction to the external table in order to avoid passing the internal cortex **FIG. 29–31**.

The outlined external table is then delicately separated on all sides **FIG. 32**. If necessary it is possible to find an area of cancellous bone. Hemostasis must be accurate, the gap sutured on each layer and the scalp sutured with clips, which are less ischemia-inducing than sutures **FIG. 33–34**. Aspiration drainage may be placed to avoid the formation of subgaleal hematomas, which can take a long time to be completely absorbed.

ADVANTAGES

The advantage of using the calvaria as a bone source lies in the fact that it is simple to harvest and the cortical nature of the membranous bone makes it optimal for jaw bone grafts, especially in the mandible and in the anterior areas in general. Resorption is minimal, especially if compared to other donor sites. This is due to the type of membranous ossification that makes the cortex extremely compact, with few cells, and therefore less prone to significant osteoclastic stimulation (Frodel 1996).

DISADVANTAGES

There are few disadvantages, being in most cases hematomas and seromas that may form under the galeal plane. With regards to major complications, the most feared are dural tears in the event of accidental harvesting of the internal cortex, or encephalic damage caused by infection or hematomas. However, the authors' experience, together with the studies reported, shows extremely low percentages of complications (Kline & Wolfe 1995).

The true limit of the calvaria is the thinness of the cortex; however, it is an excellent graft for appositional grafting (Sadove et al. 1990), but less useful when interpositional grafts are needed, or when significant increases in bone are required. The overlapping of several cortical strips, required to achieve significant

increases, unfortunately means that the last strip may not revascularize and that some scar tissue will penetrate between one strip and another, which would make the reconstruction mechanically unsuitable. The amount of bone that can be harvested is also limited; in major reconstructions it is often necessary to resort to a second harvest site.

REVASCULARIZED BONE

The degrees of maxillary atrophy and the mechanisms by which it progresses have been investigated and classified. There are not many classifications in the literature that correlate the degree of atrophy and the type of bone reconstruction to be carried out. For this reason, we herein propose a classification that allows a quick decision on the most suitable type of reconstruction for each case. In the event of severe atrophy, with extensive resorption of the basal bone, the use of grafts is often not the most appropriate choice. This is due to resorption that is not always predictable, as well as to the increase in local complications, related to the difficulties in obtaining a stress-free mucosal coverage in extensive reconstruction areas. For this reason, especially in the last 5 years, revascularized bone transplantation techniques have been proposed. The bone is transplanted in the maxillae, together with the vascular bundle that permeates it; the latter is then anastomized using microsurgical techniques to cervical host vessels. This revascularizes the graft immediately, making it resistant to infection and not subject to significant resorption **FIG. 35**.

Although revascularized bone transplants are widely used today, they are a last resort, and should only be used in selected cases. Also, patients must be extremely motivated in order to undergo this type of surgery.

FREE FIBULAR FLAP

The free fibula flap was introduced into cranial reconstruction surgery at the end of the 1980s, and is now also used successfully in the rehabilitation of severe atrophy of the jaw (Lee et al. 2004).

The harvesting technique is standardized and safe. After assessing the absence of vascular anomalies in the leg artery system, which would be a contraindication, using echo-color Doppler and angiography tests, dissection is carried out with the limb in ischemia, obtained by placing a tourniquet around the upper part of the thigh, pumped to 350 mmHg and with leg and foot flexed to about 90 degrees.

The fibula outline can be viewed on the cutaneous surface using a straight line that joins the lateral malleolus to the femur epicondyle. The cutaneous incision is made along the entire length of the leg with a 90-degree flexion.

The incision is then deepened until it severs the fascia surrounding the peroneal muscle. By following the perioneal fascia posteriorly, the septum that separates the capus longus of the peroneal muscle and the posterior part of the gastrocnemius muscle is isolated. In the septum there are some perforating vessels that can be severed during bone harvesting.

The peroneus longus and brevis muscles and the flexor hallucis longus muscle are identified and their insertions are completely detached using a cold or electric scalpel. Once the top of the bone's external cortex has been reached, proceeding in the anterior section where the deep peroneal nerve, the anterior tibial artery and the anterior tibial vein can be isolated. By freeing the last muscle insertions, the interosseous membrane can be seen, and then sectioned **FIG. 36–37**.

Osteotomies are performed on the inferior and superior border of the fibula; the interosseous artery can be seen distally, with the accompanying veins that are tied and sectioned. The vascular bundle is highlighted distoproximally, carefully sectioning the flexor hallucis longus muscle and tibialis posterior muscles.

The peroneal artery and accompanying veins are freed up to the fork with the posterior tibial artery **FIG. 38**.

After disinserting the tricepis surae insertion, the anatomic unit, made up of fibula and artery and vein vessels, is ready to be detached from the donor site, modeled, transposed and revascularized at the host site **FIG. 39–40**.

35 → FREE FIBULA FLAP.

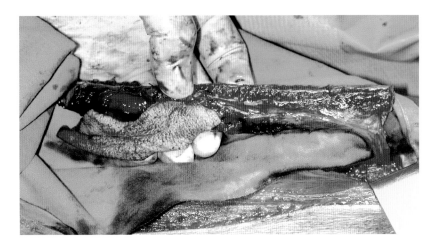

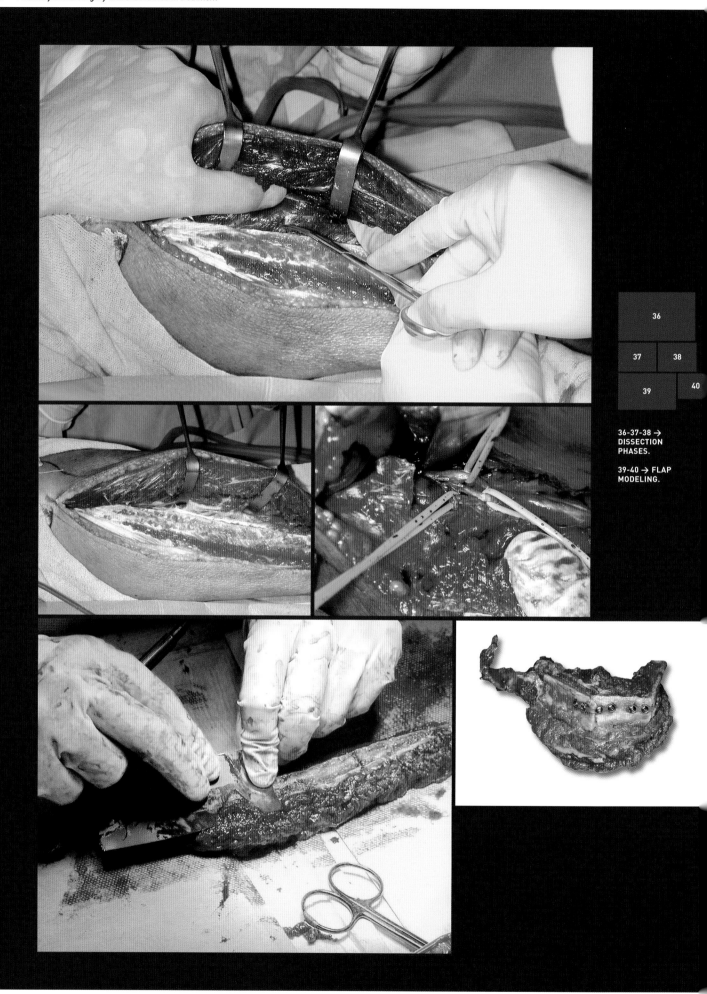

36-37-38 →
DISSECTION
PHASES.

39-40 → FLAP
MODELING.

ADVANTAGES

The greatest advantage of this technique is the high success rate (96 to 98%) and the possibility of correcting severe atrophies, due to the great amount of bone available **FIG. 41–43**. Moreover, the revascularized bone has the ability to resist infection, similar to other host vascularized tissues.

For major reconstructions using grafts, it is not the amount of bone that can be placed, but the possibility of achieving flap closure to prevent bacterial infection that is important to allow its revascularization. By using revascularized flaps, it is possible to add revascularized soft tissue (such as fascia or muscle) which will help to cover the bone portion that can also be left exposed in the oral cavity, and will heal by secondary intention.

DISADVANTAGES

The main disadvantage is the sophistication of the surgery, which means longer hospitalization, and an operation that typically lasts from 6 to 10 hours, three times longer than classic grafts, and has a higher morbidity at the harvest site. In fact, the leg needs a long time for full functional recovery and the scar of a lower limb may be an esthetic problem, especially in females **FIG. 44** (Urken et al. 1990).

The muscular part of the flap often requires further surgery for remodeling and for the sculpting of a new alveolar crest, suitable for placing implants.

For the above reasons and due to the considerable postsurgery compliance required of the patient, this reconstructive technique must be the final option, and should only be used in strongly motivated patients.

TIBIA HARVESTING

An alternative to extraoral harvesting from the iliac crest is harvesting from the lateroproximal portion of the tibia.

This technique is used when a cancellous bone graft is necessary. The operation allows considerable amounts of marrow bone to be harvested, between 20 to 40 cm^3 (Catone et al. 1992). It can be carried out under conscious sedation in day surgery (Jakse et al. 2001; Marchena et al. 2002).

The advantages for the patient are the following:
- Reduced operating time: about 30 minutes.
- Minimum blood loss, around 45 ml with a range of 25 to 122 ml.
- No drainage is needed.
- Reduced postsurgery discomfort.
- Reduced postsurgery morbidity. The onset of complications varies from 1.3% to 3.8%, compared to iliac harvesting which has a range of 8.6% to 9.2% (O'Keefe et al. 1991).
- The possibility of normal walking after surgery.

The contraindications for this type of surgery are:
- patient under 21 years of age
- previous knee surgery
- systemic pathologies, such as rheumatoid arthritis
- bone metabolism disorders or bone metastases.

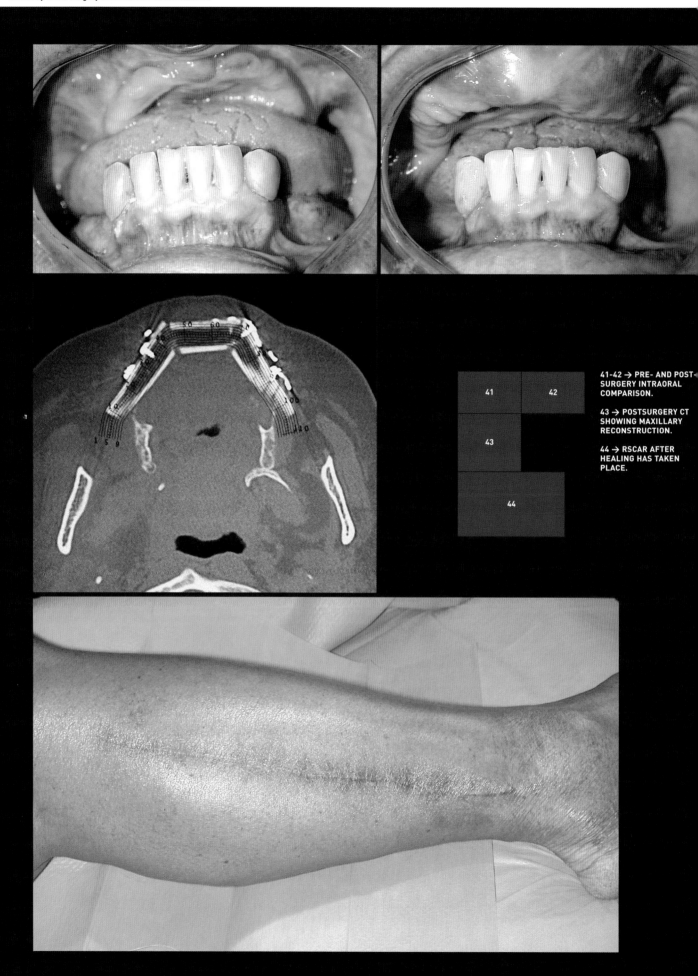

41-42 → PRE- AND POST-SURGERY INTRAORAL COMPARISON.

43 → POSTSURGERY CT SHOWING MAXILLARY RECONSTRUCTION.

44 → RSCAR AFTER HEALING HAS TAKEN PLACE.

ANATOMY

The genicular area is characterized by a complex weave of both muscular and neurovascular structures. The area involved in surgery is located in the lateral part of the tibia diaphysis and can be found as a bone prominence, called Gerdy's tubercle or anterior tibial tubercle, which is oblique in a craniocaudal and lateromedial direction.

The muscle and fiber structures present are listed below.

- Tibialis anterior muscle that is inserted in the lateral condyle of the tibia and runs in a caudal direction with insertion through a tendon on the medial side of the foot; its fibers cover the anterior tibial vascular fascia and the deep peroneal nerve. This nerve arises from the fork of the common peroneal nerve of the tibial region, between the fibula and the long peroneal muscle.

- Extensor longus digitorum muscle (long extensor muscle of the toes), which starts from the tibial lateral condyle and the peroneal epiphysis and which runs laterally to the anterior tibia, entering the last four toes.

- The fasciae latae runs between the bone plane and the subcutaneous layer, next to the tubercle, which becomes thicker in the ileotibial section.

45 → BEFORE PREPARING THE SURGICAL FIELD, THE ANATOMIC STRUCTURES ARE PALPATED AND THE INCISION LINE IS DRAWN ALONG THE CUTANEOUS PLANE, PARALLEL TO GERDY'S TUBERCLE.

46 → AFTER THE FIRST INCISION, THE FASCIA ARE DISSECTED, CONTINUING IN THE DIRECTION OF THE BONE PLANE.

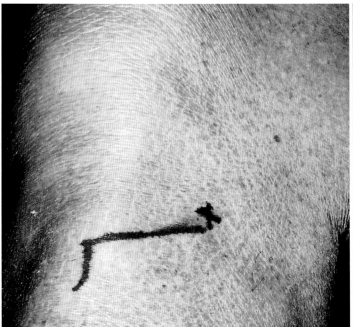
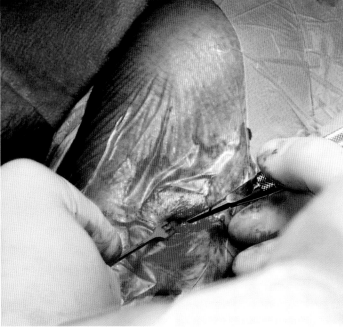

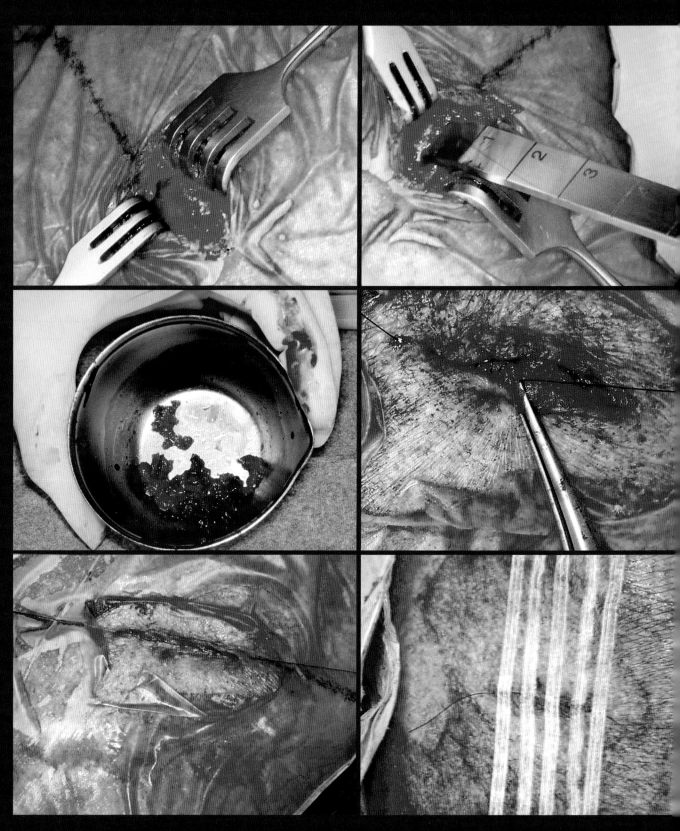

47	48
49	50
51	52

47 → DISSECTION IS COMPLETED ON THE BONE PLANE WHERE THE PERIOSTIUM IS CUT AND COMPLETELY DETACHED. THE FLAPS ARE KEPT OPEN BY RETRACTORS.

48 → CORTICAL OSTEOTOMY (2 CM X 2 CM) IS PERFORMED USING A FISSURE BUR ON A STRAIGHT HANDPIECE WITH COPIOUS IRRIGATION, THROUGH WHICH THE MARROW IS ACCESSED FOR HARVESTING.

49 → THE GRAFT IS HARVESTED USING SPECIFIC CURETTES.

50 → SUTURING IS PERFORMED BY RESTORING THE PREVIOUSLY SECTIONED FASCIA USING VICRYL 3-0.

51 → INTRADERMAL SUTURES ARE PERFORMED WITH PROLENE 5-0 ON THE OCCLUSAL PLANE.

52 → THE WOUND IS BLOCKED WITH ADHESIVE STERI-STRIPS.

Other muscles are present in the genicular region, but they are not involved in the surgical area, as they are either in the epiphysis area or the posterior area of the knee.

Joint structures present are the patellar ligament, which connects the quadriceps femoris muscle with the tibial tuberosity, mesially to Gerdy's tubercle; and the joint capsule, which enters the glenoid fossae cranially to Gerdy's tubercle.

Some vascular branches in the area originate from the upper genicular and upper lateral genicular artery, from where the inferior lateral genicular artery starts. The latter runs laterally to Gerdy's tubercle. Other vascular structures are the peroneal artery and anterior tibial artery, which is a branch of the popliteal artery. This vessel gives rise to branches such as the posterior and anterior tibial recurrent arteries that run caudally to Gerdy's tubercle.

Innervation involved in the surgery is the common peroneal nerve, that splits into two terminal branches, superficial and deep, which run cranially and laterally to Gerdy's tubercle.

SURGICAL TECHNIQUE

The patient is supine, and a soft ipsolateral support is placed under the knee and hip to allow better access to the lateroproximal portion of the tibia.

For both surgeries carried out under conscious sedation and those carried out under general anesthesia, local anesthesia is performed through subcutaneous infiltration and another subperiosteal 1 to 2 ml of lidocaine with adrenalin 1:100,000 to obtain an analgesic and hemostatic effect. Alternatively, it is possible to use bupivacaine 0.5%, which increases the postoperative analgesic effect.

A dermographic pen is used to draw the patella, the fibula, Gerdy's tubercle, the ileotibial section and the anterior tibial muscle **FIG. 45**.

Palpating the tubercle is a simple maneuver, as the subcutaneous plane is shallow.

Bleeding from cutaneous vessels can be controlled by electrocauterization. Any hematoma or seroma may increase the risk of postoperative infection of the treated area.

The vessels at greatest risk are the anterior tibial recurrent artery and the inferior lateral genicular artery.

The peroneal nerve can be damaged if the incision is made too far posteriorly.

Correct identification of Gerdy's tubercle is essential to avoid invasions of the knee joint area.

The area involved in surgery is delimited cranially by the insertion of the joint, mesially by the lateral edge of the patellar tendon and along the lateral-inferior side by the anterior tibial muscle.

The primary incision, 2 to 3 cm in length, is made obliquely to Gerdy's tubercle.

The direction of the fibers in the ileotibial section represent the incision axes: craniocaudal and lateromedial. The incision is made through the skin, the subcutaneous layers and the fasciae latae that remain adhered to the periosteum and which must be severed and detached.

A correct incision allows tissues to be closed easily during suturing.

Compact bone tissue (1 to 2 cm) is removed using a straight handpiece and a fissure bur, together with sterile irrigation, to expose the marrow area.

Bone is harvested using Molt bone curettes (starting with sizes 2 and 4) and then continued with orthopedic curettes, in a caudal direction. The final angled curette must be used carefully and deeply, avoiding cranial rotation movements that may superficially undermine the cortex of the tibial plate.

The donor site can be filled with plateletrich plasma (PRP) to promote hemostasis and regeneration of the harvested area.

Uncontrolled bleeding will cause infiltration along the fasciae planes with hematomas up to the more sloping areas.

The periosteum is sutured with vicryl 3–0, the muscle layer with chromic catgut 4–0. Closure is compulsory to avoid blood loss. The use of an intradermal suture, prolene 5-0, is recommended for the cutaneous plane. The wound is blocked by steri-strips. A medicated gauze is placed over the wound.

In the first 24 hours, rest with periods in which the patient keeps the leg lifted is recommended.

This harvest site can be used when a marrow graft is necessary and may be a less invasive technique than that from the iliac crest site. It has a low incidence of complications and is well tolerated by the patient **FIG. 46–52**.

REFERENCES

1 Ahlmann E., Patzakis M.
Comparison of anterior and posterior iliac crest bone grafts in terms of harvest-site morbidity and functional outcomes.
J. Bone Joint Surg. Am. 2002; 84-A: 716-20.

2 Beirne J.C., Barry H.J., Brady F.A., Morris V.B.
Donor site morbidity of the anterior iliac crest following cancellous bone harvest.
Int. J. Oral Maxillofac. Surg. 1996; 25: 268-71.

3 Bosworth D.M.
Repair of herniae through iliac crest defects.
J. Bone Joint Surg. Am. 1955; 37: 1069-73.

4 Boustred A.M., Fernandes D., van Zyl A.E.
Minimally invasive iliac cancellous bone graft harvesting.
Plast. Reconstr. Surg. 1997; 99: 1760-4.

5 Canady J.W., Zeitler D.P., Thompson, S.A., Nicholas C.D.
Suitability of the iliac crest as a site for harvest of autogenous bone grafts.
Cleft Palate Craniofac. J. 1993; 30: 579-81.

6 Catone G.A., Reimer B.L., McNeir D., Ray R.
Tibial autogenous cancellous bone as an alternative donor site in maxillofacial surgery: a preliminary report.
J. Oral Maxillofac. Surg. 1992; 50: 1258-63.

7 Frodel J.L.
Harvesting cranial bone.
Plast. Reconstr. Surg. 1996; 98: 753.

8 Frodel J.L. Jr, Marentette L.J., Quatela V.C.
Calvarial bone graft harvest. Techniques, considerations, and morbidity.
Arch Otolaryngol. Head Neck Surg. 1993; 119: 17-23.

9 Grillon G., Gunther S.F.
A new technique for obtaining iliac bone grafts.
J. Oral Maxillofac. Surg. 1984; 42: 172-6.

10 Kline R.M. Jr., Wolfe S.A.
Complications associated with the harvesting of cranial bone grafts.
Plast. Reconstr. Surg. 1995; 95: 5-13.

11 Kurz L.T., Garfin S.R., Booth R.E.
Harvesting autogenous iliac bone grafts: a review of complications and techniques.
Spine 1989; 14: 1324-31.

12 Jakse N., Seibert F.J., Lorenzoni M., Eskici A., Pertl C.
A modified technique of harvesting tibial cancellous bone and its use for sinus grafting.
Clin. Oral Implants Res. 2001; 12: 488-94.

13 LaRossa D., Buchman S., Rothkopf D.M., Mayro R., Randall P.
A comparison of iliac and cranial bone in secondary grafting of alveolar clefts.
Plast. Reconstr. Surg. 1995; 96: 789-97.

14 Laurie S.W.S., Kaban B., Mulliken J.B., Murray J.E.
Donor site morbidity after harvesting rib and iliac bone.
Plast. Reconstr. Surg. 1984; 73: 933–8.

15 Lee J.H., Kim M.J., Choi W.S.
Concomitant reconstruction of mandibular basal and alveolar bone with a free fibular flap.
Int. J. Oral Maxillofac. Surg. 2004; 33: 150-6.

16 Marchena J.M., Block M.S., Stover J.D.
Tibial bone harvesting under intravenous sedation: Morbidity and patient experiences.
J. Oral Maxillofac. Surg. 2002; 60: 1151-4.

17 Marx R.E., Morales M.J.
Morbidity from bone harvest in major jaw reconstruction: a randomized trial comparing the lateral anterior and posterior approaches to the ilium.
J. Oral Maxillofac. Surg. 1988; 46: 196-203.

18 McCarthy, Patel R.R., Wragg P.F., Brook I.M.
Dental implants and onlay bone grafts in the anterior maxilla: analysis of clinical outcome.
Int. J. Oral Maxillofac. Implants 2003; 18: 238-41.

19 McGurk M., Barker G., Grime P.
The trephining of bone from the iliac crest: An anterior approach.
Int. J. Oral Maxillofac. Surg. 1993; 22: 87-90.

20 Mrazik J., Amato C., Leban S., Mashberg A.
The ilium as a source of autogenous bone for grafting: Clinical considerations.
J. Oral Surg. 1980; 38: 29-32.

21 O'Keefe R.M. Jr, Riemer B.L., Butterfield S.L.
Harvesting of autogenous cancellous bone graft from the proximal tibial metaphysis. A review of 230 cases.
J. Orthop. Trauma. 1991; 5: 469-74.

22 Puri R., Moskovich R., Gsmorino P., Shott S.
Bupivacaine for postoperative pain relief at the iliac crest bone graft harvest site.
Am. J. Orthop. 2000; 29: 443-6.

23 Sadove A.M., Nelson C.L., Eppley B.L., Nguyen B.
An evaluation of calvarial and iliac donor sites in alveolar cleft drafting.
Cleft Palate J. 1990; 27: 225-8.

24 Shepard G.H., Dierberg W.J.
Use of the cylinder osteotome for cancellous bone grafting.
Plast. Reconstr. Surg. 1987; 80: 129-32.

25 Urken M.L., Weinberg H., Vickery C., Buchbinder D., Biller H.F.
Using the iliac crest free flap.
Plast. Reconstr. Surg. 1990; 85: 1001-2.

26 Wolfe S.A., Kawamoto H.K.
Taking the iliac bone graft: A new technique.
J. Bone Joint Surg. Am. 1978; 60: 411.

27 Wilson P.A.
Pain relief following iliac crest bone harvesting.
Br. J. Oral Maxillofac. Surg. 1995; 33: 242-3.

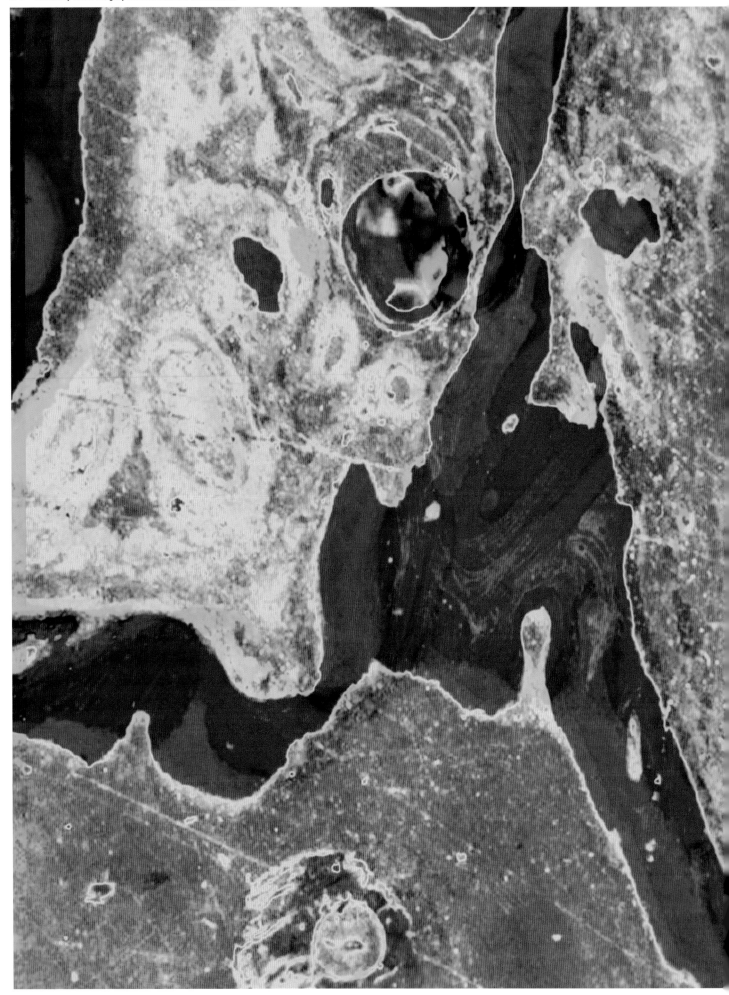

M. DEL FABBRO
F. ZUFFETTI

The use of platelet rich plasma in maxillary sinus augmentation. Biologic principles and clinical studies

18

18

INTRODUCTION

The success of a bone graft depends on the efficacy of the regeneration process, which begins immediately after the graft material is placed and over time completely replaces it with newly formed bone. The synthesis and regeneration of any type of tissue is a complex biologic process that requires a series of strictly controlled interactions between cells, extra-cellular matrix components, signal molecules and growth factors produced in loco or deriving from the systemic circulation. The identity of a particular tissue is defined by the biochemical nature of the extracellular matrix and the phenotype of the cells contained in it, which are positioned in a defined spatial relation to each other and the surrounding tissues. The key to the bone regeneration process lies in stimulating a series of cascade events in order to obtain a correct, coordinated integration between the various cellular and molecular components that lead to neo-osteogenesis. In recent years, various biologic approaches have been developed to induce and accelerate the new formation of bone tissue. In particular, the importance of specific growth factors (platelet-derived growth factor [PDGF], transforming growth factors [TGF-ß1 and TGF-ß2],

insulin-like growth factor 1 [IGF-1], etc.) was highlighted, which can influence the biologic process significantly (Canalis et al. 1991; Baylink et al. 1993; Giannobile 1996; Lind 1996, 1998; Schliephake 2002). A reserve of these growth factors is contained in the platelets that locally release several polypeptides that stimulate the healing process during blood coagulation (for example in a surgical wound). It therefore appears reasonable that a high concentration of platelets can increase the number of growth factors released locally, accelerating the tissue regeneration process during the healing phase (Marx et al. 1998; Marx 1999, 2001, 2004; Marx & Garg 1999).

PDGF and TGF-ß are the main platelet growth factors that are important for bone regeneration. The biology, structure and action of these factors has been studied for several years and there are numerous reviews that fully describe their properties and clinical fields of application (Antoniades & Williams 1983; Ross et al. 1986; Wenstermark 1990). In brief, from a molecular point of view, PDGF is a dimer, made up of the products of two genes (PDGF-A and PDGF-B) that join together as a homodimer (PDGF-AA, PDGF-BB) or a heterodimer (PDGF-AB). It was initially found in the alpha granules of platelets, but it was discovered that many cell types can synthesize PGDF (monocytes, macrophages, smooth muscular cells and endothelial cells). PDGF induces the proliferation of mesenchymal and endothelial cells; this activity is increased by the presence of other growth factors such as IGF-1. Also, PDGF has chemotactic and activation properties on macrophages, fibroblasts and leukocytes.

TGF-ß1 and TGF-ß2 are produced by platelets, monocytes/macrophages, neutrophils and T lymphocytes and their cellular targets are fibroblasts, stem cells, endothelial cells, epithelial cells and pre-osteoblasts.

These growth factors may stimulate chemotaxis and proliferation actions on marrow mesenchymal stem cells, fibroblasts and osteoblasts, and also induce angiogenesis and stimulate the deposition of bone matrix and collagen.

IGF-1 at the bone level has similar functions to TGF-ß1, stimulating the formation and deposition of bone matrix and the replication of osteoblasts and their precursors. It may act as both an autocrine and a paracrine factor, and together with PDGF can speed up and improve the quality of wound healing (Lind 1996, 1998; Schliephake 2002; Sanchez et al. 2003).

Other factors found in platelets are: PDEGF (platelet-derived epidermal growth factor), which has mitogenic and stimulating effects on keratinocytes, on endothelial cells and on fibroblasts; PDAF (platelet-derived angiogenic factor), which acts mainly on endothelial cells, stimulating angiogenesis and increasing vascular permeability; and PF-4 (platelet factor-4), produced exclusively by platelets, which has chemotactic action on neutrophils and fibroblasts (Lind 1996, 1998; Schliephake 2002; Sanchez et al. 2003).

Autogenous bone is generally considered to be the best graft material (gold standard), due to its osteogenetic, osteoinductive and osteoconductive properties (Misch & Dietsch 1993; Marx & Garg 1999; Marx 2001; Garg 2001). In addition to containing all organic and inorganic matrix elements, autogenous bone preserves part of the vital cellular component in the marrow portion. Osteoblasts and their precursors, as shown by Marx (Marx 1999, 2001; Marx & Garg 1999), possess receptors for platelet growth factors on the cell membrane, thus allowing the initiation of cell proliferation and differentiation processes, which are the basis of the formation of new tissues that make up the graft.

Graft healing is divided into two phases. During the first phase, immature bone tissue (woven bone) is formed, while in the second phase, the immature bone is progressively replaced by the lamellar bone tissue that guarantees graft compactness and solidity (Marx & Garg 1999).

These events, which take place naturally during the regeneration process after bone grafting, would be promoted by platelet-rich plasma (PRP) in the first minutes after surgery. The action of platelet factors is very short-lasting. It has been reported that the half-life of PDGF and IGF applied to periodontal defects in dogs, for example, lasted for 3 to 4 hours, while 96% of the two growth factors were removed within 4 days (Cohen et al. 1990; Lynch et al. 1991). However, the activation of macrophages, which is induced by the same factors, can trigger a cascade of chain reactions that may last for several weeks, controlling and modulating bone regeneration.

Recently, some studies published by Marx (Marx et al. 1998; Marx 1999) on the treatment of patients suffering from severe mandibular bone defects, highlighted the validity of using PRP obtained by apheresis of the patient's peripheral blood, to accelerate osteogenesis and favor the formation of bone tissue.

Marx suggested that, owing to the high concentration of growth factors contained in PRP, it is possible to obtain higher consolidation and early mineralization of the newly formed bone (Marx et al. 1998; Marx 1999, 2004; Marx & Garg 1999).

The 1998 study (Marx et al. 1998) was the first controlled clinical study on the efficacy of PRP in maxillofacial surgery. Later, other oral and maxillofacial surgeons tried to apply this technique in various clinical situations, whose common point was the need to regenerate bone tissue. One of the clinical applications for which the regenerative potential of PRP seemed to be indicated is maxillary sinus augmentation.

After the publication of Marx' study, several studies were carried out on animals (Fennis et al. 2002; Fürst et al. 2003; Jakse et al. 2003; Wiltfang et al. 2003a; Zechner et al. 2003; Roldan et al. 2004; Butterfield et al. 2005; Grageda et al. 2005; Ohya et al. 2005) and clinically (Anitua 1999; Kassolis et al. 2000; Rosenberg & Torosian 2000; Froum et al. 2002; Dugrillon et al. 2002; Maiorana et al. 2003; Rodriguez et al. 2003; Philippart et al. 2003, 2005; Wiltfang et al. 2003b; Mazor et al. 2004; Velich et al. 2004; Graziani et al. 2005; Kassolis & Reynolds 2005; Monov et al. 2005; Raghoebar et al. 2005; Steigmann & Garg 2005; Zuffetti et al. 2005; Trisi et al. 2006). Many of these studies were performed to determine the influence of PRP in the bone regeneration process, combined or not with autogenous bone or bone substitutes.

The personal experience of the authors with this technique applied in sinus augmentation procedures is presented below. Current clinical evidence on the use of PRP in sinus augmentation procedures will be discussed, by means of a critical review of the scientific literature. The aim of the study was to histologically evaluate whether the combination of autogenous bone and PRP in maxillary sinus augmentation procedures for implant purposes could accelerate the neo-osteogenesis process compared to patients treated with autogenous bone grafts only, and, at the same time, if the placement of a membrane on the osteotomic window could increase graft vitality.

MATERIALS AND METHODS

This prospective study was carried out on 8 non-smoking patients (4 males and 4 females, aged between 28 and 57 years). Four patients were completely edentulous, while the other four had partial bilateral edentulism in the maxilla. In all cases, Cawood and Howell class V maxillary bone atrophy was diagnosed (Cawood & Howell 1988).

Inclusion criteria for patients were as follows:

- residual crestal bone of less than 3 mm in the posterior maxilla
- no objective clinical patient history of cardiopathy, hemorrhage and hematological diseases, or previous radiotherapy treatment on head and neck
- absence of clinical-radiological signs of sinus pathology
- absence of clinical signs of periodontal disease
- serological negativity for hepatitis A, B, C, HIV, TPHA
- red blood cell count > 4,000,000/µl; hemoglobin > 12 g/dl; hematocrit > 37%; platelet count > 200,000/µl
- age > 18 years and body weight at least 50 kg
- non-habitual smoker
- informed consent on:
  - surgical procedure used and the need to perform bone biopsy for histologic-histomorphometric evaluation
  - blood banking process
  - PRP preparation method.

The use of platelet rich plasma in maxillary sinus augmentation. Biologic principles and clinical studies

299

All the patients underwent bilateral maxillary sinus augmentation using the Caldwell-Luc technique with cancellous graft of autogenous bone harvested from the iliac crest (anterior-medial-peritoneal side). Three months after the first surgical operation, a bone biopsy was carried out using a trephine bur, and during the same session titanium endosseous implants were inserted in the regenerated areas.

In each patient, each maxillary sinus received different treatment with different types of graft (autogenous bone with or without the addition of PRP) and application or non-use of a coverage membrane. The allocation of the type of treatment was by random number tables. The patients were divided into three groups according to the type of bone graft and the use of Resolut® membrane (W.L. Gore & Associates, Flagstaff, Arizona, USA) on the anstrotomy:

- group A: graft using autoogous bone and membrane (n = 5 sinuses)
- group B: graft using autogenous bone without membrane (n = 6 sinuses)
- group C: graft of autogenous bone with added PRP and membrane (n = 5 sinuses).

The day before the operation, the patient underwent removal of 410 ml of peripheral blood after disinfecting the skin with povidone with 10% iodine (Betadine®, Viatris, Milan, Italy) and with a needle cannula 12. The PRP was prepared the day of the operation, using a closed circuit processing technique under a hood.

According to Marx' studies (Marx et al. 1998; Marx 2004), the PRP is effective if it has a platelet count of $1500 \times 10^3/\mu l$, i.e. about 6 to 10 times its physiologic value.

Using this preparation method, it is possible to obtain a PRP with a platelet count of more than $2000 \times 10^3/\mu l$. The following were obtained from the blood removed: PRP (about 10 ml), autogenous plasma (20 ml), and cryoprecipitate autogenous plasma (10 ml). The cryoprecipitate autogenous plasma was obtained from fresh plasma frozen to $-80°C$, and then defrosted to $4°C$ using the overnight method. 5 ml were taken from the 40 ml of PRP autogenous plasma and cryoprecipitate, which were activated at the moment of use by an equal volume mix of batroxobin (Botropase®, Ravizza Farmaceutici, Muggio, Italy) and calcium chloride 10%, and mixed with autogenous bone.

Surgical re-entry for implant placement took place 3 months after the maxillary sinus augmentation. The number and size (length and diameter) of dental implants was chosen on the basis of the amount (thickness and height) of available bone, evaluated by an accurate objective examination and a careful analysis of the maxillary bone computerized tomogram (CT) carried out 3 months after the first surgical phase. During the operation, a bone autopsy was performed at the graft site, using a trephine bur.

The bioptic samples were fixed with a dedicated resin, using a 50% solution of ethanol/resin and then a 100% resin solution. The preparations were then polymerized for 48 hours. The blocks of resin obtained in this way were cut with a microtome (Remet, Italy), in order to obtain 250-μm thick sections. The sections were then reduced to 40 μm using a LS-2 grinder (Remet).

Bone tissue maturation was analyzed by the toluene blue coloring test, while basic fuchsine was used to stain the fibrous tissue in order to obtain greater contrast.

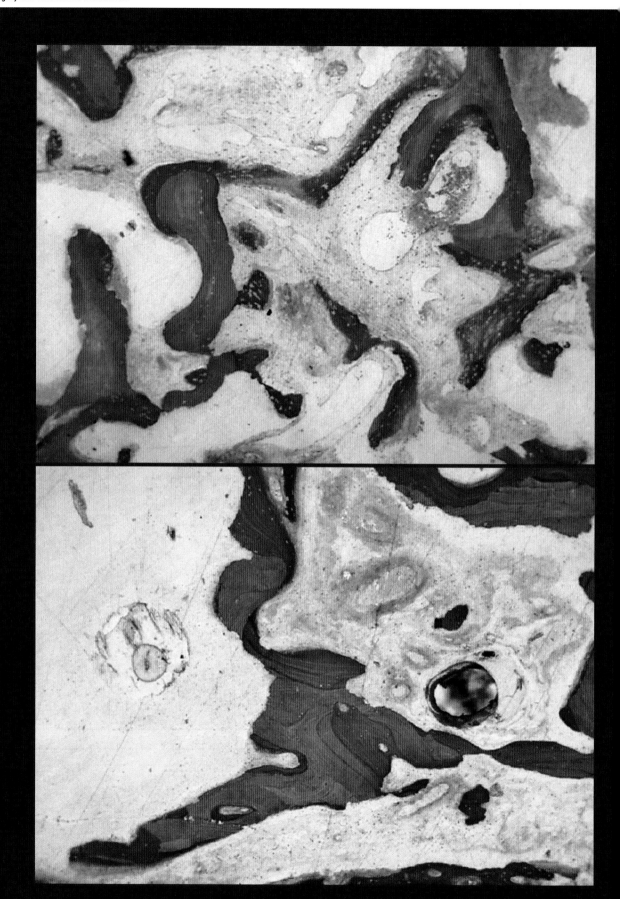

1 → AUTOGENOUS
BONE GRAFT
AFTER 3 MONTHS
OF HEALING.
ORIGINAL
MAGNIFICATION
50X.

2 → AUTOGENOUS
BONE GRAFT AND
PRP AFTER
3 MONTHS OF
HEALING.
ORIGINAL
MAGNIFICATION
50X.

The use of platelet rich plasma in maxillary sinus augmentation. Biologic principles and clinical studies

301

RESULTS

The results of the histomorphometric analysis can be seen TAB. 1.

The percentage of vital bone in bone volume in group A (autogenous bone graft only) and group C (autogenous bone graft plus PRP) is comparable. The range of bone volume % in the total volume is lower in group C than in group A.

Also, in patients with no membrane placed on the antrotomy (group B), the percentage of vital bone and the bone volume formed are lower than the groups A and C, for which a membrane was instead used.

A histologic graft preparation was made, of both autogenous bone only (group A) FIG. 1, and autogenous bone + PRP (group C) FIG. 2. The quality of newly formed bone (areas darker in colour) appears to be similar in these two histologic preparations.

DISCUSSION

One of the limits of marrow bone autogenous transplants for reconstructing large-scale maxillary deficiencies is the quality of the newly formed bone, which is often low and immature. Also, maturation and mineralization time for the bone may delay the functional rehabilitation of the area involved.

During the present study, we found no obvious difference in vital bone formation between the cases for which autogenous bone was used together with PRP and the cases for which only autogenous bone was used.

Some of the advantages we found in using PRP were the improvement in intra-surgery handling of the graft material and in obtaining better healing of soft tissues. In all the sites where PRP was used, the surgical wound healed excellently and more rapidly compared to the sites where PRP was not used. This effect on soft tissue confirms previous results (Anitua 1999; Dugrillon et al. 2002; Ghurani et al. 2000).

Histomorphometric analysis of vital bone in maxillary sinus augmentation

TAB.1

		Vital bone / bone volume	Bone volume / total volume
GROUP A	Autogenous bone graft with membrane	63.6 – 77.52%	25.10 – 26.4%
GROUP B	Autogenous bone graft without membrane	51.81 – 58.4%	20.4 – 23.96%
GROUP C	Autogenous bone graft and PRP with membrane	63.84 – 77.46%	23.26 – 25.10%

It should be remembered that PRP is not just a solution containing high levels of platelets; it also contains the three plasma proteins that can act as cellular adhesion molecules for osteoconduction. These act as a matrix for bone, connective tissue and epithelial tissue migration. These cellular adhesion molecules are fibrin, fibronectin and vitronectin (Marx 2004). The presence of these factors contributes to the plasticity and cohesion of PRP and may be important during the graft healing phase.

In this study, we also found that using a membrane on the lateral antrotomy produced a greater production of vital bone in all cases, compared to the cases treated without membrane. This confirms previous findings (Froum et al. 1998; Tarnow et al. 2000; Tawil & Mawla 2001) and we conclude that the use of a membrane should be considered for maxillary sinus augmentation procedures.

Finally, while taking into consideration the limited number of samples, the results of this histologic/histomorphometric study suggest that:

- the use of PRP does not bring about a significant difference of vital bone formation in maxillary sinus elevation with autogenous bone graft
- the application of a resorbable membrane on the lateral antrotomy increases the percentage of formed vital bone
- the use of PRP favors healing of soft tissues in all cases treated.

PRP is an autogenous preparation, and therefore does not entail risks of disease transmission or immune reactions, as may instead occur with allo- or xeno-transplants. However, there is a possibility of contamination during the preparation procedure. For this reason, the patient's blood must only be handled by qualified personnel within a hematology unit and must be prepared in a sterile environment. For greater safety, as normally happens in some hospital centers, a cell culture of the preparation should be carried out, to check for the absence of bacterial contamination.

We will now look critically at the experience of other authors in using PRP during maxillary sinus augmentation procedures **TAB. 2**.

Kassolis published a study on 15 patients who underwent maxillary sinus augmentation procedures (14 cases) and an increase of the alveolar ridge (three cases), treated with PRP and FDBA (mineralized freeze-dried bone allograft) (Kassolis et al. 2000). A total of 36 textured surface implants were placed, 29 of which during the same surgical session as the bone graft. The implant success rate after 12 months was 88.9%. Four failures were discovered on uncovering and were later replaced. The histologic investigation on two patients confirmed the presence of vital bone around the FDBA particles. The authors suggested that the use of PRP can allow the surgeon to anticipate implant placement and functional load, but, without a control group and a suitable experimental plan, these conclusions cannot be justified.

Rosenberg and Torosian (2000) described a clinical case concerning a male patient aged 70, for whom PRP was used together with an alloplastic graft, in a maxillary sinus augmentation procedure. The implants were placed 3 months after the graft. One month after implant surgery, the patient also received a temporary prosthesis on four elements, and after 5 months the permanent prosthesis was connected. Based only on this clinical case, the authors concluded that the use of PRP allows the overall duration of treatment to be halved. It is not fitting to draw conclusions on a new treatment based on the clinical results of one patient, due to the high level of variability among patients and the lack of suitable experimental outlines.

More recently, Froum published a study on three patients who underwent a bilateral maxillary sinus augmentation procedure

The use of platelet rich plasma in maxillary sinus augmentation. Biologic principles and clinical studies

303

TAB. 2

Summary of articles considered for the critical review of literature on PRP and sinus augmentation

Author and year	No. patients	No. sinuses	No. implants inserted (failed)	Residual bone height, mm	Graft material test group	Graft material for control	1-stage / 2-stage (months after graft)	Duration of follow-up (functional load)	Type of experimental design
Kassolis et al. 2000	15	14 (+3 crests)	36 (4)	<5 ≤5	FDBA+PRP	–	1-st. (29 imp.) 2-st. (6 m)	12 months	Case series
Rosenberg & Torosian 2000	1	1	4	NR	Alloplastic material	–	2-st. (3 m)	5 months	Single case
Froum et al. 2002	3	6	3 mini	NR	Bio-Oss +PRP	Bio-Oss	2-st. (7–11 m)	NR	RCT (split-mouth)
Maiorana et al. 2003	10	11	24	NR	Bio-Oss +PRP	–	2-st. (6 m)	NR	Case series
Rodriguez et al. 2003	15	24	70 (5)	< 5	Bio-Oss +PRP	–	1-st.	6–36 months	Case series
Philippart et al. 2003	18	25	58 (5)	1–3	Autogenous +rhTF +tetracycline	–	2-st. (5–7 m)	up to 5 years	Case series
Wiltfang et al. 2003	39	45	NR	2-7	b-TCP+PRP	b-TCP	2-st. (6 m)	NR	RCT
Mazor et al. 2004	105	105	276 (2)	< 5	Autogenous 30-40% + Bio-Oss 60-70% +PRP	Historical control	1-st.	16-32 (22 av.) m	Case series
Velich et al. 2004	624	810 (28 w/PRP)	1482 (81)	2-6	Various types	–	1-st. (485 cases) 2-st. (6.5 m, 325 cases)	1–5 years	Retrospective
Graziani et al. 2005	6	6	NR	2.1-7 (3.36 av.)	Autogenous bone, PRP and autogenous fibrinogenous	–	–	–	Case series
Kassolis & Reynolds 2005	10	20	NR	1-3	FDBA +PRP	FDBA +resorbable membrane	2-st (4.5-6 m)	–	RCT single-blinded
Philippart et al. 2005	3	4	30 (1)	1-4	Autogenous (calvaria)+Pep Gen P-15 + PRP + rhTF	–	2-st. (6-10m)	3m	Case series
Raghoebar et al. 2005	5	10	NR	7-9	Autogenous (iliac crest) + PRP	Autogenous (iliac crest)	2-st. (3 m)	20.2±4.3 m	Controlled split-mouth study
Steigmann & Garg 2005	20	40	NR	< 3	PRP only	Beta TCP	1-st.	6m	RCT (split-mouth)
Zuffetti et al. 2005	8	16	NR	NR	Autogenous (iliac crest) + PRP and membrane	Autogenous bone	2-st. (3 m)	NR	Case series
Trisi et al. 2006	3	3			Autogenous + Biogran +PRP (2 cases)	–	–	–	–

(Froum et al. 2002). In each patient, one of the two sinuses (test) was treated with PRP and inorganic bovine bone (Bio-Oss®), while the other sinus (control) received Bio-Oss® only. On the day of surgery, a coin was thrown to decide which of the two sinuses was to be treated with PRP. This randomizing method is not acceptable for the type of experimental design. Three miniature implants (2 mm in diameter and 10 mm long, two implants in the test side and one in the control side) were placed in one of the three patients via the crestal bone, in order to incorporate them in the graft. The permanent implants were placed in the three patients after 7, 7.5 and 11 months respectively. At the time of implant site creation, 3 mm x 10 mm long biopsies were taken using a trephine bur, through a lateral osteotomy window. The histomorphometric analysis to determine the percentage of vital bone in sinus grafts showed similar values between the experimental group and the control group. The two mini-implants placed in the test side showed a slightly higher percentage of contact between bone and implant surface (37.6% and 38.8%) compared to the implant placed in the controlateral control site (33.8%). The authors' conclusion was that the use of PRP does not make a significant difference to the production of vital bone or to contact between bone and implant surface. These conclusions also appear to be inappropriate due to the lack of a suitable experimental design and the low number of samples.

In a study published in 2003, Maiorana treated 10 patients (11 maxillary sinuses) using deproteinized bovine bone (Bio-Oss®) and PRP, using the two-stage surgical technique (Maiorana et al. 2003). Six months after grafting, 24 implants were placed and bone biopsies were carried out in the implant sites, for a histologic investigation. The authors found excellent soft tissue healing, full closure of the maxillary sinus access window and positive regenerated bone density. The authors concluded that, if compared with historical con-

trols on cases treated with Bio-Oss® only, the cases treated with added PRP have a similar amount of newly formed bone after the same period of healing, but with with higher mineralization. The authors also point out other clinical advantages of the platelet-rich gel, connected with its biologic adhesive property, such as easy handling of bone chips and good stability inside the maxillary sinus. The lack of an internal control makes the level of evidence of this study rather low. The individual variability in the graft healing process is rather high and a split-mouth experimental design would be more appropriate.

Rodriguez published a study in which PRP was used together with Bio-Oss® in maxillary sinus augmentation (Rodriguez et al. 2003). The study involved 15 patients with a residual bone height < 5 mm in the posterior region, in which 24 maxillary sinuses were treated with the lateral technique and a total of 70 implants were placed in the same surgical session as the graft (1-stage). The implants were loaded 4 months after placement and follow-up was from 6 to 36 months of functional load. A biopsy of bone graft was performed on one patient, while bone density was assessed in three patients using CT carried out 4 months after grafting. The histologic examination revealed the formation of new vital bone close to the Bio-Oss® particles. Bone density of the graft was found to be comparable or slightly higher than the surrounding native bone. The overall implant survival rate was 92.9% (five implants failed in four patients). The authors concluded that using PRP together with deproteinized bovine bone is effective in shortening the healing time by 3 to 4 times the usual period, and allowing early functional load. In this case too, due to the absence of a control group, and with only one type of histologic data, the experimental design seems to be inadequate and the conclusions are not justified.

Philippart carried out a long-term study with follow-ups of up to 5 years, investigating a graft of PRP, recombinant human tissue thromboplastin (rhTF), tetracycline and bone chips taken from the cranial calvaria (Philippart et al. 2003). With this compound graft, maxillary sinus augmentation was carried out on 18 patients (25 sinuses), inserting a total of 58 implants. The implants were inserted 5 to 7 months after grafting, and the prosthesis was applied after another 6 months. The success rate for grafts was 90.3% (three sinuses suffered a focal infection), while the implant survival rate was 91.3% (five early failures in four patients). Histologic assessment showed the presence of vascularized connective tissue rich in lamellar bone with osteocytes and surrounded by osteoblasts. The authors concluded that the mix they used was easy to handle, safe for the patient and with high bone regeneration capacity. In this case too, with no control group, these conclusions appear to be difficult to support, while confirming the good mechanical properties of PRP. Also, the addition of two elements (rhTF and tetracycline) complicates the interpretation of results as it is not possible to discern the contribution of each single factor for the healing process and bone regeneration.

Wiltfang published a randomized clinical trial (RCT) using beta tricalcium phosphate (ß-TCP) as the graft material in 39 patients (45 maxillary sinuses) (Wiltfang et al. 2003b). The test group (22 cases) were treated with ß-TCP and PRP, while the control group (23 cases) were treated with ß-TCP only. There are no details on the randomization method used. The histologic investigation did not show significant difference in the two groups, although a higher percentage of newly formed bone was found in the test group (38% with a range between 32 and 43%) compared to the control group (29%, range 25 to 37%). The graft material deterioration rate was also similar between the two groups. The authors underlined the extreme intra- and inter-individual variability in the parameters found. This lack of homogeneity, together with variability in the individual initial clinical conditions (the authors reported a range of presurgery residual bone height of 2 to 7 mm in both groups) and the uncertainty linked to randomization, reduces the reliability of the conclusions. ß-TCP was also used in the Steigmann & Garg (2005) study, but the two studies are difficult to compare due to the large differences in the experimental design and the patients' baseline characteristics.

Mazor et al. (2004) reported their experience in unilateral sinus elevation associated with the use of PRP in 105 consecutive patients, with a residual bone height of less than 5 mm in the posterior maxilla (Mazor et al. 2004). Using the Caldwell-Luc technique, the authors placed a total of 276 implants at the same time as grafting, leaving a period of 6 months before the prosthesis stage. Follow-up was between 16 and 32 months (average 22 months). Graft material was 30 to 40% of autogenous bone harvested from intraoral sites and 60 to 70% Bio-Oss®. A collagen membrane was applied to contain the graft in all cases. PRP was activated using human thrombin.

Two implants in two patients were removed due to infection and substituted after 6 months. The authors maintained that owing to the use of PRP, it was possible to anticipate the prosthesis stage by 3 months, compared to the average 9 months required in their previous experience without using PRP. However, they do not histologically document a rapid maturation of the graft. They also report improved, faster soft tissue healing, a lower postsurgical consumption of analgesics and lower local swelling. Even though this study's database is the largest of those reported so far in clinical literature, the lack of a control group reduces its intrinsic value. The special type of compound graft used in this study also makes it difficult to compare with other studies.

In a retrospective study on failures in 810 maxillary sinus augmentation operations carried out in a 5-year period (1996 to 2001) and using various materials, Velich et al. (2004) reported that, after examining orthopantographs, there was no complete resorption in combined PRP + ß-TCP grafts (28 cases) compared to an average of 2.7% in all cases. An implant failure occurred in one case only, but the cause or time of failure are not reported. Not only does the data supplied have a low significance (follow-up is not specified and is presumably not the same for everyone, it is not specified whether there was partial graft resorption, and there are no graft maturation data), but also it is not clear which of the two components brought about the positive result.

Other more recent studies have reported positive results on the use of PRP in healing after maxillary sinus augmentation, but some are case reports or case series without control groups (Graziani et al. 2005; Philippart et al. 2005; Trisi et al. 2006). Others hypothesize that neo-osteogenesis occurred in sinuses treated with PRP but only on the basis of orthopantographs, without histologic analyses (Steigmann & Garg 2005). Also, in this latter study, the residual bone height was 7 to 9 mm, much higher than the average of other studies, and this may have favored a positive result.

A radiographic study by Raghoebar et al. (2005) on five patients treated with bilateral sinus augmentation did not find differences in graft bone density between sites treated with PRP + autogenous bone from the iliac crest and sites grafted with autogenous bone only. In addition to the low number of samples, it can also be hypothesized that autogenous graft resorption masked the PRP regenerative capacity.

Finally, an RCT carried out on 10 patients who underwent bilateral sinus augmentation showed a higher percentage of vital tissue (bone and connective tissue) in the sites treated with FDBA + PRP compared to controls treated with FDBA only (78.8±8.3% vs 63.0±15.7%) (Kassolis & Reynolds 2005). The results of this study are similar to those obtained in the other RCT carried out by Wiltfang et al. (2003).

A review of the literature has shown how, as in other recent critical reviews (Sanchez et al. 2003; Freymiller & Aghaloo 2004; Boyapati & Wang 2006), research on the clinical efficacy of PRP combined with bone grafts in maxillary sinus augmentation is still in a preliminary phase.

All the studies on the use of PRP together with bone grafts consist of individual or series clinical cases, which sometimes adopt an almost experimental design. While it is acknowledged that these types of studies are the starting point, the results that emerge cannot be considered as final. In some cases, the authors used subjective indicators to measure PRP's ability to increase bone density (Marx et al. 1998) or drew conclusions based on subjective observations (Anitua 1999; Kassolis et al. 2000; Rosenberg & Torosian 2000). Owing to the lack of adequate controls and non-conventional or missing randomization techniques, the experimental designs are found to be inappropriate and the conclusions cannot be considered totally reliable. Also, the techniques used to prepare the PRP and activate it are different, and therefore, owing to the lack of standardization and homogeneity, the various works cannot be compared.

The need to use certified equipment, that can provide a final product rich in vital, active platelets is unavoidable. The use of equipment that has not been approved by bodies in charge of the control and certification of the medical field (e.g. the Food and Drug Administration in the USA, or the European Organization for Testing and Certification [EOTC] in the European Community) may be one of the primary causes for the relative failure of PRP found in some studies, as effectively pointed out by Marx in a recent article (Marx 2004). The limitations to using PRP in sinus lifts can be summarized as follows: PRP requires the presence of vital cells to carry out a beneficial action. The duration of the action of the growth factors contained therein is very brief and is only effective if the platelet count reaches high levels, at least 1 million/µl. The blood processing to obtain PRP may affect the platelet physiology, sometimes inducing the premature release of growth; if bovine thrombin is used as a coagulation activator there may be a formation of cross-reactive antibodies with potentially serious effects (Landesberg et al. 1998). Finally, the results obtained in the various studies are often conflicting and rather heterogenous and it is not possible to draw generalized conclusions.

CONCLUSIONS

In theory, treatment with growth factors is one of the best therapy approaches for bone regeneration: the growth factors released by platelets induce mesenchymal and endothelial cells to migrate, multiply, differentiate and increase blood supply, the formation of collagen and the deposition of bone matrix. Treatment with PRP was found to be effective in animal models and *in vitro* studies, where the degree of experimental condi-

tion standardization is rather high. However, when this treatment is applied to humans, the results are sometimes not as high as expected and, in addition, perhaps due to the many concurrent and hard to control variables, the actual contribution of single growth factors is difficult to quantify, also owing to the probable interaction with other factors present in the healing site.

Advantages of PRP are its safety (no transmission of illness or immune reactions) and its ease of handling (the mechanical properties of the platelet gel actually improves the plasticity of the graft).

However, when choosing the suitable therapy, it is also necessary to take into consideration additional costs, resources and the time used for the preparation of PRP, as well as the need for a hospital situation.

Serious clinical cases, with severe bone resorption in which healing proves difficult and unpredictable, may certainly benefit from the use of PRP in order to increase the possibility of safe, correct healing.

Although the great clinical potential of PRP, due to the high concentration of growth factors it contains, can be seen, the need for clinical decisions based on evidence makes it necessary for further RCTs to be carried out to establish the optimal concentration of the various growth factors and to determine whether using PRP together with various bone substitutes and/or various barrier membranes can provide a real, consistent benefit.

REFERENCES

1 **Anitua E.**
   Plasma rich in growth factors: Preliminary results of use in the preparation of future sites for implants.
   Int. J. Oral Maxillofac. Implants 1999; 14: 529-35.

2 **Antoniades H.N., Williams L.T.**
   Human platelet-derived growth factor: structure and fuction.
   Federation Proc. 1983; 42: 2630-34.

3 **Baylink D.J, Finkelman R.D, Mohan S.**
   Growth factors to stimulate bone formation.
   J. Bone Min. Res. 1993; 8 (suppl.): S565-72.

4 **Boyapati L., Wang H.-L.**
   The role of platelet-rich plasma in sinus augmentation: a critical review.
   Implant Dent. 2006; 15: 160-70.

5 **Butterfield K.J., Bennett J., Gronowicz G. et al.**
   Effect of platelet-rich plasma with autogenous bone graft for maxillary sinus augmentation in a rabbit model.
   J. Oral Maxillofac. Surg. 2005; 63: 370-6.

6 **Canalis E., McCarthy T.L., Centrella M.**
   Growth factors and cytokines in bone cell metabolism.
   Ann. Rev. Med. 1991; 42: 17-24.

7 **Cawood J.I., Howell R.A.**
   A classification of the edentolous jaws.
   Int. J. Oral Maxillofac Surg. 1988; 17: 232-236.

8 **Cohen A.M., Sodergerg C., Thomason A.**
   Plasma clearance and tissue distribution of recombinant human platelet-derived growth factor (B-chain omodimer) in rats.
   J. Surg. Res. 1990; 49: 447-52.

9 **Dugrillon A., Eichler H., Kern S., Klüter H.**
   Autologous concentrated platelet-rich plasma (cPRP) for local application in bone regeneration.
   Int. J. Oral Maxillofac. Surg. 2002; 31: 615-9.

10 **Fennis J.P.M., Stoelinga P.J.W., Jansen J.A.**
   Mandibular reconstruction: a clinical and radiographic animal study on the use of autogenous scaffolds and platelet-rich plasma.
   Int. J. Oral Maxillofac. Surg. 2002; 31: 281-6.

11 **Freymiller E.G., Aghaloo T.L.**
   Platelet-Rich Plasma: ready or not?
   J. Oral Maxillofac. Surg. 2004; 62: 484-8.

12 **Froum S.J., Tarnow D.P., Wallace S.S., Rohrer M.D., Cho S.-C.**
   Sinus floor elevation using anorganic bovine bone matrix (OsteoGraf/N) with and without autogenous bone.
   A clinical, histologic, and histomorphometric analysis.
   Part 2 of an ongoing prospective study.
   Int. J. Periodontics Restorative Dent. 1998; 18. 529-43.

13 **Froum S.J., Wallace S.S., Tarnow D.P., Cho S.-C.**
   Effect of platelet-rich plasma on bone growth and osseointegration in human maxillary sinus grafts.
   Three bilateral case reports.
   Int. J. Periodontics Restorative Dent. 2002; 22: 45-53.

14 **Fürst G., Gruber R., Tangl S., Zechner W., Haas R., Mailath G., Saronman F., Watzek G.**
   Sinus grafting with autogenous platelet-rich plasma and bovine hydroxyapatite. A histomorphometric study in minipigs.
   Clin. Oral Implants Res. 2003; 14: 500-8.

15 **Garg A.K.**
   Current concepts in augmentation of the maxillary sinus for placement of dental implants.
   Dent. Implantol. Update 2001; 11: 17-22.

16 **Ghurani R., Marx R., Monteleone K.**
   Healing enhancement of skin graft donor sites with platelet-rich plasma.
   Oral Abstract session 6. American Academy of Oral Maxillofacial Surgery, Sept. 2000.

17 **Giannobile W.V.**
   Periodontal tissue engineering by growth factors.
   Bone 1996; 19 (suppl. 1): S23-37.

18 **Grageda E., Lozada J.L., Boyne P.J., Caplanis N., McMillan P.J.**
   Bone formation in the maxillary sinus by using platelet-rich plasma: An experimental study in sheep.
   J. Oral Implantol. 2005; 31: 2-17.

19 **Graziani F., Ducci F., Tonelli M., El Askary A.S., Monier M., Gabriele M.**
   Maxillary sinus augmentation with platelet-rich plasma and fibrinogen cryoprecipitate: A tomographic pilot study.
   Implant Dent. 2005; 14: 63-9.

20 **Jakse N., Tangl S., Gilli R., Berghold A., Lorenzoni M., Eskici A., Haas R., Pertl C.**
   Influence of PRP on autogenous sinus grafts. An experimental study on sheep.
   Clin. Oral Implants Res. 2003; 14: 578-83.

21 **Kassolis J.D., Reynolds M.A.**
   Evaluation of the adjunctive benefits of platelet-rich plasma in subantral sinus augmentation.
   J. Craniofac. Surg. 2005; 16: 280-7.

22 **Kassolis J.D., Rosen P.S., Reynolds M.A.**
   Alveolar ridge and sinus augmentation utilizing platelet-rich plasma in combination with freeze-dried bone allograft: Case series.
   J. Periodontol. 2000; 71: 1654-61.

23 **Landesberg R., Moses M., Karpatkin M.**
   Risks of using platelet rich plasma gel.
   J. Oral Maxillofac. Surg. 1998; 56: 1116-67.

24 **Lind M.**
   Growth factor stimulation of bone healing.
   Effects on osteoblast, osteotomies and implant fixation.
   Acta Orthop. Scand. Suppl. 1998; 69: 2-37.

25 **Lind M.**
   Growth factors: possible new clinical tools. A review.
   Acta Orthop. Scand. 1996; 67: 407-17.

26 **Lynch S.E., Buser D., Hernandez R.A., Weber H.P., Fox C.H., Williams R.C.**
   Effects of the platelet-derived growth factor/insulin-like growth factor-1 combination on bone regeneration around titanium dental implants. Result of a pilot study in beagle dogs.
   J. Periodontol. 1991; 62: 710-6.

27 **Maiorana C., Sommariva L., Brivio P., Sigurtà D., Santoro F.**
   Maxillary sinus augmentation with anorganic bovine bone (Bio-Oss) and autologous platelet-rich plasma: preliminary clinical and histologic evaluations.
   Int. J. Periodontics Restorative Dent. 2003; 23: 227-35.

28 **Marx R.E.**
   Platelet concentrate: a strategy for accelerating and improving bone regeneration.
   In: Davies JE (ed). Bone Engineering. Toronto, Canada: Em squared, 2001: 447-52.

29 Marx R.E., Carlos E.R., Eichstaedt R.M., Schimmele S.R., Strauss J.E., Goergeff K.R.
Platelet-rich plasma: Growth factor enhancement for bone grafts.
Oral Surg. Oral Med. Pathol. Oral Radiol. Endod. 1998; 85: 638-46.

30 Marx R.E., Garg A.K.
Bone graft physiology with use of Platelet-Rich Plasma and Hyperbaric Oxygen.
In: Jensen O (Ed.). The Sinus Bone Graft. Chicago: Quintessence Publishing, 1999: 183-9.

31 Marx R.E.
Platelet-rich plasma: A source of multiple autologous growth factors for bone grafts.
In: Lynch SE, Genco RJ, Marx RE (eds). Tissue Engineering: Applications in Maxillofacial Surgery and Periodontics. Chicago: Quintessence Publishing 1999: 71-82.

32 Marx R.E.
Platelet-Rich Plasma: evidence to support its use.
J. Oral Maxillofac. Surg. 2004; 62: 489-96.

33 Misch C.E., Dietsch F.
Bone grafting materials in implant dentistry.
Implant Dent. 1993; 2: 158-62.

34 Mazor Z., Peleg M., Garg A.K., Luboshitz J.
Platelet-Rich Plasma for bone graft enhancement in sinus graft augmentation with simultaneous implant placement; patient series study.
Implant Dent. 2004; 13: 65-72.

35 Monov G., Fuerst G., Tepper G., Watzak G., Zechner W., Watzek G.
The effect of platelet-rich plasma upon implant stability measured by resonance frequency analysis in the lower anterior mandibles.
Clin. Oral Implants Res. 2005; 16: 461-5.

36 Ohya M., Yamada Y., Ozawa R., Ito K., Takahashi M., Ueda M.
Sinus floor elevation applied tissue-engineered bone. Comparative study between mesenchymal stem cells/platelet-rich plasma (PRP) and autogenous bone with PRP complexes in rabbits.
Clin. Oral Implants Res. 2005; 16: 622-9.

37 Philippart P., Brasseur M., Hoyaux D., Pochet R.
Human recombinant Tissue Factor, Platelet-rich Plasma, and tetracycline induce a high-quality human bone graft: a 5-year survey.
Int. J. Oral Maxillofac. Implants 2003; 18: 411-6.

38 Philippart P., Daubie V., Pochet R.
Sinus grafting using recombinant human tissue factor, platelet-rich plasma gel, autologous bone, and anorganic bovine bone mineral xenograft: histologic analysis and case reports.
Int. J. Oral Maxillofac. Implants 2005; 20: 274-81.

39 Raghoebar G.M., Schortinghuis J., Liem R.S., Ruben J.L., van der Wal J.E., Vissink A.
Does platelet-rich plasma promote remodeling of autologous bone grafts used for augmentation of the maxillary sinus floor?
Clin. Oral Implants Res. 2005; 16: 349-56.

40 Rodriguez A., Anastassov G.E., Lee H., Buchbinder D., Wettan H.
Maxillary sinus augmentation with deproteinated bovine bone and platelet rich plasma with simultaneous insertion of endosseous implants.
J. Oral Maxillofac. Surg. 2003; 61: 157-63.

41 Roldan J.C., Jepsen S., Schmidt C., Knüppel H., Rueger D.C., Açil Y., Terheyden H.
Sinus floor augmentation with simultaneous placement of dental implants in the presence of platelet-rich plasma or recombinant human bone morphogenetic protein-7.
Clin. Oral Implants Res. 2004; 15: 716-23.

42 Rosenberg E.S., Torosian J.
Sinus grafting using platelet-rich plasma: Initial case presentation.
Pract. Periodontics Aesthet. Dent. 2000; 12: 843-50.

43 Ross R., Raines E.W., Bowen-Pope D.F.
The biology of platelet-derived growth factor.
Cell 1986; 46: 155-69.

44 Sanchez A.R., Sheridan P.J., Kupp L.I.
Is Platelet-rich plasma the perfect enhancement factor? A current review.
Int. J. Oral Maxillofac. Implants 2003; 18: 93-103.

45 Schliephake H.
Bone growth factors in maxillofacial skeletal reconstruction.
Int. J. Oral Maxillofac. Surg. 2002; 31: 469-84.

46 Steigmann M., Garg A.K.
A comparative study of bilateral sinus lifts performed with platelet-rich plasma alone versus alloplastic graft material reconstituted with blood.
Implant Dent. 2005; 14: 261-6.

47 Tarnow D.P., Wallace S.S., Froum S.J., Rohrer M.D., Cho S.-C.
Histologic and clinical comparison of bilateral sinus floor elevations with and without barrier membrane placement in 12 patients: Part 3 of an ongoing prospective study.
Int. J. Periodontics Restorative Dent. 2000; 20: 117-25.

48 Tawil G., Mawla M.
Sinus floor elevation using a bovine bone mineral (Bio-Oss) with or without the concomitant use of a bilayered collagen barrier (Bio-Gide): a clinical report of immediate and delayed implant placement.
Int. J. Oral Maxillofac. Implants 2001; 16: 713-21.

49 Trisi P., Rebaudi A., Calvari F., Lazzara R.J.
Sinus graft with biogran, autogenous bone, and PRP: a report of three cases with histology and micro-CT.
Int. J. Periodontics Restorative Dent. 2006; 26: 113-25.

50 Velich N., Nemeth Z., Toth C., Szabó G.
Long-term results with different bone substitutes used for sinus floor elevation.
J. Craniofac. Surg. 2004; 15: 38-41

51 Wenstermark B.
The molecular and cellular biology of plateled-derived growth factor.
Acta Endocrinol. (Copenh) 1990; 123: 131-42.

52 Wiltfang J., Kloss F.R., Kessler P. et al.
Effects of platelet-rich plasma on bone healing in combination with autogenous bone and bone substitutes in critical-size defects. An animal experiment.
Clin. Oral Implants Res. 2003a; 14: 187-93.

53 Wiltfang J., Schlegel K.A., Schultze-Mosgau S., Nkenke E., Zimmermann R., Kessler P.
Sinus floor augmentation with ß-tricalciumphosphate (ß-TCP): does platelet-rich plasma promote its osseous integration and degradation?
Clin. Oral Implants Res. 2003b; 14: 213-8.

54 Zechner W., Tangl S., Tepper G., Fürst G., Bernhart T., Haas R., Mailath G., Watzek G.
Influence of platelet-rich plasma on osseous healing of dental implants: a histologic and histomorphometric study in minipigs.
Int. J. Oral Maxillofac. Implants 2003; 18: 15-22.

54 Zuffetti F., Fontanella W., Francetti L., Testori T., Del Fabbro M.
L'utilizzo delle PRP con osso autologo nel rialzo sinusale. Valutazione istologica.
Ital. Oral Surg. 2005; 4: 9-16.

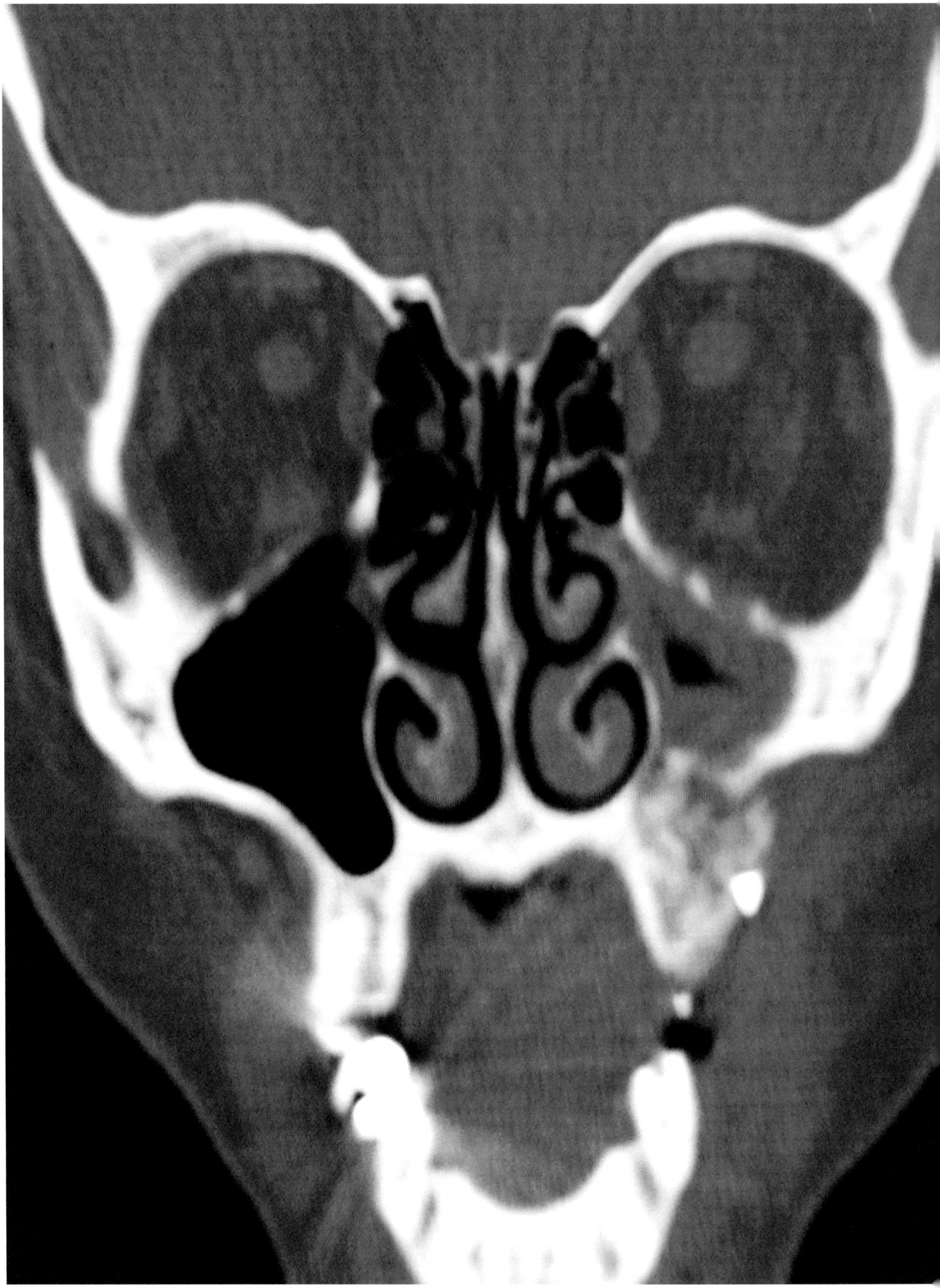

T. TESTORI
S.S. WALLACE
R. MONTEVERDI
A. BAJ
A.B. GIANNI

Complications: diagnosis and management

19

19

Although sinus elevation surgery is now a standardized and extremely predictable technique, each surgical step may give rise to complications. Incisions, elevation of the mucoperiosteal flap, antrostomy design, membrane elevation, placement of block or particulate grafts, and suturing may each give rise to complications if not performed correctly (Ulm et al. 1995; Moses & Arredondo 1997; Timmenga et al. 1997; Garg 1999; Aimetti et al. 2001).

These complications may occur intraoperatively, in the early postoperative period, or in the late postoperative period.

Early postoperative complications occur within the first 3 weeks after the surgery. Delayed complications first become evident after 3 weeks. Late complications may occur months or years after surgery and are due to improperly treated maxillary sinusitis. In this chapter, the authors describe the diagnosis and management of the main complications.

CONTRAINDICATIONS TO SINUS AUGMENTATION SURGERY

The presence of neoplastic pathologies, large maxillary cysts, and active sinusitis are contraindications for this type of surgery (Bergstrom et al. 1991; Smiler et al. 1992; Ziccardi & Betts 1999).

Further, it has been shown that patients with a history of sinus symptoms are more likely to have postoperative complications than patients with a negative history (Timmenga et al. 1997, 2001).

A complete description of all the contraindications has been addressed in Chapter 3.

IMMEDIATE INTRAOPERATIVE COMPLICATIONS

The reported frequency of complications resulting from sinus augmentation procedures is quite low. A prospective study of 100 consecutive sinus elevations (Zijderveld et al. 2008) reported an 11% incidence of membrane perforations and a 2% incidence of bleeding as intraoperative complications. It should be further noted that, had the authors of this paper utilized piezoelectric surgery for antrostomy and initial membrane elevation, the perforation rate would likely have been further reduced (Wallace et al. 2007, Blus et al. 2008).

The avoidance and handling of intraoperative complications have been discussed in previous chapters (e.g. Chapter 12). Therefore, they will only briefly be mentioned here for completion. They include:

- membrane perforation
- loss of graft material through the window
- hemorrhage from vessels supplying the sinus
- mechanical obstruction to the ostium
- neurological complications (infraorbital nerve injuries).

MEMBRANE PERFORATION

The surgical phases that most commonly result in membrane perforations are flap design, access antrostomy, sinus membrane elevation, and placement of the bone graft (Timmenga et al. 2001; Schwartz-Arad et al. 2004).

Perforations of the sinus membrane, while being an intraoperative complication, may also lead to the onset of early and late postoperative complications such as graft loss, infection, and the onset of chronic sinusitis.

Sinus membrane perforation can also be caused by excessive grafting, especially if associated with an insufficient elevation of the membrane. The placement of the graft, especially if the graft has sharp corners (single-block) or if it includes sharp bone chips (bone chips from the external calvaria or the mandibular ramus), may lead to an uncontrollable membrane perforation, dispersion of the graft into the sinus, and the possible development of sinusitis (Ulm et al. 1995; Aimetti et al. 2001). Grafting must be progressive, starting from the lateral recesses and then moving towards the center, always with controlled light to moderate pressure.

LOSS OF GRAFT MATERIAL THROUGH THE WINDOW

An increase in intra-sinus pressure as a result of postoperative inflammation or intra-sinus bleeding can result in the loss of graft material through the window. This may also occur if the patient vigorously sneezes or blows the nose. The placement of a membrane over the window will most likely prevent this occurrence. The displaced graft material is likely to cause a distention in the buccal mucosa. This can be removed with a small flap entry (not over window or membrane) or left in place and addressed at the time of implant placement. Some clinicians stabilize bioabsorbable barrier membranes with resorbable tacks or mattress sutures. The incidence of this complication is so low that most clinicians consider this to be unnecessary therapy FIG. 1.

HEMORRHAGE FROM VESSELS SUPPLYING THE SINUS

Bleeding is a consequence of injury to the internal or external branches of the posterior superior alveolar artery (PSAA)(Solar et al. 1999) FIG. 2-3.

Vascularization of the maxillary sinus occurs via three routes (Solar et al. 1999):
- Extraosseous anastomosis (EA): terminal branch of the PSAA branch of the maxillary artery (MA), with an extraosseous terminal branch of the intraorbital artery (IOA), another branch of the MA. It courses at a mean height of 23 to 26 mm from the alveolar margin. An extraosseous vestibular vascular anastomosis was observed in 44% of cases. The vessels may cause hemorrhage during flap preparation and releasing incisions.
- Intraosseous anastomosis (IA) or alveolo-antral artery: second branch of PSAA (dental branch) with the IOA. It courses at a distance of 18.9 to 19.6 mm from the alveolar margin.
- Branches of these vessels (PSAA, IOA and IA) in the sinus membrane.

The middle portion of the Schneiderian membrane is supplied by the sphenopalatine artery, the terminal branch of the MA.

MECHANICAL OBSTRUCTION TO THE OSTIUM

Mechanical obstruction of the ostiomeatal complex (OMC) may be the consequence of the migration of graft material into the maxillary sinus through a perforation, grafting the sinus to a level that physically blocks the ostium, or it may result from postoperative inflammation or infection.

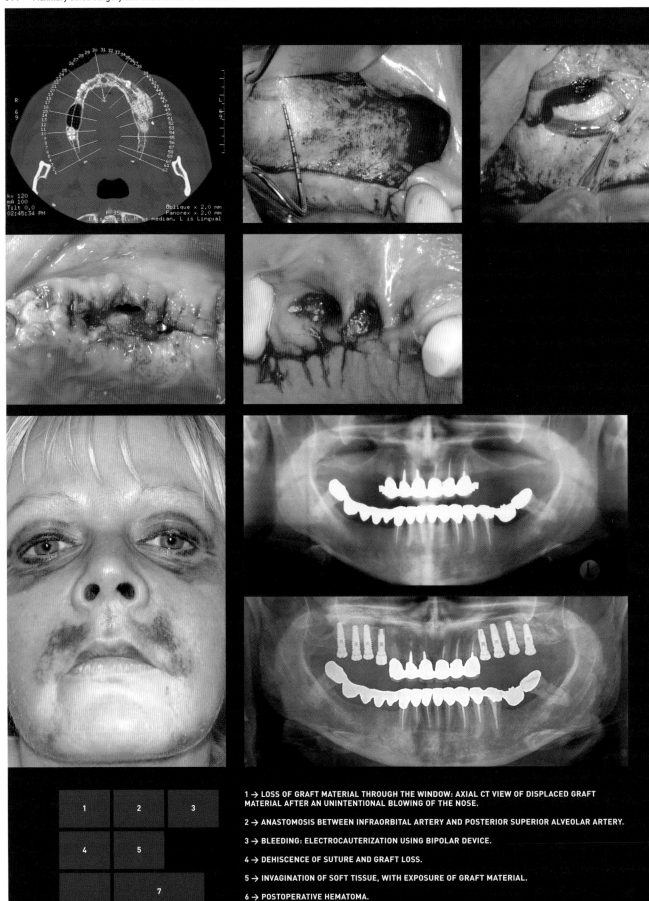

1 → LOSS OF GRAFT MATERIAL THROUGH THE WINDOW: AXIAL CT VIEW OF DISPLACED GRAFT MATERIAL AFTER AN UNINTENTIONAL BLOWING OF THE NOSE.

2 → ANASTOMOSIS BETWEEN INFRAORBITAL ARTERY AND POSTERIOR SUPERIOR ALVEOLAR ARTERY.

3 → BLEEDING: ELECTROCAUTERIZATION USING BIPOLAR DEVICE.

4 → DEHISCENCE OF SUTURE AND GRAFT LOSS.

5 → INVAGINATION OF SOFT TISSUE, WITH EXPOSURE OF GRAFT MATERIAL.

6 → POSTOPERATIVE HEMATOMA.

7 → PREOPERATIVE ORTHOPANTOGRAPH.

8 → POSTOPERATIVE ORTHOPANTOGRAPH OF SINUS AUGMENTATION AND PLACED IMPLANTS.

NEUROLOGICAL COMPLICATIONS (INFRAORBITAL NERVE INJURIES)

Blunt or pressure injury to the infraorbital nerve may result during flap retraction. If the flap extends superiorly to this position, the exit of the nerve from the bone should be visualized and retraction placed distal to it. It is also possible to injure this nerve during sharp dissection to release the flap for primary closure. The exit-point of the nerve from the skull is just below the infraorbital notch. Location of this anatomic structure is crucial prior to performing these procedures.

EARLY POSTOPERATIVE COMPLICATIONS

This group of complications occurs within 3 weeks from surgery and consists of:
- wound dehiscence and oral fistula formation
- acute graft infection
- severe postoperative hemorrhage/hematoma
- early exposure of bone graft in cases of adjunctive procedure for vertical or horizontal ridge augmentation.

WOUND DEHISCENCE AND ORAL FISTULA FORMATION

The etiology of these complications may include inadequate suturing and ulcerations caused by pressure from removable and the pontics of fixed prostheses **FIG. 4-5**. An ideal flap design that is trapezoidal in shape, full thickness preserving periosteum, with a distal and/or mesial releasing incision and a crestal horizontal incision will provide the most favorable vascular supply to the flap. In a pure sinus graft there should be no difficulty with tension-free primary closure as there has been no change in the shape of the posterior maxilla, and hence no need to increase flap mobility. This does become an issue when simultaneous ridge augmentation procedures are performed. If mucosal edges are sutured in tension, without releasing the vestibular flap using longitudinal, continuous periosteal incisions parallel to the free edge (which allow an overlap of at least 3 to 5 mm of the flap on the palatal mucosa), a passive closure will not be achieved.

In the event of non-vascularization of a simultaneous ridge augmentation graft (early dehiscence), the graft must be partially or totally removed, causing a loss of the desired crestal augmentation. An untreated or badly treated infection may result in an oroantral fistula, which will require a second surgical session for closure using transposition flaps (Moses & Arredondo 1997; Smiler 1997; Khoury 1999).

When infections are suspected, therapy should be rendered quickly, as a true sinus infection can become a pan-sinusitis if treatment is dselayed or handled improperly.

ACUTE GRAFT INFECTION

The most common causes of graft infections include contamination by pathogenic bacteria that can be present in the sinus or oral cavity or the presence of a chronic sinus infection that was not diagnosed prior to surgery.

Acute graft infections may be associated with acute sinusitis.

The main symptoms of infection are: pain, swelling, flap dehiscence, formation of fistula, and exudate that may leak from a fistula or suture line, the nose or the throat.

The preoperative diagnosis of potential sources of graft infection is invaluable as a preventive measure. Pre-existing periapical pathology, when the apices of infected teeth are in or close to the sinus, produces a reaction in the sinus that may be inflammation and/or bacterial contamination. When the membrane is elevated, these bacteria are immediately within a bone graft placed in a confined space – an ideal incubator. Localized endodontic and periodontal therapy should be completed prior to sinus grafting, and the hopeless teeth should be extracted.

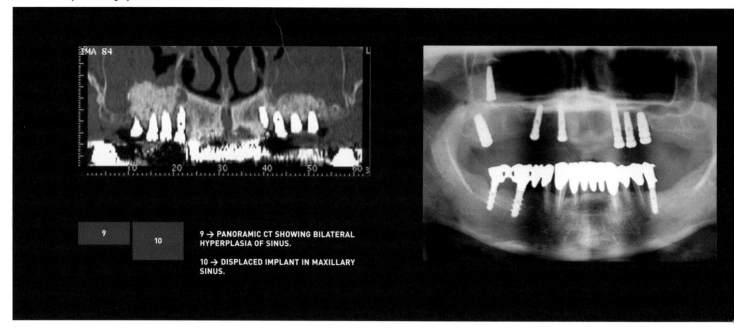

9 → PANORAMIC CT SHOWING BILATERAL HYPERPLASIA OF SINUS.

10 → DISPLACED IMPLANT IN MAXILLARY SINUS.

Simultaneous extraction of teeth that penetrate the sinus floor may open a pathway to infection, as the sinus graft is immediately connected to the oral cavity through the extraction socket, which may or may not be covered by flap release and primary closure. Sinus grafts with simultaneous ridge augmentation procedures are a further extension of the above extraction socket scenario. Barone et al. (2006) reported on 124 sinus elevations, 26 with simultaneous lateral ridge augmentations. The infection rate was 3% for the sinus graft only group (N=98) and 15.4% for the group that had simultaneous ridge augmentations (N=26). It is interesting to note that 5 of the 7 infections occurred in smokers. The cause of the infection in these cases and in other ridge augmentation studies has been attributed to the breakdown of primary soft tissue closure over the grafted site with exposure of the barrier membrane and subsequent graft infection. One should note that in a ridge augmentation procedure the incision line is directly over the barrier membrane, whereas in a properly designed sinus graft the membrane should be distant from the incision line. Soft tissue healing appears to be affected in a negative way by smoking, but smoking alone has not

been shown to be a negative factor in pure sinus grafting procedures. Onlay bone grafts had a higher complication rate in smokers than non-smokers but there was no such relationship present in pure sinus lift grafts (Levin et al. 2004).

Perforation of the Schneiderian membrane, contamination of the graft due to contact with saliva, flap dehiscence and lack of asepsis during bone graft placement are all potential risk factors for the development of a sinus infection. Hemosinus or the accumulation of antral secretion with secondary ostium obstruction causes a reduction in the partial oxygen pressure that favors the growth of anaerobic bacteria. Furthermore, the simple handling of the membrane causes an inflammatory reaction and a temporary ciliostasis (Peleg et al. 1999).

An acute sinusitis may also occur if the ostium is obstructed by postoperative edema. Pain and swelling in the maxillary region are usually resolved in about 10 to 15 days using antibiotics and endonasal decongestants. The use of vasoconstrictors and aerosol cortisone, and continuation of a suitable antibiotic therapy are recommended after surgery. If the problem is not resolved, it is advisable to send the patient to an ear, nose and throat (ENT) specialist, who will make a diagnosis by endoscopic examination and collect a sample for microbiological analysis.

Management of an acute purulent sinusitis secondary to graft material infection or hemosinus must be treated more aggressively. Symptoms include severe local pain and swelling, purulent exudate from the nose and, in severe cases, flap dehiscence and outpouring of sequestered material. In these cases hospitalization is necessary, with broad-spectrum intravenous antibiotic therapy and with likely endoscopic surgical drainage of the infection. If the problem is not resolved, a surgical reentry must be made with full, wide-ranging curettage of the maxillary sinus in order to avoid more severe complications such as venous septic thrombosis, which may involve the orbital area, with serious risk of loss of sight.

SEVERE POSTOPERATIVE HEMORRHAGE/HEMATOMA

Massive postoperative hemorrhage is extremely rare. Slight intaoperative bleeding from small endosseous vessels is more common and, if not controlled, may result in large-scale postoperative hematomas in the vestibular fornix that can predispose to graft infection.

Hematomas may occur due to the laceration of the vessels that supply the maxillary sinus **FIG. 6**.

Management of any hematomas that occur during the early postoperative phase must include an evaluation of stability (increase or decrease in size) and the use of preventive antibiotic therapy (e.g. amoxicillin with clavulanic acid, 3 g/day for 7 to 10 days). If results are unfavorable, the surgeon must consider reopening the area for surgical revision of the hematoma, ensuring the stability of the graft after removing coagulation.

EARLY EXPOSURE OF BONE GRAFT IN CASES OF ADJUNCTIVE PROCEDURE FOR VERTICAL OR HORIZONTAL RIDGE AUGMENTATION

Complications in bone graft surgery, such as inability to achieve sufficient soft tissue closure, flap necrosis, dehiscence and sometimes resorption, most often involve the soft tissue. These soft tissue complications are frequently the result of vascular compromise caused by inadequate planning, insufficient flap range or excessive surgical trauma, especially in smoking patients. Mechanical overloading of the grafted area with a removable prosthesis could also be the cause of complications, with exposure of the graft. Dehiscence may occur because of the premature separation of sutures as a result of an inadequate suture technique or tension on the flap margins. The treatment of early exposed grafted bone is very difficult and has a poor prognosis. To date, there is no predictable method to treat this type of complication. Resuturing the dehiscent area at an early stage can lead to an even larger exposed surface of grafted bone due to subsequent flap necrosis. Therefore, it is better to wait until the soft tissue matures. During this time the use of chlorhexidine solution or, even better, gel, several times a day, can be useful in reducing bacterial contamination. After a period of at least 4 weeks, the surgical closure can be performed after reducing the volume of the block graft. However, the chance of saving part or all of the grafted bone is very low.

DELAYED POSTOPERATIVE COMPLICATIONS

This group of complications occurs mainly after 3 weeks from surgery and consists of:
- chronic sinusitis with or without displacement of implants into the sinus
- delayed exposure of bone graft in cases of adjunctive procedure for vertical or horizontal ridge augmentation.

CHRONIC SINUSITIS WITH OR WITHOUT DISPLACEMENT OF IMPLANTS INTO THE SINUS

The etiology is the same as that of acute graft infection. It may remain completely asymptomatic for a long period of time **FIG. 7-9**. It is often the result of an acute infection that was not treated with a graft revision, but only with antibiotic therapy. This approach may result in a spread of the infection inside the maxillary sinus.

Some cases of delayed chronic sinusitis related to *Escherichia coli*, *Pseudomonas aeruginosa* and other anaerobic bacteria may be difficult to manage. A specific antibiotic therapy must be administered, depending on an endoscopic microbial culture, and continued for at least 3 weeks to achieve full recovery (Moses & Arredondo 1997).

In some cases a chronic sinusitis may be further complicated by the displacement of implants in the sinus. Implants can be displaced when they are placed in soft bone with 1 to 3 mm residual crestal bone with low primary stability. Excessive tissue compression on the implant head at the ridge level, caused by removable prostheses **FIG. 10** may also result in loss of primary stability.

Most clinicians reserve simultaneous implant placement for those cases that have a minimum of 4 to 5 mm of crestal bone. While simultaneous placement has been reported to be successful in 1 to 2 mm of crestal bone, one must consider the risk. If an implant is placed in 1 to 3 mm of crestal bone and primary closure is not achieved, the early formation of the biologic width will remove more than half of the supporting bone well before the maturation of the bone graft can provide support.

DELAYED EXPOSURE OF BONE GRAFT IN CASES OF ADJUNCTIVE PROCEDURE FOR VERTICAL OR HORIZONTAL RIDGE AUGMENTATION

The block graft may become exposed at a delayed date.

During the healing process, a decrease in graft volume is a normal sign of the remodeling process. As the soft tissue is attached to the underlying bone, it will also move in the direction of the resorption process. While the bone volume decreases, the fixation screws stay in their original position and may emerge through the overlying soft tissue. Usually these screws are well tolerated by the soft tissue and do not cause inflammation. In the later stages of healing or when additional screws can guarantee

proper fixation of the graft, the exposed screws can be removed. The soft tissue perforation will heal uneventfully after a couple of days.

If the dehiscence exposes vascularized crestal bone, in the presence of an appositional bone graft, second intention healing may take place, even if this increases the risk of infection. It is only possible to re-cover the part of the graft that has already been revascularized (delayed dehiscence). In other cases it may be necessary to decorticate the exposed bone until a vascularized surface is found, and to resuture the mucosal flaps prepared beforehand, by the removal of scar tissue along the edge.

If the site does not cover with soft tissue during the first two weeks after intervention, the complete graft has to be removed.

LATE COMPLICATIONS DUE TO IMPROPERLY TREATED MAXILLARY SINUSITIS

This group of complications occurs months, even years post-surgery and consists of:
* intracranial abscesses
* blindness
* aspergillosis.

Untreated chronic sinusitis may lead to even more severe complications. It is possible for a maxillary sinusitis to spread to the other paranasal sinuses (pansinusitis).

INTRACRANIAL ABSCESSES

Intracranial infections have been a major concern because of the proximity of the paranasal sinuses to the cranial cavity. Similarly, the orbital contents can become infected, because the eye shares a common wall with the ethmoid sinuses. The resulting infection can cause a loss of vision or intracranial sequelae such as severe neurologic deficiency or death. The incidence of these complications is extremely low, but when intracranial complications occur, the mortality rate may be as high as 20% (Maniglia et al. 1989).

BLINDNESS

An infrequent complication of improperly treated sinusitis is what is called by some clinicians orbital cellulitis. Preseptal cellulitis is an infection involving the soft tissues of the orbit that lie anterior to the orbital septum. Because preseptal infection is anterior to the tough tissue of the orbital septum, it does not involve the orbital contents themselves. Although these infections are 100 times more frequent than postseptal infections, they may present a diagnostic dilemma on the basis of physical examination alone.

Both preseptal cellulitis and orbital abscess/cellulitis, in their early stages, may look the same and in both conditions the eyelids may be swollen. In these cases it is strongly recommended to refer the patient immediately to an ENT specialist.

Another severe complication of untreated chronic sinusitis is represented by blindness cause by subperiosteal abscess (Patt & Manning 1991).

ASPERGILLOSIS

Aspergillosis infection is yet another late postoperative complication. It may be a more common occurrence when rough surface graft materials or implants protrude into the sinus. Cases reported to date in the literature have been related to endodontic filling material dispersed in the sinus cavity (de Foer et al. 1990). They also have been observed following sinus grafting and have been treated by a combination of antibiotic therapy and surgery by an ENT specialist. Symptoms are similar to chronic sinusitis. However, aspergillosis infections are difficult to resolve and they can become invasive, resembling a malignancy.

CONCLUSIONS

Although the complication rate following sinus elevation procedures is relatively low, it is prudent to take all possible precautions before, during, and after performing this surgically invasive procedure. Preoperative planning will inform the surgeon about conditions relative to sinus health and anatomy that may be crucial in complication avoidance. Utilizing the least complicated surgical technique that has been shown, through evidence, to give the best results will further increase the "protective umbrella" created by sound presurgical planning. When surgery has been completed it is imperative to provide the patient with proper antibiotic treatment and any additional surgical support that conditions require.

A summary of the complications is reported in **TAB.1**.

As postoperative infections may have a devastating effect on the outcome of this procedure, the following checklist is provided as a clinical guide.

Local etiology of sinus infection:
- pre-existing sinus infection (should not treat symptomatic patient)
- contamination of the surgical site
  - salivary/bacterial contamination of the graft material, instruments, or membrane
  - untreated periodontal disease
  - adjacent periapical pathology
  - lapses in the chain of sterility
  - extended surgical time
- infected simultaneous lateral ridge augmentation procedures

TAB. I

Immediate intraoperative, postoperative and late complications of maxillary sinus augmentation.

IMMEDIATE INTRAOPERATIVE COMPLICATIONS	membrane perforation
	loss of graft material through the window
	hemorrhage from vessels supplying the sinus
	mechanical obstruction of the ostium
	neurological complications (infraorbital nerve injuries)
EARLY POSTOPERATIVE COMPLICATIONS	wound dehiscence and oral fistula formation
	acute graft infection
	severe postoperative hematomas
	early exposure of bone graft in cases of adjunctive procedure for vertical or horizontal ridge augmentation
DELAYED POSTOPERATIVE COMPLICATIONS	chronic sinusitis with or without displacement of implants into the sinus
	delayed exposure of bone graft in cases of adjunctive procedure for vertical or horizontal ridge augmentation
LATE COMPLICATIONS DUE TO IMPROPERLY TREATED MAXILLARY SINUSITIS	intracranial abscesses
	blindness
	aspergillosis

The following recommendations are given as measures to reduce the incidence of post-operative infection:

- proper case selection
- proper prophylactic and therapeutic antibiotics
- chlorhexidine and/or betadine preparation of the mouth and face for surgery
- sterile draping with infection control protocol
- periodontal and endodontic problems should be addressed prior to surgery
- keep incision lines distant from window and barrier membrane
- prevent contamination of graft and barrier membrane with saliva
- sterility of all instruments being used
- keep surgical time as short as possible
- postoperative chlorhexidine rinses
- refer to an ENT specialist or maxillofacial surgeon in case of severe infections.

In a clinical case, a heavy smoker patient, who previously underwent a bilateral sinus lift and transverse increase of alveolar ridge using iliac bone grafts, came for implant placement 3 months after surgery.

After detaching the mucoperiosteal tissue, the sequestrum of the distal portion of the left transverse graft could be seen. The seqestrum was eliminated and the screw was removed. The residual bone allowed placement of the planned implants FIG. 11A-M.

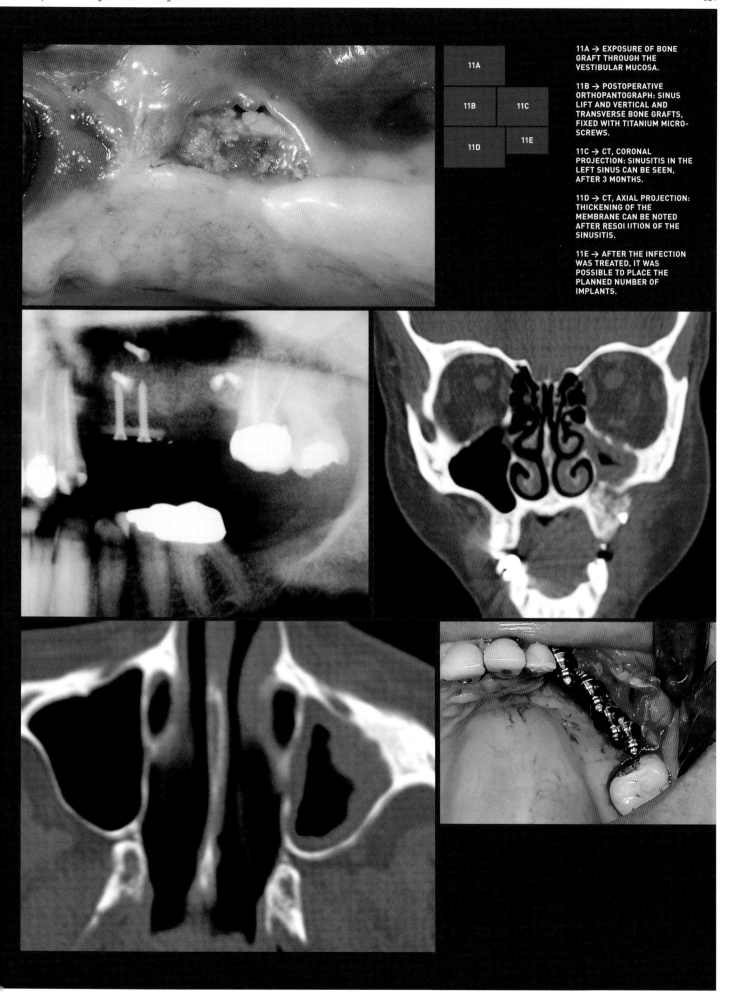

11A → EXPOSURE OF BONE GRAFT THROUGH THE VESTIBULAR MUCOSA.

11B → POSTOPERATIVE ORTHOPANTOGRAPH: SINUS LIFT AND VERTICAL AND TRANSVERSE BONE GRAFTS, FIXED WITH TITANIUM MICRO-SCREWS.

11C → CT, CORONAL PROJECTION: SINUSITIS IN THE LEFT SINUS CAN BE SEEN, AFTER 3 MONTHS.

11D → CT, AXIAL PROJECTION: THICKENING OF THE MEMBRANE CAN BE NOTED AFTER RESOLUTION OF THE SINUSITIS.

11E → AFTER THE INFECTION WAS TREATED, IT WAS POSSIBLE TO PLACE THE PLANNED NUMBER OF IMPLANTS.

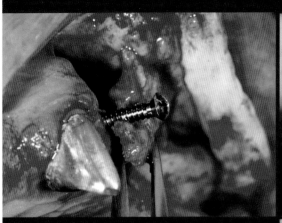

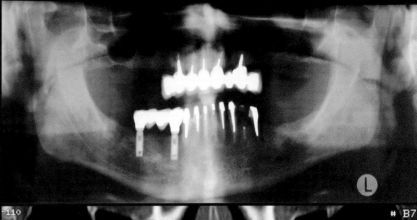

11F	11G
	11H
	11I
11L	11M

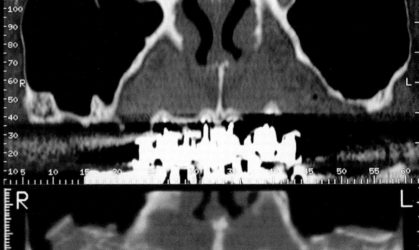

11F → REMOVAL OF BONE SEQUESTRUM.

11G → PRE-OPERATIVE ORTHOPANTOGRAPH: PRESENCE OF HYPER-PNEUMATISATION IN MAXILLARY SINUSES.

11H → PRE-OPERATIONAL CT: THE EXTENT OF MAXILLARY SINUSES CAN BE SEEN.

11I → POST-OPERATIVE CT: BILATERAL SINUS LIFT USING ILIAC BONE.

11L → PLACING OF IMPLANTS AND FILLING OF BONE DEFICIENCY WITH MIXED BOVINE BONE AND AUTOGENOUS TUBEROSITY BONE GRAFT.

11M → FINAL ORTHOPANTOGRAPH WITH PINS AND CROWNS.

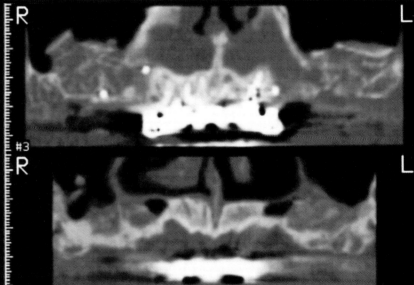

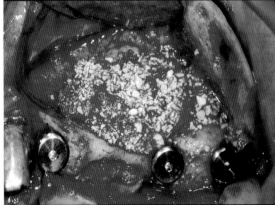

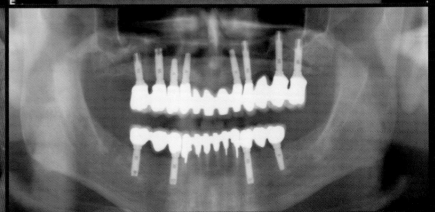

REFERENCES

1 Aimetti M., Romagnoli R., Ricci G., Massei G.
Maxillary sinus elevation: the effect of macrolacerations and microlacerations of the sinus membrane as determined by endoscopy.
Int. J. Periodontics Restorative Dent. 2001; 21: 581-9.

2 Barone A., Santini S., Sbordone L., Crespi R., Covani U.
A clinical study of the outcomes and complications associated with maxillary sinus augmentation.
Int. J. Oral Maxillofac. Implants 2006; 21: 81-5.

3 Bergstrom J., Eliasson S., Preber H.
Cigarette smoking and the periodontal bone loss.
J. Periodontol. 1991; 62. 242-6.

4 Blus C., Szmukler-Moncler S., Salama M., Salama H., Garber D.
Sinus bone grafting procedures using ultrasonic bone surgery: 5-year experience.
Int. J. Periodontics Restorative Dent. 2008; 28: 221-9.

5 De Foer C., Fossion E., Vaillant J.M.
Sinus aspergillosis.
J. Craniomaxillofac. Surg. 1990; 18: 33-40.

4 Garg A.K.
Augmentation grafting of the maxillary sinus for placement of dental implants: anatomy, physiology and procedures.
Implant Dent. 1999; 8: 36-46.

5 Khoury F.
Augmentation of the sinus floor with mandibular bone block and simultaneous implantation: a 6 years clinical investigation.
Int. J. Oral Maxillofac. Implants 1999; 14: 557-64.

6 Levin L., Herzberg R., Dolev E., Schwartz-Arad D.
Smoking and complications of onlay bone grafts and sinus lift operations.
Int. J. Oral Maxillofac. Implants 2004; 19: 369-73.

7 Maniglia A.J., Goodwin W.J., Arnold J.E., Ganz E.
Intracranial abscesses secondary to nasal, sinus and orbital infections in adults and children.
Arch. Otolaryngol. Head Neck Surg. 1989; 115: 1424-9.

8 Moses J.J., Arredondo A.
Sinus lift complications: avoiding problems and finding solutions.
Dent. Implantol. Update 1997; 8: 70-2.

9 Patt B.S., Manning S.C.
Blindness from orbital complications of sinusitis.
Otolaryngol. Head Neck Surg. 1991; 104: 789-95.

10 Peleg M., Chaushu G., Mazor Z., Ardekian L., Bakoon M.
Radiological findings of the post-sinus lift maxillary sinus: a computerized tomography follow-up.
J. Periodontol. 1999; 70: 1564-73.

11 Smiler D.G.
The sinus lift graft: basic technique and variations.
Pract. Periodont. Aesthet. Dent. 1997; 9: 885-93.

12 Smiler D.G, Johnson P.W, Lozada J.L.
Sinus lift grafts and endosseous implants: treatment of the posterior atrophic maxilla.
Dent. Clin. North Am. 1992; 36: 151-86.

13 Solar P., Geyerhofer U., Traxler H., Windisch A., Ulm G., Watzek G.
Blood supply to the maxillary sinus relevant to sinus floor elevation procedures.
Clin. Oral Implants Res. 1999; 10: 34-44.

14 Schwartz-Arad D., Herzberg R., Dolev E.
The prevalence of surgical complication of the sinus graft procedures and their impact on implant survival.
J. Periodontol. 2004; 75: 511-6.

15 Timmenga N.M., Raghoebar G.M., van Weissenbruch R., Vissink A.
Maxillary sinusitis after augmentation of the maxillary sinus floor: a report of 2 cases.
J. Oral Maxillofac. Surg. 2001; 59: 200-4.

16 Timmenga N.M., Raghoebar G.M., Boering G., van Weissenbruch R.
Maxillary sinus function after sinus lift for the insertion of dental implants.
J. Oral Maxillofac. Surg. 1997; 55: 936-9.

17 Ulm C.W., Solar P., Krennmair G., Matejka M., Watzek G.
Incidence and suggested surgical management of septa in sinus lift procedures.
Int. J. Oral Maxillofac. Implants 1995; 10: 462-5.

18 Wallace SS., Mazor Z., Froum S.J., Cho S.C., Tarnow D.P.
Schneiderian membrane perforation rate during sinus elevation using piezosurgery: clinical results of 100 consecutive cases.
Int. J. Periodontics Restorative Dent. 2007; 27: 413-9.

19 Ziccardi V.B., Betts N.J.
Complications of maxillary sinus augmentation. In: Jensen OT. The sinus bone graft.
Chicago: Quintessence Publishing 1999: 201-8.

20 Zijderveld S.A., van den Bergh, J.P.A., Schulten E.A.J.M., ten Bruggenkate C.M.
Anatomical and surgical findings and complications in 100 consecutive maxillary sinus floor elevations.
J. Oral Maxillofac. Surg. 2008; 66: 1426-38.

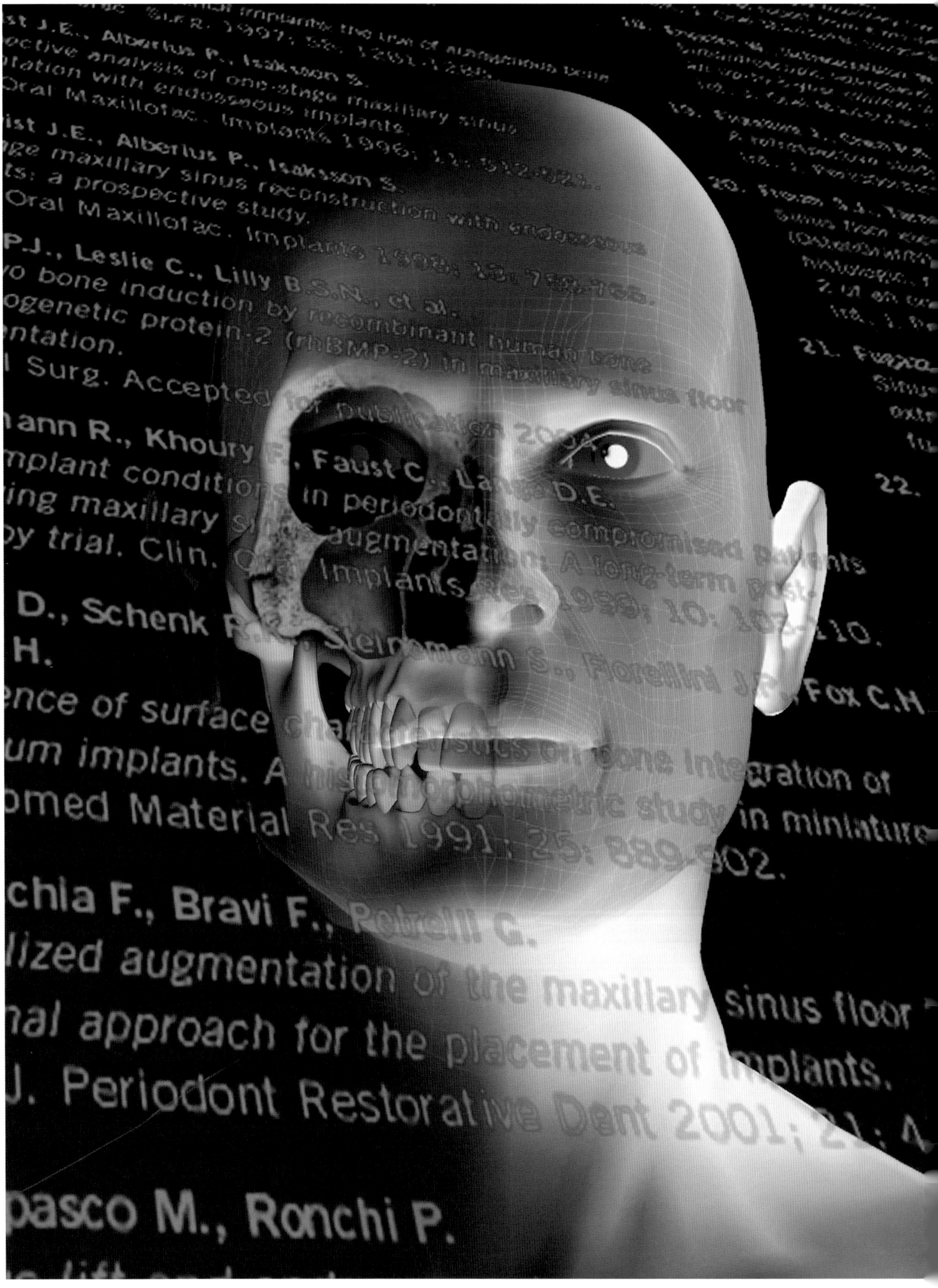

ist J.E., Alberius P., Isaksson S.
ige maxillary sinus reconstruction with endosseous
ts: a prospective study.
Oral Maxillofac. Implants 1998; 13: 758-766.
P.J., Leslie C., Lilly B.S.N., et al.
o bone induction by recombinant human bone
ogenetic protein-2 (rhBMP-2) in maxillary sinus floor
ntation.
l Surg. Accepted for publication 200
ann R., Khoury F., Faust C., Lange D.E.
nplant conditions in periodontally compromised patients
ing maxillary sinus augmentation. A long-term post
by trial. Clin. Oral Implants Res 1999; 10: 103-110.
D., Schenk R.K., Steinemann S., Fiorellini J.P., Fox C.H.
H.
ence of surface characteristics on bone integration of
um implants. A histomorphometric study in miniature
omed Material Res 1991; 25: 889-902.
chia F., Bravi F., Pobelli G.
lized augmentation of the maxillary sinus floor
nal approach for the placement of implants.
J. Periodont Restorative Dent 2001; 21:
pasco M., Ronchi P.

M. DEL FABBRO
L. FRANCETTI
S. TASCHIERI
T. TESTORI

Systematic review of the literature on maxillary sinus augmentation associated with implantation procedures

20

20

Maxillary sinus elevation for implantation purposes is a relatively recent technique that, as seen in previous chapters, has allowed implantation to be applied even to patients with extremely resorbed edentulous ridges in the posterior area of the maxilla.

As this surgical technique has only become widespread in the last 20 years, randomized controlled clinical trials (RCTs) that testify to its long-term efficacy are still rare in the medical literature. Most of the literature is instead composed of retrospective studies, case reports, and non-controlled studies. Although these types of publications have a lower scientific value than controlled prospective studies, they provide a substantial consistent quality of clinical cases, from which it is possible to obtain several useful indications on the prognosis of treatment.

In order to obtain quantitative indications on the long-term effectiveness and predictability of treatment, referring to a large number of cases treated and implants inserted, an analysis of the literature on sinus augmentation associated with implant treatment was performed.

The outcome of primary interest was the survival risk of implants placed in the bone graft, starting from the placement phase.

We also wished to evaluate whether some of the variables involved in this type of procedure may have influenced the result, in terms of implant survival rate.

The variables considered were:

- The type of material used for the graft (autogenous bone alone or combined with other substitute materials such as allogenic bone, heterologous bone, alloplastic bone, or bone substitutes used alone).

- The time when implants are placed (simultaneously to graft or later, after a maturation phase).

- The type of implant surface: smooth (machined, turned) or rough (textured) without taking into consideration the different degrees of roughness or the type of physical-chemical treatment used to obtain certain types of surface.
It has been proved that rough surfaces are more successful than smooth surfaces in risky situations such as low quality bone (Buser et al. 1991; Cochran et al. 1998; Lazzara et al. 1999; Khang et al. 2001; Kumar et al. 2002; Stach & Kohles 2003) or in smoker patients (Bain et al. 2002) or diabetics (Fiorellini et al. 2000).

- The type of surgical procedure: lateral maxillary sinus access to the sinus with creation of a bony window (Caldwell-Luc technique), or osteotomy with crestal access.

METHODS

Research was carried out using the main electronic databases (MEDLINE, EMBASE, The Cochrane Central Register of Controlled Trials), using the search engine Ovid. Scientific articles published in indexed medical journals in the period from 1986 to February 2007 were taken into consideration, without imposing restrictions on language.

As it was considered that there were too few RCTs on the subject, no restrictions were imposed on the type of experimental design, including cohort studies, retrospective studies and case series. The research on electronic databases was carried out using key words such as maxillary sinus lift, sinus augmentation, sinus floor elevation, sinus graft, bone graft, endosseous implants, and oral implants, combined with each other.

Another manual search was carried out on the sector's major journals (*International Journal of Oral & Maxillofacial Implants* (JOMI), *International Journal of Oral & Maxillofacial Surgery, Journal of Oral & Maxillofacial Surgery, International Journal of Periodontics & Restorative Dentistry, Journal of Periodontology, Clinical Oral Implants Research, Implant Dentistry, Clinical Implant Dentistry and Related Research, Journal of Oral Implantology*), and on the references of the works found, identifying potentially interesting publications.

A good reference point was also represented by previous reviews and meta-analyses, in particular those published by Tolman (1995), Tong et al. (1998), Wallace & Froum (2003) and Del Fabbro et al. (2004).

The material that was the subject of the Sinus Consensus Conference in 1996, published in 1998 in a supplement of JOMI, was also not considered. In fact, even though the analysis was of excellent quality, much of the reported data are presumably multiple publications of single clinical studies, and it is not

possible to make a distinction (Jensen et al. 1998).

The search supplied a total of 496 publications.

A screening of the articles was then carried out, bearing in mind the following inclusion criteria:

- at least 20 cases (maxillary sinuses) treated
- all patients had received endosseous "root form" implants
- less than 5% of the patients were lost at the follow-up in a period of at least 6 months
- the average duration of follow-up was at least 12 months, starting from implant placement, or an observation period of at least 24 months was reported in range
- the data on implant survival rates were explicitly reported, or could be obtained from the data presented
- no other atrophic crest augmentation procedures were carried out, such as vertical lifts or horizontal increases, simultaneous to sinus elevation
- the data reported were not duplicated by previous publications (in this case only the most recent data were taken into consideration, or data from a longer (average) observation period).

Quality assessment of each study and data extraction for the analysis was carried out by two independent observers, according to a predetermined standard sheet form in which all necessary information had to be collected, including a judgement on the overall quality of the publication.

All the studies that did not fit with one or more of the above inclusion criteria were excluded from this analysis. We also decided to exclude all non-clinical work (reviews, technical reports, animal studies).

To evaluate the influence of various factors of interest, we carried out separate analyses, subdividing the data extracted according to three main parameters. We then further divided the above groups on the basis of the average duration of follow-up (where indicated or deductible from reported data) into two subgroups: studies with an average observation period of less than or equal to 3 years and studies with an average follow-up of more than 3 years.

Before continuing, it is necessary to say that for each group and subgroup the weighted mean survival rates were calculated; calculating the arithmetic mean would not have been correct as the various studies did not all have the same statistical weight: the number of implants examined in the follow-up of each study is in fact extremely variable **TAB. 1**. It is therefore obvious that in the calculation of the average survival rate, it is not correct to assign the same weight to a study with 10 placed implants, one of which failed, as to a study with 350 placed implants and 35 failures, even if the survival rate (90%) is the same.

RESULTS

By analyzing the number of articles published in indexed journals over the years we found a progress growth **FIG. 1**, which was especially noticeable from 1996, the year in which the abovementioned Sinus Consensus Conference was held.

A total of 60 scientific publications were found to possess all the requirements for being included in the analysis, while 436 were excluded **FIG. 2**.

Overall, these 60 studies represent a period of more than 14 years, from 1993 to February 2007, and report data referring to 4184 patients, in which more than 13,600 implants were placed in bone grafts in the maxillary sinus **TAB. 1**.

The average survival rate, considering the overall number of implants placed and failures occurring, without subdivision into subgroups, was found to be 93.8%.

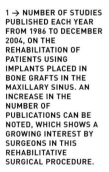

1 → NUMBER OF STUDIES PUBLISHED EACH YEAR FROM 1986 TO DECEMBER 2004, ON THE REHABILITATION OF PATIENTS USING IMPLANTS PLACED IN BONE GRAFTS IN THE MAXILLARY SINUS. AN INCREASE IN THE NUMBER OF PUBLICATIONS CAN BE NOTED, WHICH SHOWS A GROWING INTEREST BY SURGEONS IN THIS REHABILITATIVE SURGICAL PROCEDURE.

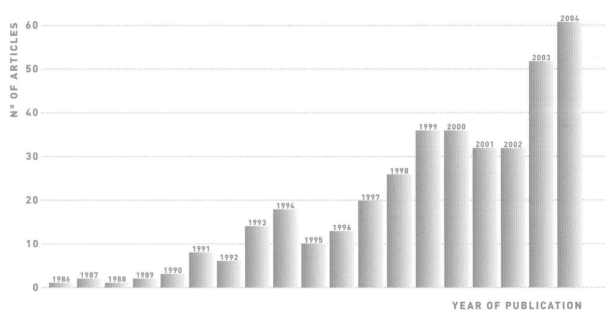

YEAR OF PUBLICATION

Studies within the inclusion criteria of this analysis, in chronological order

TAB. 1

Type of study	Reference	Year	Material from graft	No. patients	No. sinuses	No. implants in graft	Implants failed	Rate survived %	1- / 2- stage	Follow-up range (average), months
ct	Lozada et al.	1993	Compound graft	60	69	158	13	92	1/2	up to 60
cs	Keller et al.	1994	A	20	23	66	5	92.4	1	12-72
retro	Blomqvist et al.	1996	A	49	93	171	30	82.5	1	14-58 (30)
retro	Hurzeler et al.	1996	B/C/B+C/A+B	133	168	340	4	98.8	1/2	12-60 (34.3)
retro	Triplett & Schow	1996	A	50	70	145	19	86.9	1/2	>12
retro	Wheeler et al.	1996	A+B/B	24	34	64	3	95.3	1/2	12-60
cs	Zinner & Small	1996	A+B/E	50	66	215	3	98	1	7->60
retro	Block & Kent	1997	A	33	53	173	20	88.4	1	36-132 (70)
retro	Daelemans et al.	1997	A	33	44	121	8	93.4	1	up to 80 (40.2)
retro	Block et al.	1998	A	16	27	73	3	95.9	1	63-126 (75)
ct	Blomqvist et al.	1998	A	50	100-	202	32	84.2	2	9-48 (34.1)
ct	Froum et al.	1998	F/F+A/F+D/F+A+D	78	113	215	4	98.2	1/2	0-48
retro	Fugazzotto & Vlassis	1998	C/D/E/G	153	194	433	15	96.5	1/2	6-73 (32)
retro	Kaptein et al.	1998	A/B	88	132	388	46	88.1	1/2	up to 70 (55)
cs	Peleg et al.	1998	A/D	20	20	55	0	100	1	15-39 (26.4)
cs	van den Bergh et al.	1998	A	42	62	161	0	100	2	12-72 (38.2)
retro	Watzek et al.	1998	A/A+B	20	40	145	6	95.4	2	12-72 (38.8)
ct	Buchmann et al.	1999	A	50	75	167	0	100	1	>36->60
ct	De Leonardis & Pecora	1999	H	57	65	130	2	98.5	1/2	12
retro	Johansson et al.	1999	A	39	39+	131	31	75.3	1	36
retro	Keller et al.	1999	A	37	58	139	20	85.6	1/2	up to 144 (57.1)
retro	Khoury	1999	A	216	216	467	28	94	1	24-72 (49)
retro	Lekholm et al.	1999	A	55	82	280	53	81	1/2	36
retro	Peleg et al.	1999	A/D	63	63	160	0	100	1	23-48 (31)
retro	Lorenzoni et al.	2000	C	32	42	98	7	92.7	1/2	up to 60 (40.4)
RCT	Olson et al.	2000	A/B/D/B+D/A+D	29	45	120	3	97.5	1/2	up to 71 (38.2)
RCT	Tarnow et al.	2000	Various types	12	24	55	2	96.4	2	0-60
cs	van den Bergh et al.	2000	E	24	30	69	0	100	2	12-72 (34.6)
RCT	Wannfors et al.	2000	A	40	80	150	24	84	1/2	12
cs	Bahat & Fontanessi	2001	A+B/A+C	62	83	313	23	93	1/2	12-96 (37.3)
retro	Geurs et al.	2001	Various types	100	145	329	20	93.9	1/2	(38)
cs	Kahnberg et al.	2001	A	26	39	91	35	61.2	1	12->60 (39.8)
retro	Raghobaer et al.	2001	A	99	182	392	32	91.8	1/2	12-124 (59.6)
ct	Tawil & Mawla	2001	C	29	30	61	9	85.2	1/2	12-40 (22.4)
retro	Becktor et al.	2002	A	81	120	329	67	79.6	1/2	22-105 (64.2)
cs	Hallman et al.	2002	A/A+C/C	21	36	111	10	91	2	12
cs	Engelke et al.	2003	A+G	83	118	211	11	94.8	1/2	0-60 (>12)
cs	McCarthy et al.	2003	A	18	27	79	16	80.2	1/2	17-66(37.5)
cs	Philippart et al.	2003	A	18	25	58	5	91.3	2	12->48(31.5)
cs	Rodriguez et al.	2003	C+I	15	24	70	5	92.8	1	6-36 (>12)
cs	Stricker et al.	2003	A	41	66	183	1	99.5	1/2	15-40 (27.4)
retro	Valentini & Abensur	2003	C+D/C	59	78	187	10	94.5	1/2	78
RCT	Boyne et al.	2005	A/A+D/J	44+	88	219	37	83.1		>12
retro	Hallman et al.	2004a	B+K	50	71	218	12	94.5	2	6-42 (20)
ct	John & Wenz	2004	A/A+C/C	38	38+	103	4	96.1	1/2	18
cs	Itiurriaga & Ruiz	2004	A	58	79	223	0	100	2	>17
cs	Hallman et al.	2004b	A/C	20	30	108	15	86	2	60
cs	Hatano et al.	2004	A+C	191	191+	361	21	94.2	1	6-108 (27.3)
cs	Schwarz-Arad et al.	2004	A/A+C/A+D/C	70	81	212	9	95.8	1/2	24-84.8(43.6)
ct	Shlomi et al.	2004	A/A+C	63	73	253	23	90.9	1/2	24
ct	Zijderveld et al	2005	A/G	10	16	41	0	100	2	5-18(12)
cs	Simunek et al.	2005	L	24	24	45	1	97.8	1/2	12-23(16.4)
cs	Ewers	2005	M	118	209	614	27	95.6	2	fino a 156
cs	Butz & Huys	2005	A+N	20	22	56	0	100	1/2	12-84
cs	Wallace et al.	2005	A+C/C	51	64	135	3	97.8	1/2	>12
cs	Scarano et al.	2006	Various types	94	144	362	6	98.3	1	24-84(48)
ct	Testori et al.	unpub	A/A+C/A+L	22	26	63	2	96.8	1/2	24-65(44)
ct	Peleg et al.	2006	A/A+C/A+D	731	731	2132	44	97.9	1	108
ct	Karabuda et al.	2006	C/P	91		259	11	95.7	1/2	8-72(36)
cs	Mardinger et al.	2007	C	109	129	294	0	100	1/2	20
				4184	**5285+**	**13639**	**843**	**93.82**		

*A=autogenous bone, B=HA (hydroxyapatite), C=Bio-Oss®, D=DFDBA (demineralized freeze-dried bone allograft), E=FDBA (freeze-dried bone allograft), F=OsteoGraf/N, G=TCP (tricalcium phosphate), H=calcium sulfate, I=PRP (platelet-rich plasma), J=BMP-2 (bone morphogenetic protein-2), K=fibrin glue, L=BioGran®, 1=1-stage procedure, 2=2-stage procedure, RCT=randomized controlled trial, ct=controlled trial, cs=case series, retro=retrospective study.

The follow-up in these studies is extremely variable, from a minimum of 6 months to more than 10 years after implant placement; the heterogeneity of the way in which data on observation times are presented in the various studies did not always permit an estimation of the average follow-up period.

Of the 60 articles, only four were RCTs, 12 were controlled studies, 23 were case series and 21 were retrospective studies. We found, however, that by analyzing the four categories separately, studies with different levels of evidence have an overall implant survival rate. This result was also reported in another similar recent review, carried out by Wallace and Froum (2003), and in another systematic review on implant-supported fixed partial prostheses (Pjetursson et al. 2004). It would therefore seem that, according to the data available, the implant survival rate in the sinus lift is independent of the type of experimental design.

INFLUENCE OF GRAFT MATERIAL

Starting from the time when the maxillary sinus lift procedure was described and applied for the first time, the technique has evolved and progress has been made in the field of the biomaterials used for grafts.

Although autogenous bone is still considered the gold standard of graft materials the use of other biocompatible substances (that substitute autogenous bone) has become increasingly popular. The use of bone substitute limits surgical morbidity and avoids resorting to a second surgical site for bone harvesting. These graft materials can constitute of bone from a human donor (allogenic) or an animal donor (heterologous), or of biocompatible synthetic material (alloplastic). Most of these materials have morpho-structural connectivity properties similar to those of the bone matrix. They can be used alone or in combination with autogenous bone, in various proportions, to obtain the necessary graft volume.

2 → DIAGRAM SHOWING THE VARIOUS STAGES OF THE SYSTEMATIC REVIEW.

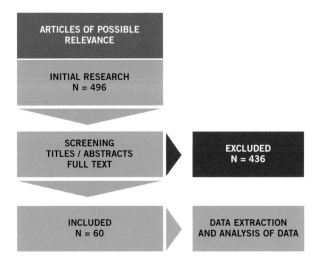

The data gathered in this analysis are divided into three groups: the first group includes autogenous bone grafts alone (blocks or particulated chips), the second group includes combined grafts (autogenous bone + bone substitute) and the third group includes all the studies that used bone substiute alone. In the combined grafts group, the following types of materials were used in association with autogenous bone: Bio-Oss® (in nine studies), DFDBA (seven studies), hydroxyapatite (HA, four studies), OsteoGraf/N (three studies), Int-200 (two studies), ß-TCP (one study), OsteoGraf/N + DFDBA (one study) and OsteoGraf/N + FDBA (one study).

MATERIAL FROM GRAFT	TIME OF OBSERVATION OF IMPLANTS	NUMBER OF PATIENTS	NUMBER OF IMPLANTS INSERTED	% SURVIVAL
AUTOGENOUS BONE	overall	1131	4027	88.95%
	≤ 36 months	337	1231	90.09%
	> 36 months	794	2796	88.45%
MIXED GRAFT	overall	939	2841	94.72%
	≤ 36 months	696	1847	96.75%
	> 36 months	232	994	90.95%
BONE SUBSTITUTES	overall	828	2706	96.08%
	≤ 36 months	628	2096	96.33%
	> 36 months	200	610	95.25%

TAB. 2

SURVIVAL RATE OF IMPLANTS PLACED IN MAXILLARY SINUS BONE GRAFTS. COMPARISON BETWEEN GRAFT MATERIALS USED: AUTOGENOUS BONE ABOVE; BONE SUSTITUTES IN COMBINATION WITH AB; (HETEROLOGOUS BONE, ALLOGENIC BONE, ALLOPLASTIC MATERIALS) TOGETHER WITH AUTOGENOUS BONE, OR ALONE.

TIMESCALE OF PLACEMENT OF IMPLANTS	TIME OF OBSERVATION OF IMPLANTS	NUMBER OF PATIENTS	NUMBER OF IMPLANTS INSERTED	% SURVIVAL OF IMPLANTS
SIMULTANEOUS	overall	2223	6480	94.85%
	≤ 36 months	771	2074	94.26%
	> 36 months	1452	4406	95.12%
DELAYED	overall	1136	4420	93.81%
	≤ 36 months	696	2252	94.59%
	> 36 months	430	1827	92.72%

TAB. 3

SURVIVAL RATE OF IMPLANTS PLACED IN MAXILLARY SINUS BONE GRAFTS. COMPARISON BETWEEN THE TWO TECHNIQUES FOR PLACING IMPLANTS: SIMULTANEOUS OR DELAYED TO BONE GRAFT SURGICAL SESSION.

SURFACE OF IMPLANTS	TIME OF OBSERVATION OF IMPLANTS	NUMBER OF PATIENTS	NUMBER OF IMPLANTS INSERTED	% SURVIVAL
SMOOTH	overall	950	3346	86.34%
	≤ 36 months	452	1273	88.22%
	> 36 months	498	2073	85.19%
ROUGH	overall	2554	8344	96.70%
	≤ 36 months	1087	3280	97.31%
	> 36 months	1349	4450	96.40%

TAB. 4

SURVIVAL RATE OF IMPLANTS PLACED IN MAXILLARY SINUS BONE GRAFTS. COMPARISON BETWEEN IMPLANT SURFACES: SMOOTH AND ROUGH.

In the group that used only bone substitutes, 14 different types of graft were used: Bio-Oss® (eight studies), DFDBA (five), HA (three), OsteoGraf/N + DFDBA (two), FDBA (one), OsteoGraf/N (one), ß-TCP (one), calcium sulfate (one), HA + DFDBA (one), DFDBA + Bio-Oss® (one), HA + Bio-Oss® (one), DFDBA + Int-200 (one), PRP+Bio-Oss® (one), bovine HA + fibrin glue, Cerasorb, phycogenic material + fluoro-hydroxyapatite, marine algae. In a randomized comparative study, bone morphogenetic protein-2 (BMP-2) carried in a resorbable collagen sponge (Boyne 2005) was used.

The substitute material most commonly used by far, and with proven efficacy in maxillary sinus augmentation, as well as in many other bone regenerative procedures, is therefore Bio-Oss® (deproteinized bovine bone) which is discussed more in detail in a previous chapter.

From the results obtained by dividing the graft materials into three groups TAB. 2, FIG. 3 it can be seen that using autogenous bone alone guarantees an average implant survival rate of 88.9% (range 61.5 to 100%) out of 4027 implants observed. If we consider the last division into subgroups, depending on the follow-up duration, the results obtained are almost comparable. If instead we consider autogenous bone in blocks or chips separately, the former has a survival rate of 82.6% (391 patients, 1487 implants) while the second has a survival rate of 93.7% (211 patients, 867 implants). When grafts composed of autogenous bone mixed with chips are used, the implant survival rate is 91% (465 patients, 1448 implants). The form of autogenous bone used therefore seems to be critical for implant survival. While during the early approaches to sinus lift aug-

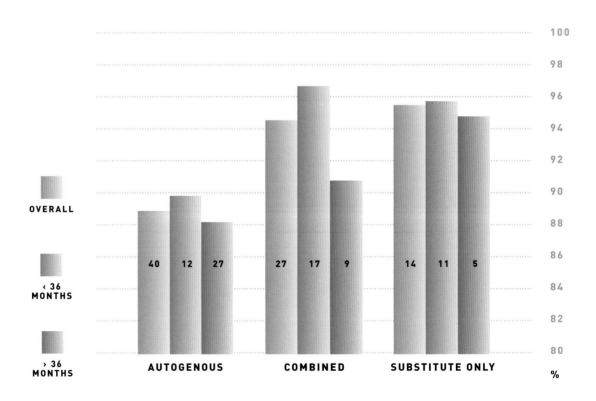

3 → SURVIVAL RATE OF IMPLANTS PLACED IN MAXILLARY SINUS BONE GRAFTS. COMPARISON BETWEEN GRAFT MATERIALS USED: ONLY AUTOGENOUS BONE AND OTHER MATERIALS (HETEROLOGOUS BONE, ALLOGENIC BONE, ALLOPLASTIC MATERIALS) TOGETHER WITH AUTOGENOUS BONE, OR ALONE. THE NUMBER OF RELATIVE ARTICLES IS SHOWN ON THE BARS.

OVERALL

‹ 36 MONTHS

› 36 MONTHS

AUTOGENOUS   COMBINED   SUBSTITUTE ONLY

40   12   27   27   17   9   14   11   5

%

mentation, autogenous bone blocks were mostly used, bone chips are now increasingly used and the block form is reserved for severe cases with extremely resorbed edentulous ridges or in the case of preoperation if the Schneiderian membrane has been perforated.

The studies in which autogenous bone was used together with other materials or where other materials were used alone, reported a better overall survival rate than autogenous bone, but in line with that of autogenous bone chips. It is necessary to point out that most of these studies have a short- to mid-term follow-up. There are still relatively few studies with follow-ups of more than 36 months compared with the autogenous bone subgroup.

At this point it is necessary to make some observations. The quality and quantity of residual bone are important factors in the choice of surgical procedure and graft material, and in the predictability of treatment. When the residual bone is quantitatively low, an autogenous bone graft is preferred, as this has been considered to be the gold standard, preferred material for many years, and provides greater chance of long-term success. It has also been suggested by some authors that the implant survival rate depends on the height of residual bone (Geurs et al. 2001): the thinner the bone the higher the implant failure rate.

Comparative randomized clinical studies between autogenous bone and other graft materials for the treatment of extremely atrophic edentulous maxillae are extremely scarce. Also, not all the studies report precise data about the bone vertical thickness. Therefore it is not possible to correlate residual bone height and the success/survival rate, for each graft material used.

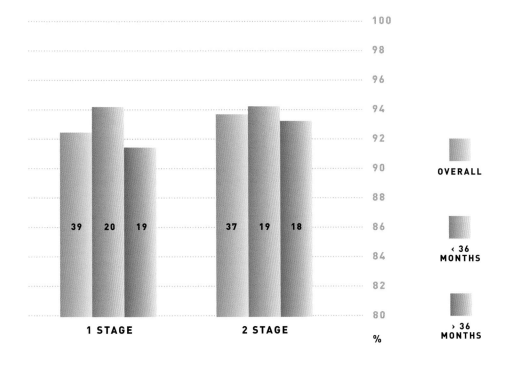

4 → SURVIVAL RATE OF IMPLANTS PLACED IN MAXILLARY SINUS BONE GRAFTS. COMPARISON BETWEEN THE TWO TECHNIQUES FOR PLACING IMPLANTS: SIMULTANEOUS (1 STAGE) OR DELAYED TO BONE GRAFT SURGICAL SESSION (2 STAGE). THE NUMBER OF RELATIVE ARTICLES IS SHOWN ON THE BARS.

INFLUENCE OF IMPLANT PLACEMENT TIME COMPARED TO GRAFT (SIMULTANEOUS VS. DELAYED PROTOCOL)

The results of the comparison between simultaneous vs delayed procedures have been summarized **TAB. 3, FIG. 4**.

In the first group, the average implant survival rate was found to be 94.85% (range 61.5 to 100%) in 2223 patients and 6480 implants observed. In the studies with follow-ups of less than 36 months, the survival rate is slightly higher than that of follow-ups with observation of more than 36 months. The difference is not, however, significant.

In the group with delayed implant placement, the average implant survival rate was found to be 93.87% (range 84.2 to 100%) in 1136 patients and 4420 implants observed. No differences were found depending on the duration of the follow-up.

There is therefore a substantial equivalence between the two procedures in terms of implant survival, which is excellent in both cases, whatever the duration of the observation period.

We must note that the choice of simultaneous or delayed implant placement (with the bone graft) is mainly dictated by the size (height) of the residual bone. If it is sufficient to ensure good primary implant stability, then the simultaneous technique can be carried out, reducing the number of surgical sessions required, and therefore patient discomfort.

INFLUENCE OF TYPE OF IMPLANT SURFACE

This analysis aims to compare predictability of treatment if smooth or rough surface implants are used. According to recent studies, it seems that the latter have provided better results than smooth surface implants, when

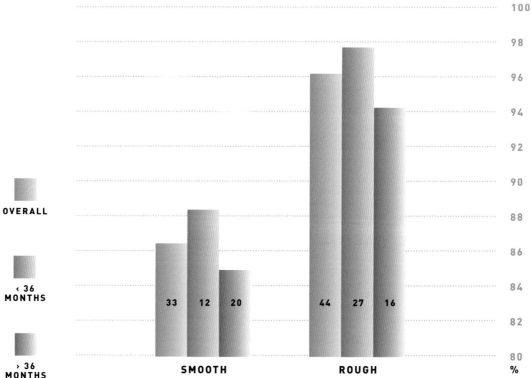

5 → SURVIVAL RATE OF IMPLANTS PLACED IN MAXILLARY SINUS BONE GRAFTS. COMPARISON BETWEEN IMPLANT SURFACES: SMOOTH AND ROUGH. THE NUMBER OF RELATIVE ARTICLES IS SHOWN ON THE BARS.

OVERALL

‹ 36 MONTHS

› 36 MONTHS

used in poor quality bone and/or in patients with risky conditions for implant therapy, such as smokers (Bain et al. 2002). In this analysis **TAB. 4, FIG. 5**, we found that smooth surfaces have a survival rate of 86.3% (in 950 patients and 3346 implants), much lower than rough surfaces (95.9% in 1306 patients and 4406 implants). The superiority of rough surfaces compared to smooth surfaces can be found in both the short and long term. Whereas in excellent quality bone the success of implant treatment does not depend on the type of implant surface, in the posterior maxilla in elderly edentulous patients with atrophic ridges, the use of osteoinductive and/or osteoconductive surfaces can favor the success of treatment.

A combined analysis was carried out between autogenous bone grafts in blocks or chips and smooth or rough implant surfaces. It was discovered that the worst implant survival rate occurs combining smooth surfaces with block grafts (82.6% in 391 patients and 1487 implants), while the best performance is offered by the combination of chip grafts and rough surface (95.3% in 141 patients and 624 implants). Of implants placed in autogenous bone, 72.8% had smooth surfaces, accounting for 86% of the total number of implant failures observed in the autogenous bone subgroup.

INFLUENCE OF SURGICAL TECHNIQUE

Maxillary sinus surgical techniques other than the Caldwell-Luc technique are effectively described by Cordioli and Mazjoub in a Chapter 15, and in recent systematic reviews (Wallace & Froum 2003; Emmerich et al. 2005). In this review, we found that although the results of these recent techniques are rather promising, (implant success range between 88.6 and 100%), there are still very few clinical studies available for a reliable analysis with an adequate statistical strength, concerning mid- to long-term efficacy. The studies that adopted the Summers osteotomy technique or similar techniques have therefore been excluded from this analysis.

DISCUSSION

Systematic reviews of literature and meta-analyses are used more and more frequently in the medical-scientific field. Meta-analysis is a statistical technique that combines and summarizes the results of similar multiple studies published on a given subject as part of a systematic review, and describes the real clinical effects of specific treatments, pharmacological therapies, and surgical techniques in a much more accurate manner than single clinical studies can do. It is therefore a powerful decision-making tool for validating or not validating procedures, treatment, materials, drugs etc.

As the number of patients involved in a clinical trial is mostly rather low, single studies often do not achieve a sufficiently high statistical power to validate statistical relations between causes and effects reported in the studies. By combining the results of multiple studies, the statistical power can be increased significantly, thus allowing slight but clinically significant differences to be found that cannot be evidenced in each individual study. It must, however, be said that meta-analysis can only be applied if the various studies to be grouped together are adequately homogenous with each other. Otherwise it is not possible to statistically validate the results of a systematic review.

The strategies used for systematic reviews of literature intend to limit systematic errors (bias) as far as possible during the identification stages of potentially interesting scientific studies, during their collection, critical evaluation, and summarizing of data coming from all the relevant publications on the subject being examined. If adequate homogeneity is found, the statistical methods for combining and summarizing the results of various studies together are then applied. This is particularly useful for sorting through an enormous amount of information on the given subject, which can often cause confusion and be misleading. Through this strict identification process of all the existing relevant data on a subject, the systematic review can be useful in quantifying the current level of knowledge, identifying those fields in which the necessary answers to possible questions have been provided and those which need to be studied further. It can therefore also prove useful for planning future research.

Many systematic reviews base their conclusions on RCT analyses only. Due to the rigorous methods with which they are carried out, these studies represent the highest level of evidence. They are by nature comparative and are generally based on the comparison between a test group and a control group. RCTs are particularly useful, for example, for evaluating the efficacy of a new therapy compared to conventional therapy, under strictly controlled experimental conditions.

These studies, however, are rather difficult to perform as they require the scrupulous observation of a usually complex, detailed protocol, they often last for a long period of time, use up a considerable amount of human and financial resources and for these reasons are generally carried out by universities or specialized research centers.

For the average professional, it may be just as important to know the long-term success rate of a given therapy, when it is used in daily clinical practice. This is what may be defined as the effectiveness of a therapy.

To obtain information on the effectiveness of a therapy and the influence of some variables on it, it may be just as useful to carry out a systematic review of literature, referring to several studies published in peer-reviewed journals that report the experiences of patients treated by the same clinical protocol, even if the experimental design is different from an RCT.

Well performed non-comparative studies may in fact provide useful indications in terms of treatment prognosis, especially if they have long follow-up periods, and must be taken into consideration. In this way, a larger patient database can be obtained and, if the information provided by each study is sufficiently complete, generalizable conclusions can be drawn.

However, very often in systematic reviews (also in those that consider RCTs only), the heterogeneity between the various articles (often due to various primary objectives of the different studies) is such that it does not permit a formal quantitative statistical analysis (or a meta-analysis). Therefore a qualitative analysis is carried out, reporting the data concerning each single article that was selected by means of precise inclusion criteria. The overall weighted averages for each variable examined can be calculated, but no attempt should be made to evaluate the statistical significance of any differences observed.

In this way, useful indications are provided for the surgeon who, depending on the summary data obtained, can himself judge the weight of certain variables on the performance of a treatment.

With regards to this analysis, the main limit is represented by the lack of homogeneity between the various studies. This lack of homogeneity, also found in other systematic reviews on maxillary sinus augmentation procedures (Graziani et al. 2004; Esposito et al. 2006) was found in the study goals, in the patients' initial condition, in the experimental design, in the criteria of success/survival used, in the way of reporting data, in results, in the duration of follow-up and in the materials.

It is rather difficult to compare studies that sometimes have completely different aims and characteristics, such as for example histologic studies to evaluate the maturation of a graft or comparative studies between different implant systems, different graft materials, or comparisons between smokers and non-smokers based on the survival rate. All the selected studies reported results concerning patients who underwent maxillary sinus augmentation using the Caldwell-Luc technique, and who received implants in the posterior maxilla, but the primary variable under examination in each study is often different in each one.

Usually, due to the main goal of each investigation, statistical details of implant survival rates are not present in the publications considered, or are reported simply and rather heterogenously in the various studies. Only six of the 60 publications included in the analysis have well-organized life table analyses, indicating the cumulative implant survival percentages. However, there are also differences in the method of these studies, in the initial goal and in the results, which mean that not even the life table analyses are perfectly comparable with each other. It is therefore not possible to draw up a global life table analysis that includes all the cases examined in the works considered, due to the abovementioned heterogeneity in the presentation of results. Weighted averages were therefore calculated in each subgroup, based on the number of implants and the average follow-up time reported in each work. The observation period extremes (minimum and maximum), for example a range of 12 to 120 months, is often only indicated, although it was almost always possible to obtain an average value of follow-up duration. The actual follow-up average may, however, be different from the simple arithmetic average between minimum and maximum: in one of the excluded works, for example, while the range was from 12 to 24 months, the average follow-up clock time was only 18 months, and this work would therefore come under the subgroup with a follow up of < 36 months, even though some of the cases reported had a long-term follow-up.

The patient's initial condition, in particular the amount of residual bone, is an important factor that may influence the success of treatment; it normally determines the choice of implant insertion timing planning. If thickness of residual bone is less than 5 mm, the delayed procedure is normally preferred, as a bone that is too thin does not guarantee suitable primary stability and it is better to wait for the consolidation and maturation of the graft before placing implants. The bone thickness may also influence the choice of graft material: autogenous bone, or a composite graft, a combination with autogenous bone, is often preferred (due to the wealth of osteogenetic elements) if a sinus floor elevation must be carried out with extremely thin residual bone available.

The use of resorbable or non-resorbable membranes may influence graft maturation, as suggested in a recent RCT in which 12 patients underwent bilateral grafts, and a membrane was used in only one of the two sinuses (Tarnow et al. 2000). Froum et al. (1998) and Tawil and Mawla (2001) found a better implant survival rate and better graft quality in patients in whom coverage membranes had been used compared to the control group. In contrast, other studies reported no particular advantages when the graft was covered by a membrane. There is not sufficient scientific evidence or enough data to draw statistically reliable conclusions on the importance or non-importance of the use of membranes. We therefore decided not to consider this variable in the present analysis.

Other factors that were not taken into consideration but which may influence the result of treatment (especially from the biomechanical point of view) are: the type of prosthetic reconstruction, the type of occlusal antagonist, and the characteristics of macro-geometry (shape, size) of implants. Further factors of possible importance are the duration of the graft maturation period, the presence of concurring grafts, and the patient's characteristics such as age, gender, smoking habits, presence of other possible systemic pathologies, and intake of drugs that interfere with bone metabolism.

This systematic review has provided the following conclusions:
- The maxillary sinus elevation procedure associated with implant treatment is nowadays a predictable technique.
- The lateral sinus approach is well documented; the other techniques using crestal approaches are promising but still need further clinical evidence.

- Autogenous bone is still the most commonly used, reliable material but some bone substitutes now available (both alone and combined with autogenous bone) can provide just as positive if not better results, at least in the short to mid term. In a recent Cochrane review, Esposito et al. (2006) reported that materials such as Bio-Oss® and Cerasorb® can effectively substitute autogenous bone in the sinus augmentation procedure. The choice of using autogenous bone rather than an alternative material may depend on the patient's clinical situation.
- Implants with a rough surface have a better success rate than those with a smooth surface.
- Simultaneous and delayed procedures give equivalent results.
- Many other variables can influence treatment predictability, but their contribution cannot currently be quantified.

Although the number of publications on the subject is constantly increasing, most of them report short- to mid-term experiences in which the results are rather promising and provide hope for a greater diffusion of the use of sinus augmentation in patients with atrophic maxillae who require implant treatment, while observing its indications and contraindications.

The performance of high-quality RCTs, with long-term follow-up and large sample size, carried out thoroughly, abiding by the set protocols and defined according to current guidelines, may certainly in the future provide more precise answers to the subjects addressed in this analysis.

REFERENCES

1 Bahat O., Fontanessi R.V.
Efficacy of implant placement after bone grafting for three-dimensional reconstruction of the posterior jaw.
Int. J. Periodont. Restorative Dent. 2001; 21: 221-31.

2 Bain C.A., Weng D., Meltzer A., Kohles S.S., Stach R.M.
A meta-analysis evaluating the risk for implant failure in patients who smoke.
Compend. Contin. Educ. Dent 2002; 23: 695-9.

3 Becktor J.P., Eckert S.E., Isaksson S., Keller E.
The influence of mandibular dentition on implant failures in bone-grafted edentulous maxillae.
Int. J. Oral Maxillofac. Implants 2002; 17: 69-77.

4 Block M.S., Kent J.N.
Sinus augmentation for dental implants: the use of autogenous bone.
J. Oral Maxillofac. Surg. 1997; 55: 1281-6.

5 Block M.S., Kent J.N., Kallukaran F.U., Thunthy K., Weinberg R.
Bone maintenance 5 to 10 years after sinus grafting.
J. Oral Maxillofac. Surg. 1998; 56: 706-14.

6 Blomqvist J.E., Alberius P., Isaksson S.
Retrospective analysis of one-stage maxillary sinus augmentation with endosseous implants.
Int. J. Oral Maxillofac. Implants 1996; 11: 512-21.

7 Blomqvist J.E., Alberius P., Isaksson S.
Two-stage maxillary sinus reconstruction with endosseous implants: a prospective study.
Int. J. Oral Maxillofac. Implants 1998; 13: 758-66.

8 Boyne P.J., Leslie C., Lilly B.S.N. et al.
De novo bone induction by recombinant human bone morphogenetic protein-2 (rhBMP-2) in maxillary sinus floor augmentation.
J. Oral Maxillofac. Surg. 2005; 63: 1693-1707.

9 Buchmann R., Khoury F., Faust C., Lange D.E.
Peri-implant conditions in periodontally compromised patients following maxillary sinus augmentation: A long-term post-therapy trial.
Clin. Oral Implants Res. 1999; 10: 103-10.

10 Buser D., Schenk R.K., Steinemann S., Fiorellini J.P., Fox C.H., Stich H.
Influence of surface characteristics on bone integration of titanium implants. A histomorphometric study in miniature pigs.
J. Biomed. Material Res. 1991; 25: 889-902.

11 Butz SJ, Huys LW.
Long-term success of sinus augmentation using a synthetic alloplast: a 20 patients, 7 years clinical report.
Implant Dent. 2005; 14: 36-42.

12 Cochran D.L., Schenk R.K., Lussi A., Higginbottom F.L., Buser D.
Bone response to unloaded and loaded titanium implants with sandblasted and acid etched surface: a histometric study in the canine mandible.
J. Biomed. Material Res. 1998; 40: 1-11.

13 Daelemans P., Hermans M., Godet F., Malevez C.
Autologous bone graft to augment the maxillary sinus in conjunction with immediate endosseous implants: a retrospective study up to 5 years.
Int. J. Periodontics Restorative Dent. 1997; 17: 27-39.

14 De Leonardis D., Pecora G.E.
Augmentation of the maxillary sinus with calcium sulfate: one-year clinical report from a prospective longitudinal study.
Int. J. Oral Maxillofac. Implants 1999; 14: 869-78.

15 Del Fabbro M., Testori T., Francetti L., Weinstein R.L.
Systematic review of survival rates for implants placed in grafted maxillary sinus.
Int. J. Periodontics Restorative Dent. 2004; 24: 565-77.

16 Emmerich D., Att W., Stappert C.
Sinus floor elevation using osteotomes: a systematic review and meta-analysis.
J. Periodontol. 2005; 76: 1237-51.

17 Engelke W., Schwarzwäller W., Behnsen A., Jacobs HG.
Subantroscopic laterobasal sinus floor augmentation (SALSA): an up-to-5-year clinical study.
Int. J. Oral Maxillofac. Implants 2003; 18:1 35-143.

18 Esposito M., Grusovin M.G., Worthington H.V., Coulthard P.
Interventions for replacing missing teeth: bone augmentation techniques for dental implant treatment.
Cochrane Database Syst Rev 2006; 1: CD003607.
DOI:10.1002/14651858.CD003607.pub2.

19 Ewers R.
Maxilla sinus grafting with marine algae derived bone forming material: a clinical report of long-term results.
J. Oral Maxillofac. Surg. 2005; 63: 1712-23.

20 Fiorellini J.P., Chen P.K., Nevins M., Nevins M.L.
A retrospective study of dental implants in diabetic patients.
Int. J. Periodontics Restorative Dent. 2000; 20: 366-73.

21 Froum S.J., Tarnow D.P., Wallace S.S., Rohrer M.D., Cho S.-C.
Sinus floor elevation using anorganic bovine bone matrix (OsteoGraf/N) with and without autogenous bone: a clinical, histologic, radiographic, and histomorphometric analysis. Part 2 of an ongoing prospective study.
Int. J. Periodontics Restorative Dent. 1998; 18: 529-43.

22 Fugazzotto P.A., Vlassis J.
Long-term success of sinus augmentation using various surgical approaches and grafting materials.
Int. J. Oral Maxillofac. Implants 1998; 13: 52-8.

23 Geurs N.C., Wang I.-C., Shulman L.B., Jeffcoat M.K.
Retrospective radiographic analysis of sinus graft and implant placement procedures from the Academy of Osseointegration Consensus Conference on sinus graft.
Int. J. Periodontics Restorative Dent. 2001; 21: 517-23.

24 Graziani F., Donos N., Needleman I., Gabriele M., Tonetti M.
Comparison of implant survival following sinus floor augmentation procedures with implants placed in pristine posterior maxillary bone: a systematic review.
Clin. Oral Implants Res. 2004; 15: 677-82.

25 Hallman M., Hedin M., Sennerby L., Lundgren S.
A prospective 1-year clinical and radiographic study of implants placed after maxillary sinus floor augmentation with bovine hydroxyapatite and autogenous bone.
J. Oral Maxillofac. Surg. 2002; 60: 277-84.

26 Hallman M., Nordin T.
Sinus floor augmentation with bovine hydroxyapatite mixed with fibrin glue and later placement of nonsubmerged implants: a retrospective study in 50 patients.
Int. J. Oral Maxillofac. Implants 2004a; 19: 222-7.

27 Hallman M. Zetterqvist L.
A 5-year prospective follow-up study of implant-supported fixed prostheses in patients subjected to maxillary sinus floor augmentation with an 80:20 mixture of bovine hydroxyapatite and autogenous bone.
Clin. Impl. Dent. Relat. Res. 2004b; 6: 82-9.

28 Hatano N., Shimizu Y., Ooya K.
    *A clinical long-term radiographic evaluation of graft height
    changes after maxillary sinus floor augmentatin with a 2:1
    autogenous bone/xenograft mixture and simultaneous
    placement of dental implants.*
    Clin. Oral Implants Res. 2004; 15: 339-45.

29 Hürzeler M.B., Kirsch A., Ackermann K.L., Quinones C.R.
    *Reconstruction of the severely resorbed maxilla with dental
    implants in the augmented maxillary sinus: a 5-year clinical
    investigation.*
    Int. J. Oral Maxillofac. Implants 1996; 11: 466-75.

30 Itiurriaga M.T.M., Ruiz C.C.
    *Maxillary sinus reconstruction with calvarium bone grafts and
    endosseous implants.*
    Int. J. Oral Maxillofac. Surg. 2004; 62: 344-47.

31 Jensen O.T., Shulman L.B., Block M.S., Iacono V.J.
    Report of the Sinus Consensus Conference of 1996.
    Int. J. Oral Maxillofac. Implants 1998; 13(suppl.): 11-32.

32 Johansson B., Wannfors K., Ekenback J., Smedberg J.I.,
    Hirsch J.
    *Implants and sinus-inlay bone grafts in a 1-stage procedure on
    severely atrophied maxillae: surgical aspects of a 3-year follow-up
    study.*
    Int. J. Oral Maxillofac. Implants 1999; 14: 811-8.

33 John H.D., Wenz B.
    *Histomorphometric analysis of natural bone mineral for
    maxillary sinus augmentation.*
    Int. J. Oral Maxillofac. Implants 2004; 19: 199-207.

34 Kahnberg K.E, Ekestubbe A., Gröndahl K., Nilsson P.,
    Hirsch J.M.
    *Sinus lifting procedure. I. One-stage surgery with bone
    transplant and implants.*
    Clin. Oral Implants Res. 2001; 12: 479-87.

35 Kaptein M.L.A., de Putter C., de Lange G.L., Blijdorp P.A.
    *Survival of cylindrical implants in composite grafted Maxillary
    sinuses.*
    J. Oral Maxillofac. Surg. 1998; 56: 1376-80.

36 Karabuda C., Arisan V., Hakan O.
    *Effects of sinus membrane perforations on the success of
    dental implants placed in the augmented sinus.*
    J. Periodontol. 2006; 77: 1991-7.

37 Keller E.E., Eckert S.E., Tolman D.E.
    *Maxillary antral and nasal one-stage inlay composite bone
    graft: preliminary report on 30 recipient sites.*
    J. Oral Maxillofac. Surg. 1994; 52: 438-47.

38 Keller E.E, Tolman D.A., Eckert S.E.
    *Maxillary antral-nasal inlay autogenous bone graft reconstruction
    of compromised maxilla: a 12-year retrospective study.*
    Int. J. Oral Maxillofac. Implants 1999; 14: 707-21.

39 Khang W., Feldman S., Hawley C.E., Gunsolley J.
    *A multi-center study comparing dual acid-etched and
    machined-surfaced implants in various bone qualities.*
    J. Periodontol. 2001; 72: 1384-90.

40 Khoury F.
    *Augmentation of the sinus floor with mandibular bone block
    and simultaneous implantation: a 6-year clinical investigation.*
    Int. J. Oral Maxillofac. Implants 1999; 14: 557-64.

41 Kumar A., Jaffin R.A., Berman C.
    *The effect of smoking on achieving osseointegration of
    surface-modified implants: a clinical report.*
    Int. J. Oral Maxillofac. Implants 2002; 17: 816-9.

42 Lazzara R., Testori T., Trisi P., Porter S.S., Weinstein R.L.
    *A human histologic analysis of Osseotite and machined
    surface using two-surfaced implants.*
    Int. J. Periodontics Restorative Dent. 1999; 19: 117-29.

43 Lekholm U., Wannfors K., Isaksson S., Adielsson B.
    *Oral implants in combination with bone grafts. A 3-year
    retrospective multicenter study using the Brånemark implant
    system.*
    Int. J. Oral Maxillofac. Surg. 1999; 28: 181-87.

44 Lorenzoni M., Pertl C., Wegscheider W., Keil C., Penkner K.,
    Polansky R., Bratschko R.O.
    *Retrospective analysis of Frialit-2 implants in the augmented
    sinus.*
    Int. J. Periodontics Restorative Dent. 2000; 20: 255-67.

45 Lozada J.L., Emanuelli S., James R.A., Boskovic M., Lindsted K.
    Root-form implants placed in subantral grafted sites.
    J. Calif. Dent. Assoc. 1993; 21: 31-5.

46 Mardinger O., Manor I., Mijiritsky E., Hirshberg A.
    *Maxillary sinus augmentation in the presence of antral pseudo-
    cyst: a clinical approach.*
    Oral Surg. Oral Med. Oral Pathol. Oral Radiol. Endod. 2007;
    103: 180-4.

47 McCarthy C., Patel R.R., Wragg P.F., Brook I.M.
    *Sinus augmentation bone grafts for the provision of dental
    implants: report of clinical outcome.*
    Int. J. Oral Maxillofac. Implants 2003; 18: 377-82.

48 Olson J.W., Dent C.D., Morris H.F., Ochi S.
    *Long-term assessment (5 to 71 months) of endosseous dental
    implants placed in the augmented maxillary sinus.*
    Ann. Periodontol. 2000; 5: 152-6.

49 Peleg M., Garg A.K., Mazor Z.
    *Predictability of simultaneous implant placement in the severely
    atrophic posterior maxilla: A 9-year longitudinal experience
    study of 2132 implants placed into 731 human sinus grafts.*
    Int. J. Oral Maxillofac. Implants 2006; 21: 94-102.

50 Peleg M., Mazor Z., Chaushu G., Garg A.K.
    *Sinus floor augmentation with simultaneous implant
    placement in the severely atrophic maxilla.*
    J. Periodontol. 1998; 69: 1397-1403.

51 Peleg M., Mazor Z., Garg A.K.
    *Augmentation grafting of the maxillary sinus and simultaneous
    implant placement in patients with 3 to 5 mm of residual
    alveolar bone height.*
    Int. J. Oral Maxillofac. Implants 1999; 14: 549-56.

52 Philippart P., Brasseur M., Hoyaux D., Pochet R.
    *Human recombinant tissue factor, platelet-rich plasma, and
    tetracycline induce a high-quality human bone graft: a 5-year
    survey.*
    Int. J. Oral Maxillofac. Implants 2003; 18: 411-6.

53 Pjetursson B.E., Tan K., Lang N.P., Brägger U., Egger M.,
    Zwahlen M.
    *A systematic review on the survival and complication rates of
    fixed partial dentures (FPDs) after an observation period of at
    least 5 years. I. Implant-supported FPDs.*
    Clin. Oral Implants Res. 2004; 15: 625-42.

54 Raghobaer G.M., Timmenga N.M., Reintsema H., Stegenga B.,
    Vissink A.
    *Maxillary bone grafting for insertion of endosseous implants:
    results after 12-124 months.*
    Clin. Oral Implants Res. 2001; 12: 279-86.

55 Rodriguez A., Anastassov G.E., Lee H., Buchbinder D., Wettan H.
Maxillary sinus augmentation with deproteinated bovine bone and platelet rich plasma with simultaneous insertion of endosseous implants.
J. Oral Maxillofac. Surg. 2003; 61: 157-63.

56 Scarano A., Degidi M., Iezzi G., Pecora G., Piattelli M., Orsini G., Caputi S., Perrotti V., Mangano C., Piattelli A.
Maxillary sinus augmentation with different biomaterials: a comparative histologic and histomorphometric study in man.
Implant Dent. 2006; 15: 197-207.

57 Schwarz-Arad D., Herzberg R., Dolev E.
The prevalence of surgical complications of the sinus graft procedure and their impact on implant survival.
J. Periodontol. 2004; 75: 511-6.

58 Shlomi B., Horowitz I., Kahn A., Dobriyan A., Chaushu G.
The effect of sinus membrane perforation and repair with Lambone on the outcome of maxillary sinus floor augmentation: a radiographic assessment.
Int. J. Oral Maxillofac Implants 2004; 19: 559-62.

59 Simunek A., Cierny M., Kopecka D., Kohout A., Bukac J., Vahalova D.
The sinus lift with phycogenic bone substitute. A histomorphometric study.
Clin. Oral Implants Res. 2005; 16: 342-8.

60 Stach R.M., Kohles S.S.
A meta-analysis examining the clinical survivability of machined-surfaced and Osseotite implants in poor quality bone.
Implant Dent. 2003; 12: 87-96.

61 Stricker A., Voss P.J., Gutwald R., Schramm A., Schmelzeisen R.
Maxillary sinus floor augmentation with autogenous bone grafts to enable placement of SLA-surfaced implants: preliminary results after 15-40 months.
Clin. Oral Implants Res. 2003; 14: 207-12.

62 Tarnow D.P., Wallace S.S., Froum S.J., Rohrer M.D., Cho S.-C.
Histologic and clinical comparison of bilateral sinus floor elevations with and without barrier membrane placement in 12 patients: part 3 of an ongoing prospective study.
Int. J. Periodontics Restorative Dent. 2000; 20: 117-25.

63 Tawil G., Mawla M.
Sinus floor elevation using a bovine bone mineral (Bio-Oss) with or without the concomitant use of a bilayered collagen barrier (Bio-Gide): a clinical report of immediate and delayed implant placement.
Int. J. Oral Maxillofac. Implants 2001; 16: 713-21.

64 Tolman D.
Reconstructive procedures with endosseous implants in grafted bone: A review of the literature.
Int. J. Oral Maxillofac. Implants 1995; 10: 275-94.

65 Tong D.C., Rioux K., Drangsholt M., Beirne O.R.
A review of survival rates for implants placed in grafted maxillary sinuses using meta-analysis.
Int. J. Oral Maxillofac. Implants 1998; 12: 175-82.

66 Triplett R.G., Schow S.R.
Autologous bone grafts and endosseous implants: complementary techniques.
J. Oral Maxillofac. Surg. 1996; 54: 486-94.

67 Valentini P., Abensur D.
Maxillary sinus grafting with anorganic bovine bone: A clinical report of long-term results.
Int. J. Oral Maxillofac. Implants 2003; 18: 556-60.

68 van den Bergh J.P.A., ten Bruggenkate C.M., Krekeler G., Tuinzing D.B.
Maxillary sinus floor elevation and grafting with human demineralized freeze dried bone.
Clin. Oral Implants Res. 2000; 11: 487-93.

69 van den Bergh J.P.A., ten Bruggenkate C.M., Krekeler G., Tuinzing D.B.
Sinusfloor elevation and grafting with autogenous iliac crest bone.
Clin. Oral Implants Res. 1998; 9: 429-35.

70 Wallace S.S., Froum S.J.
Effect of maxillary sinus augmentation on the survival of endosseous dental implants as compared to the survival of implants placed in the non-grafted posterior maxilla: an evidence-based literature review.
Ann. Periodontol. 2003; 8: 328-43.

71 Wallace S.S., Froum S.J., Cho S.C., Elian N., Monteiro D., Kim B.S., Tarnow D.P.
Sinus augmentation utilizing anorganic bovine bone (Bio-Oss) with absorbable and nonabsorbable membranes placed over the lateral window: histomorphometric and clinical analyses.
Int. J. Periodontics Restorative Dent. 2005; 25: 551-9.

72 Wannfors K., Johansson B., Hallman M., Strandkvist T.
A prospective randomized study of 1- and 2-stage sinus inlay bone grafts: 1-year follow-up.
Int. J. Oral Maxillofac. Implants 2000; 15: 625-32.

73 Watzek G., Weber R., Bernhart T., Ulm C., Haas R.
Treatment of patients with extreme maxillary atrophy using sinus floor augmentation and implants: preliminary results.
Int. J. Oral Maxillofac. Surg. 1998; 27: 428-34.

74 Wheeler S.L., Holmes R.E., Calhoun C.J.
Six-year clinical and histologic study of sinus-lift grafts.
Int. J. Oral Maxillofac. Implants 1996; 11: 26-34.

75 Zijderveld S.A., Zerbo I.R., van den Bergh J.P., Schulten E.A., ten Bruggenkate C.M.
Maxillary sinus floor augmentation using a beta-tricalcium phosphate (Cerasorb) alone compared to autogenous bone grafts.
Int. J. Oral Maxillofac. Implants 2005; 20: 432-40.

76 Zinner I.D., Small S.A.
Sinus-lift graft: Using the maxillary sinuses to support implants.
J. Am. Dent. Assoc. 1996; 127: 51-7.

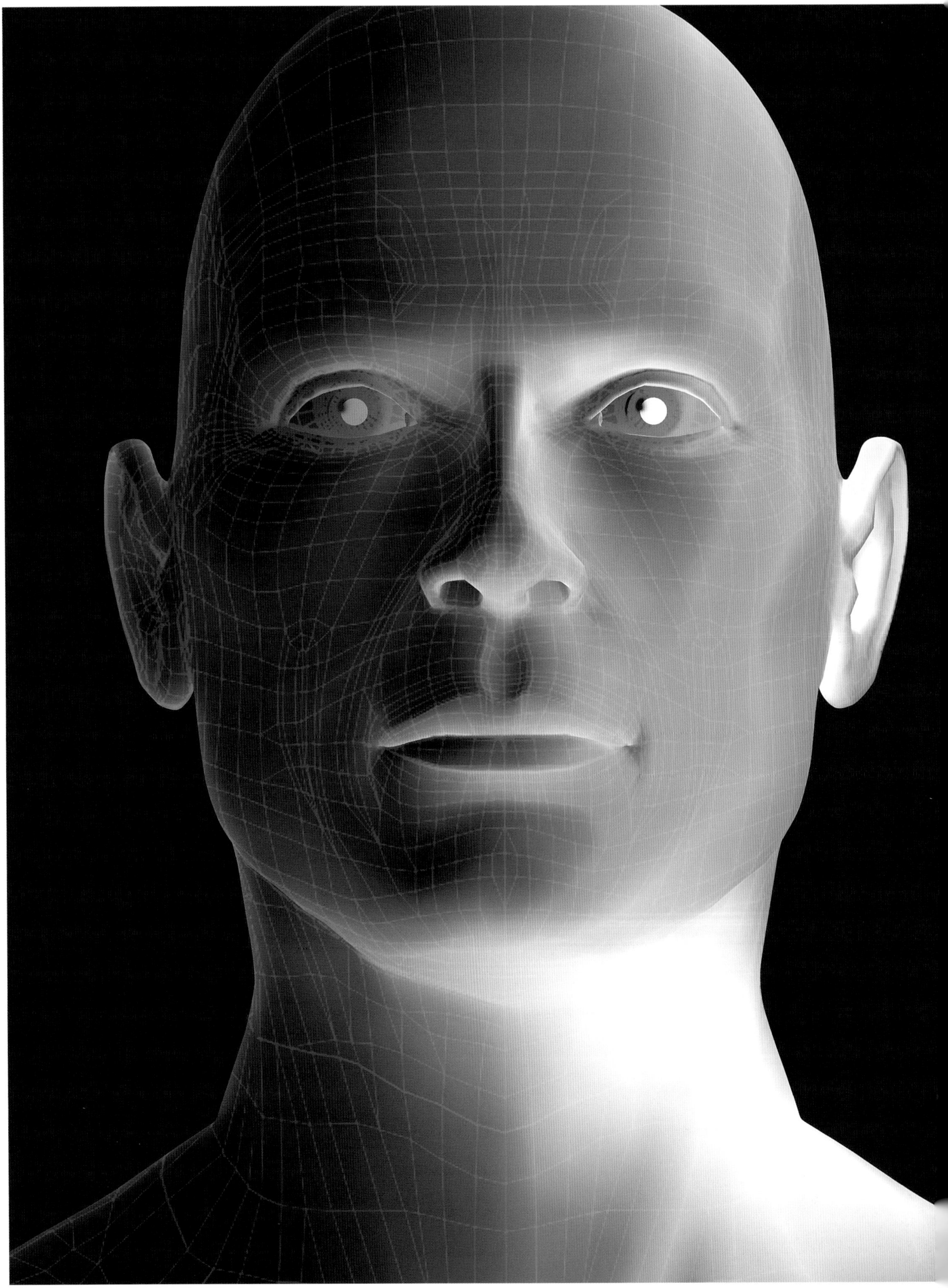

S.S. WALLACE
M. DEL FABBRO
T. TESTORI

Future developments in maxillary sinus surgery

21

21

Sinus augmentation surgery has become the subject of great attention since it was first introduced in 1977 by Hilt Tatum. The systematic review of literature reported in the previous chapter found 496 articles on implants inserted in the maxillary sinus, most of which were published in the last 6 or 7 years. Since the technique was adopted, there have been changes to the surgical procedure, different graft materials have been introduced, membranes are now used over the antrostomy and there have been alterations to the macro- and micro-geometry of the implants. Surgeons must be informed about the existence of these changes and their effects, so that they can make the right choices and the patient can benefit from improved techniques and more appropriate materials for the specific clinical situation.

Two recent systematic analyses of the literature concerning sinus elevations, carried out independently (Wallace and Froum, 2003; Del Fabbro et al. 2004), reported that only one randomized controlled trial (RCT) was actually carried out with scientific thoroughness (Boyne et al. 2005), and very few other RCTs have been found. Out of the publications included in the respective analyses, only a small number were controlled studies, while most of them were clinical case series or retrospective analyses. These last two types of experimental design are considered to have a low level of evidence.

While the data obtained from these studies are most certainly useful for gaining experience, changing our therapeutic choices and improving results, it is necessary to approach clinical research radically, to conform to medical evidence-based research models.

This change in research protocol is additionally necessary because of the new types of biomaterials that we have only recent begun to study.

Latest generation biomaterials are available thanks to the continuous progress in research on materials, genetics and molecular biology, and deeper knowledge of the molecules involved in the processes of complex biological mechanisms.

Developments in medical treatment are increasingly directed towards 'molecular' medicine, which can use specific molecules to stimulate specific functions.

For example, bone morphogenetic proteins (in particular BMP-2 and BMP-7), described for the first time by Urist (1965) and available in a recombinant form since 1988 (Wozney et al. 1988), are the most powerful osteoinductive factors known. Their efficacy is well documented and they are currently used in for orthopedic applications (in particular non-consolidated tibia fractures and spinal fusions). However, use in oral and maxillofacial surgery is currently limited to few (although encouraging) experimental findings on animals and rare clinical experiments. A few of the latter refer to sinus lifts, but the only study with a high incidence level is the Boyne study indicated above. This study analyzed the effect of different doses of BMP-2, obtained with recombinant DNA technology (rh-BMP-2) on bone growth in the maxillary sinus. Preliminary studies on the safety and efficacy of BMP-2 in various animal species were carried out, as usual, before tests on humans. Boyne's study on humans was conducted at an analysis level never encountered before in maxillary sinus research and the results referred to the patients, rather than to the implants. In other words, the following questions were asked: Did the graft procedure allow implant placement which permitted prosthesis construction that proved effective under functional load? Or: Was the treatment positive for the patient?

This is one of the key points of modern evidence-based dentistry (EBD), i.e. to consider the patient rather than the single tooth or the implant as the analysis unit. Research has begun to use recombinant growth factors such as rhPDGF (recombinant human platelet-derived growth factor) in periodontal surgery and regenerative therapy in recent years (Nevins et al. 2003), and studies are currently ongoing to optimize the use of genic therapy for the regeneration of bone defects. One of these studies was recently published by the research group led by William Giannobile, which successfully used the *Bmp7* gene in periodontal regeneration (Jin et al. 2003). Virus carriers that transport the *Bmp* or *PDGF* gene in loco can permit the induction of a powerful, long-lasting local regenerative response, stimulating specific biological processes, with minimum discomfort for the patient. Further studies on BMPs, growth factors and stem cell technology are needed to keep up with the times and benefit from modern biomolecular technologies and tissue engineering progress.

As well as this need, experimental and clinical research require protocols with extremely high standards, so that they are safe, efficient and dose-dependent and can be assessed thoroughly and reliably. It can be hypothesized that in the next few years, the use of recombinant growth factors in periodontal and implant regenerative therapy will continue to increase, on the condition that their cost, which is currently prohibitive, decreases

to a point that allows widespread use by surgeons. Evidence-based literature reviews have proved that implants placed in the maxillary sinus after sinus augmentation procedures have an average survival rate of 92% (more than 9000 implants in about 2700 patients), and the prosthesis success rate is even higher.

We have also experimented with new sinus surgery, such as the Summers technique, which, under suitable residual crestal bone conditions, has a 93.5% implant survival rate (445 implants in more than 250 patients). The wide implant survival rate range reported by various studies, from 61.2% to 100% using a lateral antrostomy approach and from 88.6% to 100% using the osteotomy technique, would suggest that we are still in the perfecting phase of the research.

Our objective for the future must therefore be multi-factorial and must include the following goals:

1. Past scientific works must be analyzed again, and more thoroughly, with particular attention paid to surgical protocol and graft materials. The diagnostic choices made further to this analytic process should lead to higher survival rates and a narrowed variability range in results.

2. Research must be started in new directions, and new technologies and surgical techniques must only be adopted after evidence of an increase in success is scientifically obtained.

3. We must also open our minds, allow changes in our cultural baggage and accept the use of these new techniques and technologies, even when they seem to go against what we were taught in the past and what we have always tried to put into practice.

4. Finally, we must understand, as researchers and clinicians, that our ultimate aim is to provide the patient with the utmost level of quality in healthcare. Our responsibility is therefore to develop, improve and use therapies that guarantee maximum pre-

dictability to the patient. However, as providers of healthcare services, we must do this taking into account the patient's needs and expectations, adopting the most simple and the least expensive solution, and always carefully assessing the cost-benefit ratio of new therapy possibilities.

Our future is nearer than we believe and we must be ready to face it in the best way possible, maintaining scientific thoroughness and setting our patients' health as our primary objective.

REFERENCES

1 **Boyne P.J., Leslie C., Lilly B.S.N., et al.**
   De novo bone induction by recombinant human bone morphogenetic protein-2 (rhBMP-2) in maxillary sinus floor augmentation.
   J. Oral Maxillofac. Surg. 2005; 12: 1693-707.

2 **Del Fabbro M., Testori T., Francetti L., Weinstein R.**
   Systematic review of survival rates for implants placed in grafted maxillary sinus.
   Int. J. Periodontics Restorative Dent. 2004; 24: 565-77.

3 **Jin Q.M., Anusaksathien O., Webb S.A., Rutherford R.B., Giannobile WV.**
   Gene therapy of bone morphogenetic protein for periodontal tissue engineering.
   J. Periodontol. 2003; 74: 202-13.

4 **Nevins M., Camelo M., Nevins M.L., Schenk R.K., Lynch S.E.**
   Periodontal regeneration in humans using recombinant human platelet-derived growth factor-BB (rhPDGF-BB) and allogenic bone.
   J. Periodontol. 2003; 74: 1282-92.

5 **Urist M.R.**
   Bone: formation by autoinduction.
   Science 1965; 150: 893-9.

6 **Wallace S.S., Froum S.J.**
   Effect of maxillary sinus augmentation on the survival of endosseous dental implants as compared to the survival of implants placed in the non-grafted posterior maxilla: an evidence-based literature review.
   Ann. Periodontol. 2003; 8: 328-43.

7 **Wozney J.M., Rosen V., Celeste A.J. et al.**
   Novel regulators of bone formation: molecular clones and activities.
   Science 1988; 242: 1528-34.

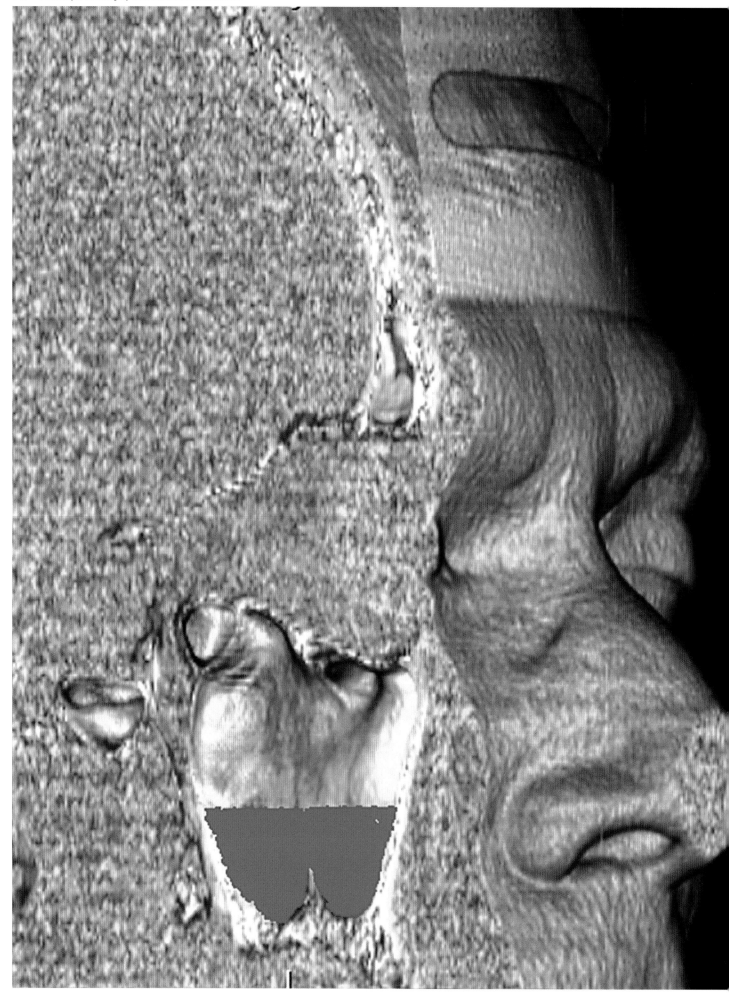

F. PERONA
G. CASTELLAZZI

Advanced imaging techniques in sinus surgery

22

22

INTRODUCTION

Recent implant techniques can be applied in patients with partial edentulism in the posterior area of the maxillary arch, where alveolar bone resorption is more evident, giving crucial support to clinical treatment. In these situations, implant-supported prosthetic rehabilitation carried out by the augmentation of the sinus floor is increasingly required **FIG. 1**.

Given the morphology of the maxillary sinus and of the corresponding dental arch, a correct preoperative diagnostic examination able to resolve the 3D anatomical structure in a radiological context is extremely useful (Casap et al. 2004; Kan et al. 2006).

It is clear that diagnostic imaging plays a crucial role, confirmed by its dramatic development in the last 30 years supported by a tremendous enhancement in the complexity of conventional investigations, as well as by the emergence of new generation imaging techniques such as computerized tomography (CT) and magnetic resonance (MR) (Tsai and Hsieh, 2005). Moreover, recently developed software, such as Ris/Pacs, enable professionals to set up very large easy-to-manage digital archives in a safe way, without risks for data recovery (Canadè et al. 2003).

This growing development has considerably increased the diagnostic capability of radiological imaging. It has allowed a very precise revision of diagnostic protocols, with new possibilities for non-invasive evaluations in a highly specialized field such as that of implant prosthesis treatment. Radiographic evaluation is the main source of information necessary to plan a proper preoperative protocol in the implantation treatment area (Schmitt 2006). Data are obtained from the classical 2D intraoral to orthopanoramic examinations, as well as from the 3D CT imaging: the latter technology allows the design of guide masks that support a very accurate implant placement planned to reach optimal clinical results.

The need for an exact correspondence between the guide mask indications and the anatomy of the interventional area has prompted the development of computerized technologies able to link the CT imaging data with those of a proper virtual surgery and to design intraoperative guides corresponding to optimal therapeutic treatment programs.

Recent virtual simulation techniques allow further development both in the clinic and in educational areas.

A number of new software programs have been developed to set up 3D images exactly overlapping the anatomic structures involved in the interventional treatment: the procedure used to reach this goal, independently of the type of software, is based on three major steps:

- image acquisition of anatomic components in axial sections and further digitalization either by CT or MR
- data transfer to computerized workstations
- re-elaboration of raw data in 3D environments in order to obtain realistic images of the anatomic structures under study.

In our clinical department, we use a Dextroscope machine (Volume Interactions, Singapore). It consists of a workstation able to perform a very sophisticated 3D elaboration of different body areas: the normally sitting operator is equipped with glasses that allow 3D vision; by using proper tools (i.e. pen with a localization sensor) the operator is able to modify the volume appearing in the front-standing screen with his/her hands, selecting a panel of different functions such as cutting, rotation and threshold variation as if the operator was working on real objects. The operator can explore the best access points, removing bone structures or tissues, studying the optimal way to approach the treatment area **FIG. 2–4**.

This application, previously used only for neurosurgery, is now compatible with other surgical disciplines, such as implantology or vascular surgery, and is endowed with the following characteristics:

- The CT/MR images are DICOM (digital imaging and communications in medicine) converted and their processing, from acquisition to visualization, takes 15 to 40 seconds.
- Different images can be superimposed according to the "transparency principle", adding a number of volumes, even from distinct examinations both in terms of mode (coronal, axial) or of physical principle used (MR, CT), in order to obtain the highest level of detail.
- The 3D model is visualized by combining the slices obtained through the original investigation, and re-elaborated for each visualization angle in real-time.
- Whole basal information obtained is experimentally evaluated using the preset function that allows detection or the alternative deletion of certain anatomic structures.

- Proportions and dimensions are maintained in case of standard mode importation using a reference matrix such as DICOM.
- Interface is easy-to-understand while drives are self-explanatory and of strict radiological pertinence (e.g. transparency, gray threshold).
- The main functions that allow differentiation of the distinct anatomic structures are transparency, threshold level, reduction and contrast, detail, zoom, and color table.
- The 3D stereoscopic visualization is highly realistic.

The advantage of using Dextroscope is therefore in the setting up of an adequate preoperative study. The treatment plan is derived from the different views visualized in the volume of interest. Another advantage is the educational support it provides for students.

Confirmation of the convenience of a 3D stereoscopic vision technique comes mainly from neurosurgeons working at the Johannes Gutenberg Neurosurgery Clinic, University of Mainz, Germany, who were able to modify the operative procedure in 20% of cases by using Dextroscope. In addition, Dr. Benjamin Carson, neurosurgeon at the Johns Hopkins University, Baltimore, MD, USA, says "It was fantastic. When I put those glasses on and went into the virtual workstation it was like I had them right in front of me." Moreover, "When working with tailored approaches of the keyhole strategy, the Dextroscope is currently the only system to provide a real detailed 3D model of patients' individual patho-anatomy", confirmed Prof. Axel Perneczky, University of Mainz, Germany. "This enables you to plan and explain the individual surgery of each patient. Due to its unique interactive operation, the Dextroscope is also very useful for neurosurgeon teaching education and training."

1 → THREE-DIMENSIONAL RECONSTRUCTION OF MAXILLARY SINUSES. TRANSVERSE SECTION. AN UNDERWOOD SEPTUM CAN BE SEEN IN THE RIGHT SINUS.

2 → RECONSTRUCTION WITH SECTION ON FRONTAL PLANE, PASSING THROUGH MAXILLARY SINUS AND NASAL CAVITY.

Different types of software for preoperative planning in the implantation area are now available: SimPlant (Materialise Dental, Leuven, Belgium), Vimplant (CyberMed, Seoul, Korea), NobelGuide (Nobel Biocare, Zurich, Switzerland), DentalVox (BioMax, Germany), ImplantMaster (iDent Imaging, Ft. Lauderdale, FL, USA). They allow the correct, rapid insertion of implants.

SimPlant is the first virtual planning system launched on the market. It enables the control of the implant virtual positioning in different projections and allows the evaluation of the bone tissue quality in the area of interest. By using SimPlant, it is possible to simulate reconstructive interventions in order to modify the existing bone mass, in case it was insufficient to support the implantation treatment. This characteristic has supported such a wide diffusion of the software in the world to lead to the establishment of the "SimPlant Academy" (www.simplantacademy.org), a non-profit virtual community of professionals who deal with this system at various levels, in order to exchange their personal experience.

Vimplant is similar to SimPlant, but includes an extra system for the automatic identification of the alveolar nerve and of nervous structures.

NobelGuide allows prosthesis virtual realization before the true intervention through the possibility of 3D patient anatomy reproduction coming from CT data in DICOM format.

DentalVox enables planning of the operative strategy and therefore the virtual execution of the program, depending on optimal prosthetic results; it uses a specific processing system that leads to elimination of distortions present in all images obtained with conventional DentaScan systems. Moreover, this software is interconnected with a robot (Centrax), which is able to set up a surgical guide based on a plaster model, perfectly corresponding to implant direction and depth.

Finally, ImplantMaster is specific implantation planning-oriented software.

The use of the present systems does not rule out the possibility of complications during the interventional procedure. Perfect preoperative planning is not the only factor for success in clinical practice: in the presence of anatomic variations, the use of grafts may be necessary, and surgeons are sometimes induced to modify the original protocol and to depart from the strict use of a pre-constituted prosthesis.

VIRTUAL PLANNING SYSTEMS

Virtual planning systems have been developed to counteract the above-described possibilities. These methods, including IGI (Den X, Jerusalem, Israel), RoboDent (Berlin, Germany) and Artma Virtual Implant System (Medlibre, Munich, Germany), enable verification of the accuracy of the treatment plan during the intervention, as there is constant evaluation of the anatomic structures under study. This type of approach allows monitoring of the relationship between the implant virtual planning and the subsequent realization during the interventional procedure.

The innovation of this system is based on the following crucial points:
- the need for a dynamic intraoperative control of treatment protocol accuracy
- the management of intraoperative events
- the constant control of anatomic structures in the absence of direct view, using minimally invasive approaches
- real-time visualization of adjustments to be applied to the treatment protocol
- the possibility of online support from remote experienced professionals.

IGI includes a workstation, very sophisticated image acquisition and a localization system: a 3D model of the dental arch of interest is created and used to plan and monitor the pre-established virtual treatment protocol in real time.

RoboDent's characteristics are comparable to those of IGI, as they are directly equivalent in terms of machinery. However, RoboDent is used exclusively by maxillofacial surgeons and in the implantation area. It includes an extra function, the so called "navigated control", which makes a constant check of the burs, whose function is automatically stopped in cases of potential damage to the anatomic structures close to the implantation area.

Artma Virtual Implant System differs from the previous software due to the presence of a display attached to the operator glasses. This device can visualize at the same time both the area of intervention and the virtual plan appearing on the screen in order to superimpose the real optical plane and the virtual one, to follow the operator's head movements: the surgeon, therefore, can visualize the real anatomic structures and the projections of the virtual interventional protocol.

VIRTUAL SIMULATORS

For over a century, American educational methods in the surgical field have been strictly bound to the "see it, do it, teach it" way (Roberts et al. 2006). In other words, they have been restricted to the observation of a single surgical movement carried out by an experienced professional and to its exact replication by the observing beginner. This is a time-consuming method, and limited to only one student, which can be potentially dangerous for the patient. The recent introduction of minimally invasive surgery (MIS) has greatly modified this approach (Gallagher et al. 2005). The operator movements are, in fact, limited to a

very small area such as that of the abdominal laparoscopy field: they are, therefore, very difficult to reproduce while, at the same time, the 2D image visualization on a screen is more difficult than the 3D visualization. Furthermore, operators must be experienced in the utilization of the sophisticated devices, which are completely different from those classically employed in conventional surgery. However, these requirements are met by the new virtual technologies that allow surgical education to be performed in a safer way: each movement of the operator can be repeated and learned by the use of complex machinery and software, working on a virtual patient. Specific simulators are also now available in the medical field, and are ready for wide distribution. They can perfectly reproduce the surgeon's movements in a context faithful to real operating conditions, increasing the capability of the surgeon using a virtual method with no risks for patients due to lack of experience of the professional. These methods are based on the same principles used to train pilots using flight simulators.

In 1999, the Accreditation Council of Graduate Medical Education (ACGME; USA) established that a physician should be expert in at least five different areas (Canadè et al. 2003):

- patient care
- knowledge of medicine
- learning and implementing basic clinical signs
- interpersonal communication
- "systems-based practice".

An investigation carried out in 2001 confirmed that the vast majority of general surgery program directors are in favor of a surgical training not done in vivo on the patients. The availability of virtual technology has enforced these basic learning principles, becoming part of the training programs planned for the students; moreover, it has been demonstrated that surgeons who experience virtual training are able not only to obtain more satisfactory

3-4→ VIRTUAL PLANNING
PHASES. VOLUMETRIC STUDY
OF MAXILLARY SINUS IN FULL
(RED) AND OF BONE GRAFT
AREA (BLUE) THAT WILL BE
PLACED DURING SURGERY.

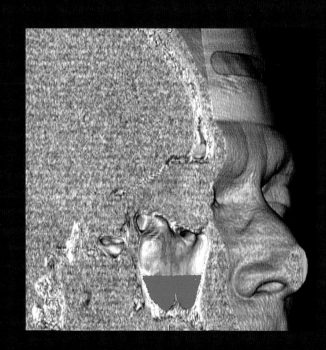

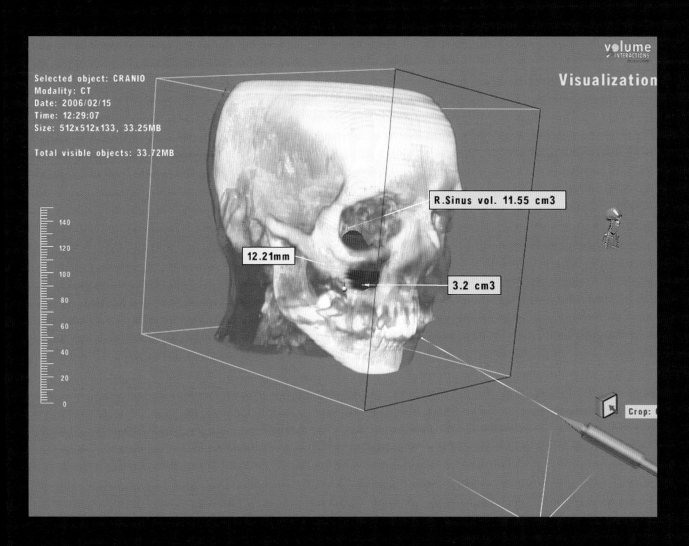

results, but also to reach optimal knowledge and expertise more rapidly than with the conventional educational methods (Ratiu et al. 2003).

In this chapter we have discussed "surgery simulators", but how can we define this? It is a mixture of sophisticated systems of virtual navigation and proper applicative manual devices (pens with volume sensors, 3D glasses, specific screens) able to reproduce the real conditions of the surgical phase on a screen and that can be used interactively by the operator who can, therefore, act as if he/she was in the operating theater, doing all the typical movements of the real practice such as cutting, suturing and placing clips.

Another advantage of this technology is the possibility of recording operator performances in terms of execution time, used devices and manual skills, during each training session. Through this procedure the educator can read the recorded files and evaluate the learning level of his/her own students, and, moreover, set the software differently in order to reduce or increase the difficulty level of each training session (Gould 2007).

Procedural simulators are designed to reproduce the anatomy of specific areas, allowing training in the main surgery fields: different simulators have been set up to support sinus endoscopic intervention, bronchoscopy, gastrointestinal endoscopy and stent placement.

For endoscopic surgery of the maxillary sinus, the best-known simulator is the Endoscopic Sinus Simulator (ESS; Lockeed Martin, Moorestown, NJ, USA). It allows navigation inside paranasal cavities and supports a detailed study of these complex anatomic structures during the training sessions, avoiding damage to proximal areas at the same time. The learning surgeon moves a sinusal endoscope inserted in the nose of a specifically designed model in order to visualize its nasal cavities. This promising system is undergoing various feasibility studies, as Marvin P. Fried,

MD, chairman of Otolaryngology at Montefiore Medical Center, USA, described. "We are using the most advanced surgery simulators and their virtual reality technology to train and improve the endoscopic skills of surgeons and, most importantly, to detect errors in techniques and near misses before surgeons operate on patients." He added, "Our study is important because, until now, there has been no objective way to measure and monitor improvements in the technical skills of surgeons being trained in minimally invasive sinus surgery."

CONCLUSIONS

More and more complex and sophisticated devices and procedures are being developed and updated to simplify the setting up of implantation guides. Radiologists are being challenged to know in detail the new implant technologies, and to understand the possibility of reproducing them in a virtual way. Progress in biotechnology is consistently followed by dramatic developments in diagnostic imaging techniques, specially designed for preoperative evaluations or for simulation in an educational context or in preoperative planning.

In conclusion, radiology and new imaging techniques, combined with a new concept for surgical skills training, are undergoing a dramatic transformation in clinical practice. Modern technologies and training techniques are making the teachers of surgery reconsider previously held principles. Radiological multimodal acquisition in its current form can facilitate the improvement of maxillofacial surgical skills and operating room performance of surgical operators and residents.

An innovative and progressive approach, learning from the experiences of other technological fields, can provide a new way of looking at sophisticated techniques such as maxillary sinus elevation. As the technology develops, the way we practice will continue to evolve, to the benefit of physicians and patients.

REFERENCES

1   Canadè A., Palladino F., Pitzalis G., Campioni P., Marano P.
    Web-based radiology: a future to be created.
    Rays. 2003; 28: 109-17.

2   Casap N., Wexler A., Lustmann J.
    Image-guided navigation system for placing dental implants.
    Compend. Contin. Educ. Dent. 2004; 25: 783-4.

3   Gallagher A.G., Ritter E.M., Champion H. et al.
    Virtual reality simulation for the operating room. Proficiency-based training as a paradigm shift in surgical skills training.
    Ann. Surg. 2005; 241: 364-72.

4   Gould D.A.
    Interventional radiology simulation: prepare for a virtual revolution in training.
    J. Vasc. Interv. Radiol. 2007; 18: 483-90.

5   Kan J.Y., Rungcharassaeng K., Oyama K., Chung S.H., Lozada J.L.
    Computer-guided immediate provisionalization of anterior multiple adjacent implants: surgical and prosthodontic rationale.
    Pract. Proced. Aesthet. Dent. 2006; 18: 617-23.

6   Ratiu P., Hillen B., Glaser J., Jenkins D.P.
    Visible human 2.0 – the next generation.
    Stud. Health Technol. Inform. 2003; 94: 275-81.

7   Roberts K.E., Bell R.L., Duffy A.J.
    Evolution of surgical skill training.
    World J. Gastroenterol. 2006; 12: 3219-24.

8   Schmitt S.
    Virtual diagnostics using cone beam CT.
    Dent. Today 2006; 25: 90-1.

9   Tsai M.D., Hsieh M.S.
    Volume manipulations for simulating bone and joint surgery.
    IEEE Trans. Inf. Technol. Biomed. 2005; 9: 139-49.

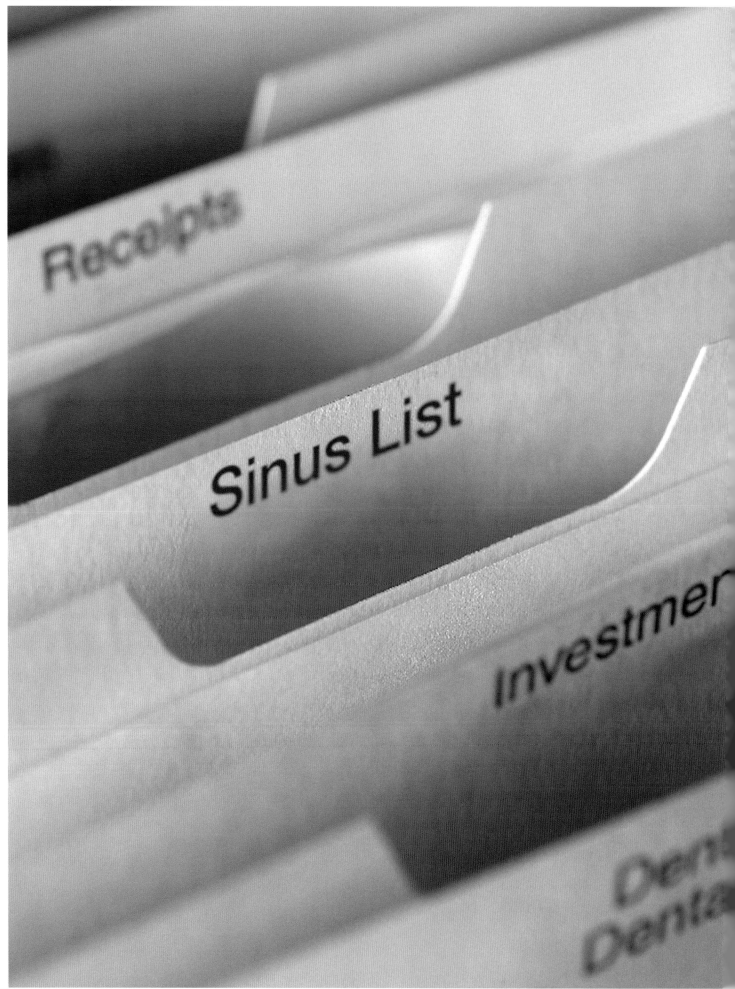

M. DEL FABBRO
F. BIANCHI
F. GALLI
T. TESTORI

Appendix: collection of clinical records, files, patient monitoring and data reporting

23

23

From the perspective of a modern concept of dental surgery, we believe it useful to accompany our clinical practice with careful data collection, using a method that is as standardized as possible.

The documentation is advantageous for evaluating the value of our work and for possibly correcting some procedures. It is also mandatory for carrying out clinical studies, which will then be followed by a scientific publication.

An essential prerequisite for collecting clinical data and/or for clinical investigations is the total transparency and truthfulness of the data.

Before proceeding with data collection, it is necessary to define the type of clinical study that is to be performed. Distinguishing whether the study will be retrospective, case-control, randomized or prospective, for example, helps to guide the timeline for evaluating patients and drawing up a suitable data-collecting protocol. The desire to obtain histologic data must be decided immediately in order to plan the biopsies.

The standardization is important. This is an aspect often neglected by clinicians. Taking time to fill in a patient's medical records allows us to collect a large amount of information on the initial condition and individual characteristics, which are extremely valuable for both the decision-making phase of treatment planning and later, to assess healing progress and compare the outcome with the initial condition. Ideally, medical records should be easy to fill in, preferably based on pre-set multiple choice questions so that the person filling in the records only has to select the appropriate box, or insert a short text in the section "other". This formula speeds up the filling-in procedure, helping the surgeon, who is always short of time, and aids comparison of different records.

With regards to documentation concerning maxillary sinus surgery and the placement of implants, there is a large amount of data relating to both basal bone conditions and the surgical procedure selected.

The quality and quantity of residual crestal bone, and the possible presence of septa are useful for planning the operation, and for assessing the extent of the elevation over time.

The type of surgical procedure used must be described, indicating: the type of incision, the size of the antrostomy, the type of graft material, the harvest site, the graft volume, the Schneiderian membrane perforation, the use or non-use of a membrane in antrostomy and the type of covering suture used.

Any perforation of the sinus membrane and other intrasurgical complications must be specified, referring to both their occurrence and to how they are dealt with.

Pre- and post-surgery pharmacological therapy must also be noted.

A collection of uniformly completed medical records is also essential for drawing up a scientific report, in order to have all the necessary information available for a quantitative analysis of results and/or for the research of any correlation between clinical parameters and individual characteristics. It is also extremely important that the records are filled in immediately and not postponed, as some important information may be forgotten.

The objective of a scientific publication must be to provide sufficient basic information that allows the reader to understand and assess the research results, and thus allow them to be reproduced by others.

There are some fundamental criteria for writing a scientific article, which are summarized in documents elaborated and updated regularly buy the ICMJE (International Committee of Medical Journal Editors; 2003). Such documentation are guidelines for the conducting and reporting of randomized clinical trials (RCTs), the clinical studies at the top of the hierarchy of scientific evidence (Altman et al. 2001). These guidelines may also be used as a model for simple RCT studies, which should have a degree of scientific thoroughness.

Generally speaking, some basic advice can be given to anyone who wants to report the results of his own studies in the form of a scientific publication. The *title* must be as concise as possible but must accurately describe the topic being addressed. The *introduction* must contain:

- a general view of the research and the problem
- a short bibliographical review that guides the reader to the current state of knowledge
- a clear goal and a working hypothesis that will be verified.

In the section *Materials and Methods*, it will be necessary to include sufficient details to allow the clinical study to be reproduced by others; therefore, the contents of this section must be precise and detailed.

When preparing to present the *Results*, it may be good practice to keep the following saying in mind: "The fool collects data, the wiseman selects them" (John Wesley Powell). It is essential to discriminate and select the data that are of interest to the reader. It is necessary to use appropriate tables and graphs, but to avoid the repetition of data already reported in the text. Tables and graphs should be self-explanatory, i.e. immediately comprehensible for the reader. The artwork should be kept to a necessary minimum for adequate documentation of the important stages of the procedures, taking care to choose clean, high-quality clinical images. Low-quality figures can provide a negative impression to an otherwise valuable work. The results of any statistical analyses must be presented concisely, providing values of significance in terms of P (probability).

A critical analysis of what has been found must be carried out in the *Discussion* section. Even excellent results may lose part of their value if not provided with a suitable analysis. It is necessary to follow some essential points:

- make generalizations based on results
- explain incompatible data
- define points and matters that have not been dealt with (if present) and the reasons why they have not been taken into consideration
- compare results obtained with previous studies and justify any discrepancies
- clarify any theoretical and practical implications of the research, discussing the limitations
- present arguments to support any generalizations
- limit any type of speculation not supported by evidence as far as possible.

At the end of the discussion, any new hypotheses can be proposed, obviously identifying them as such. Finally, the *Conclusions* must report the essential parts of the discussion in a few clear, precise points. This last section is important if one considers the fact that many "lazy" readers first read the title and then skip most of the text and go directly to read the conclusions.

As they are usually conducted according to a rigorous predefined methodology, meta-analyses and systematic reviews of literature are considered to be the scientific work with the highest level of evidence; they combine the results of several clinical studies and therefore analyze a much larger database compared with single studies. The better the quality of the studies that are analyzed, the higher the level of evidence from these reviews. As mentioned above, RCTs are the most reliable clinical studies because the protocol is designed to reduce systematic errors to a minimum. They are therefore the preferred studies for a meta-analysis. However, the single RCTs often provide their results in terms of measures of centrality and dispersion (e.g. averages and standard deviations), two of the most used parameters for describing synthetically the outcomes of a study, i.e. they group together original data to provide summary information for the reader. Individual patient data is rarely reported in an RCT. Although the grouped data allows conclusions to be drawn from a single RCT, they are not suitable for a further analysis such as a meta-analysis of literature, especially when it is necessary to look for a relationship between the effect of a treatment and the individual characteristics of patients. A meta-analysis performed using only assembled data is unreliable and may produce misleading results, especially if the assembled data are treated as though they were individual data (Berlin et al. 2002; Nieri et al. 2003). Having individual medical records available is necessary to analyze the relationship between clinical variables correctly and to compare different studies. Knowing the individual characteristics of the patients in each single study, even if they differ, may in fact allow an estimation of the weight of these differences in the final result, and the analysis will be more reliable. Having the individual data available is therefore the only system for reliably investigating the relationship between patient characteristics and the effect of treatment, if several different studies must be grouped together. The ideal situation may derive from the creation of "*clinical registries*", i.e. collections of medical records that are as standardized as possible, and can be consulted freely or on request, for scientific purposes (Weyant 2003). These clinical registries have been created in the United States and in Sweden and have formed the basis of long-term multi-center studies, which require a high number of samples, on dental implants (Albrektsson et al. 1988; Department of Veterans Affairs 1991). Some journals have begun publishing tables of individual patient data compiled from single medical records, available online, in combination with the full text article (Clauser et al. 2003). The fact that these data are available could make a crucial difference to the accuracy of systematic reviews, and could be included in the criteria to evaluate the quality of individual articles. This may be a further incentive to publish more complete, detailed works, that therefore correspond as much as possible to the criteria of evidence-based medicine.

REFERENCES

1 **International Committee of Medical Journal Editors.**
   Uniform Requirements for Manuscripts Submitted to Biomedical Journals: Writing and Editing for Biomedical Publication. Updated November 2003. Available at: www.ICMJE.org

2 **Altman D.G., Schultz K.F., Moher D., et al. for the CONSORT Group.**
   The revised CONSORT statement for reporting randomized trials: explanation and elaboration.
   Ann. Intern. Med. 2001; 134: 663-94.

3 **Albrektsson T., Dahl E., Enbom L., et al.**
   Osseointegrated oral implants: a Swedish multicenter study of 8139 consecutively inserted Nobelpharma implants.
   J. Periodontol. 1988; 59: 287-96.

4 **Berlin J.A., Santanna J., Schmid C.H., Szczech L.A., Feldman H.I.**
   Individual patient- versus group-level data meta-regressions for the investigation of treatment effect modifiers: ecological bias rears its ugly head.
   Statist. Med. 2002; 21: 371-87.

5 **Clauser C., Nieri M., Franceschi D., Pagliaro U., Pini Prato G.**
   Evidence-based mucogingival therapy. Part 2: ordinary and individual patient data meta-analyses for surgical treatment of recession using complete root coverage as the outcome variable.
   J. Periodontol. 2003; 74: 741-56.

6 **Department of Veterans Affairs.**
   Dental implant registry history and findings.
   Int. J. Oral Implantol. 1991; 8: 81-92.

7 **Nieri M., Clauser C., Pagliaro U., Pini Prato G.**
   Individual patient data: a criterion in grading articles dealing with therapy outcomes.
   J. Evid. Base Dent. Pract. 2003; 3: 122-6.

8 **Weyant R.J.**
   Short-term clinical success of root-form titanium implant systems.
   J. Evid. Base Dent. Pract. 2003; 3: 127-30.

MAXILLARY SINUS AUGMENTATION USING OSTEOTOMY TECHNIQUE

DATE _____

2ND SURGICAL OPERATION	PROSTHESIS MOLD

EXPIRY DATE _____   JANUARY FEBRUARY MARCH APRIL MAY JUNE JULY AUGUST SEPTEMBER OCTOBER NOVEMBER DECEMBER   20_____

PATIENT: _____   Date of birth: _____
Address: _____   Tel. _____

Time patient enters operating theatre: _____
Premedication (type and dosage of medicinal product): _____
Anesthesia (type and dose): _____
Type of incision (with any releases): _____

TYPE OF GRAFT MATERIAL _____
Harvest site: _____

RESIDUAL BONE and BONE QUALITY (1, II, III) IN RIDGE

		17	16	15	14	24	25	26	27
CRANIOCAUDAL	mm								
PALATAL VESTIBULAR	mm								
BONE QUALITY									

PRESENCE OF SEPTA   NO ❑   YES ❑   direction _____   height from floor mm: _____

AMOUNT OF MEMBRANE ELEVATION (approximately)
Cranio/caudal mm _____

PERFORATION OF MEMBRANE   NO ❑   YES ❑

GRAFT VOLUME (initial volume minus residual) cm^3
Bio-Oss 0.5 g with particle size 0.5–1 mm hydrated becomes 1.1 cm^3

IMPLANTS

N°	SITE	TYPE: using adhesive inside packages	Bone quantity: - I dense - II normal - III soft	CT bone quality	Newton primary stability	ISQ	NOTES
1							
2							
3							
4							
5							

Complications during surgery: _____
_____
_____

• Type of suture: _____
• Pharmacological therapy administered immediately after operation: _____
_____
• Postsurgery pharmacological therapy: _____
• Type of planned prosthesis: _____
• Data and time of patient's discharge: _____

1ST SURGEON: _____	2ND SURGEON: _____

• SURGICAL WOUND HEALING INDEX

❑ 1. Complete closure absence of fibrin   ❑ 2. Complete closure thin line of fibrin   ❑ 3. Complete closure presence of fibrin   ❑ 4. Incomplete closure dehiscence   ❑ 5. Incomplete closure necrosis

MAXILLARY SINUS ELEVATION WITH LATERAL ANTROSTOMY

IMMEDIATE IMPLANTS ☐	DEFERRED IMPLANTS ☐

1ST OPERATION: DATE _____

2ND OPERATION ☐	PROSTHESIS MOLD ☐

EXPIRY DATE: _____ JANUARY FEBRUARY MARCH APRIL MAY JUNE JULY AUGUST SEPTEMBER OCTOBER NOVEMBER DECEMBER 20_____

PATIENT:_____ Date of birth: _____

Address: _____ Tel. _____

Time patient enters operating theatre: _____

Premedication (type and dosage of medicinal product): _____

Anesthesia (type and dose): _____

Type of incision (with any releases): _____

TYPE OF GRAFT MATERIAL _____

Harvest site: _____

RESIDUAL BONE and BONE QUALITY (1, II, III) IN RIDGE

		17	16	15	14	24	25	26	27
CRANIOCAUDAL	mm								
PALATAL VESTIBULAR	mm								
BONE QUALITY									

Anstrotomy size in c/c direction: mm _____   M / D mm _____

PRESENCE OF SEPTA   NO ☐   YES ☐   direction _____   height from floor mm: _____

SIZE OF MEMBRANE ELEVATION (approximately)
     A / C mm _____   M / D mm _____   V / P mm _____   Volume _____

PERFORATION OF MEMBRANE   NO ☐   YES ☐   size mm _____   site _____

GRAFT VOLUME (initial volume minus residual) cm^3_____
Bio-Oss 0.5 g with particle size 0.5–1 mm hydrated becomes 1.1 cm^3

USE OF MEMBRANE during antrostomy   NO ☐   YES ☐   type _____   design _____

fixation method _____

IMPLANTS

N°	SITE	TYPE: using adhesive inside packages	Bone quantity: - I dense - II normal - III soft	CT bone quality	Newton primary stability	ISQ	NOTES
1							
2							
3							
4							
5							

Complications during surgery: _____

_____

_____

- Type of suture: _____
- Pharmacological therapy administered immediately after operation: _____

_____

- Postsurgery pharmacological therapy: _____
- Type of planned prosthesis: _____
- Data and time of patient's discharge: _____

1ST SURGEON: _____	2ND SURGEON: _____

INFORMED CONSENT

PATIENT: _____   Date of birth: _____

Address: _____   Tel. _____

Date: _____

I the undersigned hereby authorize and request the practice of Dr. _____
and his collaborators to carry out the following procedures:

A) ORAL SURGERY OPERATION ....

The details of the operation and any alternative therapy solutions have been described to me.
More specifically, I have been informed about the risks connected with the operation:

- early or late implant failure
- infections
- neurological lesion
- hematoma

I have understood that the result of the operation cannot be guaranteed as response of my body is decisive for the success of the operation, which cannot be foreseen in advance.

It has, however, also been explained to me that my general and oral state of health permits the prediction of a favorable, long-lasting result.

I have also been informed about the importance of maintenance therapy, which consists of periodical professional check-ups.

The most common complications that can occur during the operation and in the healing period have been explained to me and I have understood them.

I give my consent to being photographed before, during and after surgery, and to the use of this documentation, the property of the dental surgeon, for the following reasons (listed as an example, and not limited to):

1. Scientific publications
2. Projection or other presentation methods, during courses and conferences.

I CERTIFY THAT I HAVE READ AND UNDERSTOOD THIS INFORMED CONSENT
AND THAT EACH SPACE WAS FULLY FILLED IN BEFORE I WAS ASKED TO SIGN IT

PATIENT'S signature: _____   date _____

(as consent can be revoked, it is necessary to renew it before surgery)

PATIENT'S signature: _____   date _____

N.B. a signed copy must be attached to the patient's medical records

NOTES

Index

Index